Rheumatology: Prevention, Diagnosis and Treatment

Rheumatology: Prevention, Diagnosis and Treatment

Editor: Sullivan Princeton

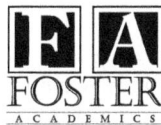

FA
FOSTER
ACADEMICS

www.fosteracademics.com

www.fosteracademics.com

FA **FOSTER**
ACADEMICS

Cataloging-in-Publication Data

Rheumatology : prevention, diagnosis and treatment / edited by Sullivan Princeton.
  p. cm.
Includes bibliographical references and index.
ISBN 978-1-63242-807-3
1. Rheumatology. 2. Rheumatism--Diagnosis. 3. Rheumatism--Treatment.
4. Rheumatism--Prevention. I. Princeton, Sullivan.
RC927 .R445 2019
616.723--dc23

Foster Academics,
118-35 Queens Blvd., Suite 400,
Forest Hills, NY 11375, USA

ISBN 978-1-63242-807-3 (Hardback)

Contents

Preface

Rheumatic disorders are the conditions that cause chronic and intermittent pain, and affect the joints and connective tissue. Some rheumatic disorders are osteoarthritis, tendinitis, back pain, capsulitis, palindromic rheumatism, etc. Some rheumatic diseases are autoimmune in origin such as rheumatoid arthritis, scleroderma, systemic lupus erythematosus, ankylosing spondylitis, etc. Different rheumatic disorders have varied causes and all of these require different kinds of treatment. The diagnosis of rheumatic disorders is done through a physical examination and specialized laboratory and imaging tests. The initial therapy of rheumatological diseases is usually through analgesics, such as non-steroidal anti-inflammatory drugs (NSAIDs), disease-modifying anti-rheumatic drugs (DMARDs), etc. Physiotherapy and occupational therapy are other recommended treatment techniques. The study of such conditions and the development of therapeutic interventions for these disorders are under the scope of rheumatology. This book elucidates the concepts and innovative models around prospective developments with respect to rheumatology. The topics included in this book on the prevention, diagnosis and treatment of rheumatic diseases are of utmost significance and bound to provide incredible insights to readers. Through this book, we attempt to further enlighten the readers about the new concepts in this field.

The researches compiled throughout the book are authentic and of high quality, combining several disciplines and from very diverse regions from around the world. Drawing on the contributions of many researchers from diverse countries, the book's objective is to provide the readers with the latest achievements in the area of research. This book will surely be a source of knowledge to all interested and researching the field.

In the end, I would like to express my deep sense of gratitude to all the authors for meeting the set deadlines in completing and submitting their research chapters. I would also like to thank the publisher for the support offered to us throughout the course of the book. Finally, I extend my sincere thanks to my family for being a constant source of inspiration and encouragement.

Editor

The extra-articular impacts of rheumatoid arthritis: moving towards holistic care

I. C. Scott[1,2]* (iD), A. Machin[1], C. D. Mallen[1] and S. L. Hider[1,2]

Abstract

Although treat-to-target has revolutionised the outcomes of patients with rheumatoid arthritis (RA) there is emerging evidence that attaining the target of remission is insufficient to normalise patients' quality of life, and ameliorate the extra-articular impacts of RA. RA has a broad range of effects on patient's lives, with four key "extra-articular" impacts being pain, depression and anxiety, fatigue and rheumatoid cachexia. All of these are seen frequently; for example, studies have reported that 1 in 4 patients with RA have high-levels of fatigue. Commonly used drug treatments (including simple analgesics, non-steroidal anti-inflammatory drugs and anti-depressants) have, at most, only modest benefits and often cause adverse events. Psychological strategies and dynamic and aerobic exercise all reduce issues like pain and fatigue, although their effects are also only modest. The aetiologies of these extra-articular impacts are multifactorial, but share overlapping components. Consequently, patients are likely to benefit from management strategies that extend beyond the assessment and treatment of synovitis, and incorporate more broad-based, or "holistic", assessments of the extra-articular impacts of RA and their management, including non-pharmacological approaches. Innovative digital technologies (including tablet and smartphone "apps" that directly interface with hospital systems) are increasingly available that can directly capture patient-reported outcomes during and between clinic visits, and include them within electronic patient records. These are likely to play an important future role in delivering such approaches.

Keywords: Rheumatoid arthritis, Pain, Fatigue, Mental health, Cachexia

Background

The current treatment paradigm for patients with rheumatoid arthritis (RA) is "treat-to-target" (T2T) [1]. This involves measuring a patient's disease activity, using composite scores like the disease activity score on a 28-joint count (DAS28), and escalating disease-modifying anti-rheumatic drug (DMARD) therapy until the targets of remission, or low disease activity (LDA) are attained. The T2T strategy is based on the extensive evidence that patients attaining remission have better health related quality of life (HRQoL) and function, and lower rates of radiological damage, when compared to patients in higher disease activity states [2–6].

RA has many impacts on patients' lives not directly addressed by reducing disease activity using T2T strategies. Four key examples are [1] pain, [2] depression and

anxiety, [3] fatigue, and [4] muscle loss. Although controlling disease activity and achieving remission benefits patients it usually fails to normalise HRQoL [5, 7] and ameliorate pain [8] and fatigue [9, 10]. This is particularly true of those individuals with established disease, with two independent studies showing that short-form 36 (SF-36) health profiles – measuring health across 8 domains, each of which is scored from 0 to 100, with higher scores representing better health – are worse in patients with established RA in remission, compared with the normal general population (Fig. 1) [5, 7]. The first study by Radner et al. [5], compared SF-36 health profiles in 356 German RA patients at a single time-point stratified by disease activity status (captured using the simplified disease activity index) to those observed in the healthy German population; lower HRQoL was seen in all 8 domains in patients in remission compared with the healthy population. The second study, by Scott et al. [7], compared SF-36 health profiles in 205 English RA patients enrolled to the TACIT trial

* Correspondence: i.scott@keele.ac.uk
[1]Research Institute for Primary Care & Health Sciences, Primary Care Sciences, Keele University, Newcastle-under-Lyme, Staffordshire, UK
[2]Department of Rheumatology, Haywood Hospital, High Lane, Burslem, Staffordshire, UK

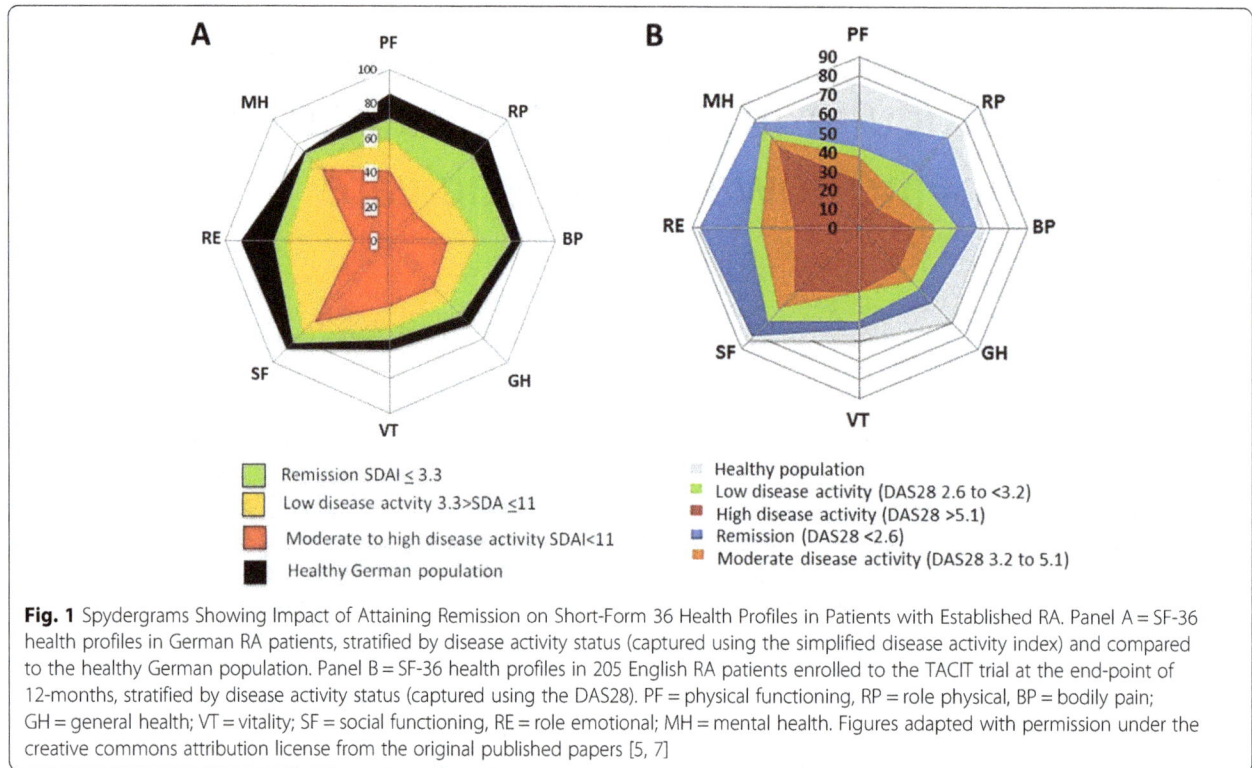

Fig. 1 Spydergrams Showing Impact of Attaining Remission on Short-Form 36 Health Profiles in Patients with Established RA. Panel A = SF-36 health profiles in German RA patients, stratified by disease activity status (captured using the simplified disease activity index) and compared to the healthy German population. Panel B = SF-36 health profiles in 205 English RA patients enrolled to the TACIT trial at the end-point of 12-months, stratified by disease activity status (captured using the DAS28). PF = physical functioning, RP = role physical, BP = bodily pain; GH = general health; VT = vitality; SF = social functioning, RE = role emotional; MH = mental health. Figures adapted with permission under the creative commons attribution license from the original published papers [5, 7]

(of combination DMARDs vs. anti-TNF) at the trial end-point of 12-months, stratified by disease activity status (captured using the DAS28); lower HRQoL was seen in all domains in patients in remission, with the exception of mental health. The impact of RA on HRQoL is likely to be minimised by extending the focus of disease management beyond synovitis, to incorporate the evaluation of issues like pain, depression and anxiety.

In this review we will provide an overview of pain, depression and anxiety, fatigue, and muscle loss in patients with RA. We have focussed on these four "extra-articular" impacts as they are a diverse group of features, which have been studied in detail, are relatively common, improve with readily available interventions, have negative impacts on patients' lives including reducing their HRQoL, and cannot be resolved simply by achieving remission. We will summarise their prevalence, aetiology, assessment tools, and treatment strategies. We will also outline the ways in which they can be assessed within routine practice settings.

Pain

Definition

The conventional definition of pain from the International Association for the Study of Pain. defines it as "an unpleasant sensory and emotional experience associated with actual or potential tissue damage, or described in terms of such damage [11]". This broad definition reflects the multidimensional nature of pain, which is purely subjective, harbours an emotional element, and can occur in the absence of actual tissue damage. At the same time, it is important to appreciate that there are divergent views on how to define pain. For example, McCaffery defined pain to be "whatever the experiencing person says it is, existing whenever the experiencing person says it does" [12].

Assessing pain

A broad range of patient reported outcome (PRO) instruments have been developed and used to capture pain in patients with RA. Burkhardt and Jones have published a detailed summary of their assessment of the key measures [13]. An overview of these is provided in Table 1. They span quick and simple unidimensional instruments of pain intensity such as the pain VAS [14], generic multidimensional instruments such as the McGill Pain Questionnaire [15, 16] (capturing information on many pain dimensions across a range of adult populations), and disease-specific instruments like the RA pain scale (RAPS) [17] (gaining information on pain most relevant to patients with RA).

The simplest to use within a busy, routine clinical setting is the pain VAS [14]. This comprises one horizontal or vertical line, commonly 10 cm long, that has the verbal descriptors "no pain" and "pain as bad as it could be" at either end (although variations in verbal end-points are often observed). Patients place a line perpendicular to the VAS line at the point best representing

Table 1 Key Methods to Assess Pain in Patients with Rheumatoid Arthritis

Measure	Population	Content	Completion time (minutes)	Scoring time (minutes)
McGill Pain Questionnaire [15, 16]	For use in adults with chronic pain problems	78 words describing the sensory, affective and evaluative aspects of pain, alongside a 5-point present pain intensity scale.	5–15	1–2
Rheumatoid Arthritis Pain Scale [17]	Adults with RA	24 items measuring descriptions of pain, it's severity and interference.	5	2
Pain Visual Analogue Scale [14]	Any adult population	Usually one horizontal line, measuring 10 cm, anchored with verbal descriptors "no pain" and "pain as bad as it could be".	< 1	< 1
Verbal Descriptive Scale [14]	Any adult population	Similar to pain visual analogue scale, replacing whole numbers with verbal descriptors of pain (e.g. no pain, slight pain, mild pain, moderate pain, severe pain, very severe pain, the most intense pain imaginable).	< 1	< 1
Numeric rating scale [123]	Any adult population	Segmented version of pain visual analogue scale, with patients selecting a whole number (0–10 integers) that best reflects their pain intensity	< 1	< 1
Short-Form 36 Bodily pain [124]	Any adult population	A 2-item scale in which patients rate: [1] the intensity of their pain (6-point scale ranging from "none" to "very severe"), and [2] extent to which pain interferes with their work (5-point scale ranging from "not at all" to "extremely")	< 2	1

their current pain, with the score ranging from 0 to 100 (if scored in mm). The pain VAS has been shown to have high test-retest reliability in patients with RA, although it is higher in literate ($r = 0.94$) than illiterate ($r = 0.71$) people [18]. The optimal cut-off to define an "acceptable" level of pain has been defined as ≤2.0 units, and the minimal clinically important change for pain in observational studies reported as being 1.1 units [19]. Whilst the pain VAS is easy to score and interpret, as it is a unidimensional measure it cannot fully capture the multidimensional nature of patients' pain.

Prevalence in RA

Pain represents a key symptom in patients with RA. In the earliest stages of the disease process, it is the dominant reason why people initially seek a review by their physician, with a recent qualitative study of patients with newly diagnosed RA reporting pain to be central to their symptom experience [20].

In patients with established RA, pain is also an important issue. In two multi-national RA patient surveys – the "Good Days Fast" survey, which explored the impact of RA on the lives of women, and the "Getting to Your Destination Faster" survey, which explored patients' treatment goals – pain was identified as being of paramount importance [21]. In the "Good Days Fast" survey, from 1958 women surveyed, 63% reported experiencing pain every day, with 75% taking analgesics. Despite the high prevalence of pain, however, many patients reported problems discussing it with their health care provider, with 55% feeling too shy to talk about how much pain they experienced, and 73% reporting they feel like they are complaining when discussing their pain

symptoms. In the "Getting to Your Destination Faster" survey, from the 1829 patients surveyed, 70% agreed that pain relief was the most important aspect of their management. A further third survey, of 1024 patients with RA in Norway, showed similar findings. In this study, 69% of patients reported pain as their preferred area for improvement [22], despite which over one-third of patients were not receiving analgesics. Taken together, these three patient surveys provide good evidence that improving pain is a crucial, patient-centred treatment goal in RA.

Aetiology of RA pain

Pain in patients with RA is multifactorial. Synovitis, systemic inflammation [23], and joint damage [24] all play roles in both the initiation and perpetuation of pain. However, pain also often occurs in the absence of synovitis or joint damage, highlighting the importance of peripheral sensitisation (hypersensitivity of the nociceptive primary afferent neurons in the peripheral nervous system) and central sensitisation (hyperexcitability of nociceptive neurons in the central nervous system) [25].

High levels of pain are generally observed in patients with highly active disease, and improve with the use of intensive synthetic and biologic DMARD therapy [26]. Although reducing synovitis with intensive DMARD treatment improves pain, in many patients clinically significant levels of pain remain in the absence of synovitis. This is demonstrated in an analysis of the North American Brigham and Women's Hospital RA Sequential study (BRASS), by Lee et al. [8]. In this analysis, the 154 patients in DAS28-CRP defined sustained remission over 12 months were evaluated; 11.9% had clinically significant pain at baseline (defined as a multi-dimensional health assessment (MDHAQ) pain score of ≥4) and 12.5% after 1 year of follow-up. Pain scores were observed to be significantly and positively associated with fatigue and sleep disturbance (evaluated using the MDHAQ), and significantly and negatively associated with self-efficacy (evaluated using the arthritis self-efficacy score). No significant association with inflammatory markers or seropositivity was reported. Other studies have also reported pain scores above those seen in the normal population in patients with RA in remission [5, 7].

There is strong clinical and experimental evidence that peripheral and central sensitisation play crucial roles in RA-related pain. This has led to the use of the term "fibromyalgic RA", in which fibromyalgia and RA co-exist in the same patient [27]. The prevalence of co-existing fibromyalgia in people with RA is high; a large study of 11,866 patients with RA identified 1731 (17.1%) as also having fibromyalgia, the presence of which associated with increased medical costs, more severe RA, and a worse HRQoL [28]. Animal studies provide further evidence for the role of pain pathway aberrancies in inflammatory arthritis, with these seeming to occur prior to the onset of clinical signs of synovitis. Nieto et al. evaluated this issue in two separate studies of female rodents with a collagen-induced arthritis. In the first study, allodynia of the rodent hind paw developed concomitantly with articular inflammatory cell infiltration, activation of joint nociceptors, and spinal microgliosis; these changes took place prior to the onset of visible synovitis. When paw swelling finally developed, a significant number of primary afferent neurons innervating tissues external to the joint were also activated [29]. In the second study, they reported that mechanical allodynia was evident prior to the development of visible paw swelling, worsened as swelling developed, and was associated with reactive spinal microgliosis [30]. Microglial cells are resident macrophages in the central nervous system [31], which rapidly respond to a broad range of stimuli. They appear critical to the development of chronic pain and central sensitisation [32], with activated microglia secreting pro-inflammatory and pro-nociceptive mediators, such as TNF and IL-18, which modulate synaptic transmission and pain [33, 34].

Whilst it is often perceived that joint damage is a contributor to pain, the evidence for this is, at best, limited. Sokka et al. evaluated the relationship between Larsen scores and function (assessed using the health assessment questionnaire (HAQ)) and pain (assessed using the pain visual analogue scale (VAS)) in 141 patients with established RA [35]. Larsen scores had a signification association with HAQ ($r = 0.277$, $P = 0.001$) but not pain VAS ($r = 0.008$, $P = 0.929$). Sarzi-Puttini et al. also evaluated associations between cross-sectional pain VAS, and disease characteristics and outcomes in 105 patients with established RA [24]. In a multivariate regression model, Larsen scores explained only 2.1% of the variation in pain VAS.

Treatment of pain in RA

The multifactorial and multidimensional nature of pain suggests that a multifaceted approach to its management is needed that combines pharmacological strategies, with psychological and physical therapies, which have been demonstrated across a range of trials to have beneficial effects on reducing RA pain.

DMARDs and biologics reduce pain in active RA, and optimising immunosuppressive therapy to control RA is important in this regard. In addition, both simple analgesics such as paracetamol and non-steroid anti-inflammatory drugs (NSAIDs) also reduce pain levels, although their effects are generally small-to-modest. Hazelwood et al. systematically reviewed the evidence for the efficacy of paracetamol in inflammatory arthritis, identifying 12 trials and 1 observational study [36]. There was weak evidence of a benefit of paracetamol over placebo. However, most of the included studies were reported 20–50 years ago, and some evaluated atypical paracetamol dosing (such as 2 g of paracetamol over 24-h [37]). Additionally, they had high-risks of bias due to incomplete reporting of details surrounding sequence generation, allocation concealment, and blinding, alongside incomplete outcome data with high dropout rates and lack of intention-to-treat analysis. NSAIDs are commonly used in patients with RA, with clinical trials supporting their efficacy [38, 39]. Whilst clinicians and patients prefer to use NSAIDs over paracetamol in RA, the relative analgesic merits of NSAIDs compared with paracetamol are uncertain [40].

Opiates are prescribed to a substantial minority of patients with RA. One observational study from North America found over one-third of RA patients used opiates in some form [41]. In more than a tenth use was chronic, with opiate use increasing in recent years. However, there is limited evidence for their efficacy. Whittle et al. systematically reviewed the literature for trials comparing opiates vs. another intervention or placebo in patients with RA. Eleven studies were identified, all of which were of a short duration (< 6 weeks). Although opiates were more likely to improve the patient-reported global impression of change in pain, they were also more likely to cause adverse events, with no difference in net efficacy after adjustment for adverse events observed between opioids and placebo [42].

Tricyclic anti-depressants and neuromodulators (such as nefopam) are also often used, particularly if patients have poor sleep or fibromyalgic RA. As with opiates, the evidence supporting their efficacy is weak, with systematic reviews reporting limited evidence that oral nefopam and topical capsaicin are superior to placebo at reducing pain in patients with RA [43], and inconclusive evidence about the efficacy of tricyclic antidepressants [44].

When these limited benefits are weighed against the toxicity profiles of these analgesics – with both paracetamol and NSAIDs associating with an increased risk of myocardial infarction, renal impairment, and upper GI bleeds [45–47], and nefopam and tricyclic antidepressants frequently causing side-effects – it appears vital to ensure that patients are fully informed of the risks and benefits of their analgesic treatment, and that they are used cautiously, for the shortest duration possible, and stopped if patients are failing to gain clinical benefit.

Exercise is encouraged in patients with RA, due to its wide-ranging impacts on general health and well-being. Exercise is defined as any activity that improves physical fitness. It can vary in type and intensity. Several trials have evaluated the impact of dynamic exercise (defined as activities with sufficient intensity, duration, and frequency to improve stamina or muscle strength) on pain in RA [48]. A systematic review reported small benefits on pain scores in patients receiving short-term, land-based aerobic capacity and muscle strength training, with patients receiving dynamic exercise rating their pain to be 0.5 units lower (on a 0–10 scale) at 12-weeks, compared to those not receiving the intervention [48]. However, this change is below the minimal clinically important difference for pain [49].

Psychological interventions are also a vital component of managing chronic musculoskeletal pain. These focus on empowering patients to self-manage their pain. Three commonly employed psychological strategies comprise: [1] stress management training, which helps patients cope with functional problems resulting from RA; [2] education, helping patients make informed decisions about self-managing their condition; and [3] cognitive-behavioural therapy (CBT), which teaches patients methods to manage their pain. Knittle et al. evaluated the effects of such face-to-face psychological interventions by undertaking a systematic review and meta-analysis of relevant randomised controlled trials. Small, but statistically significant effects were seen on improving physical activity, pain, disability and depression at follow-up evaluations [50]. Similar findings were reported in another systematic review of psychological interventions in RA, undertaken by Astin et al [51]; it found significant but small pooled effect sizes post-intervention for pain of 0.22.

Anxiety and depression

Definition

Anxiety disorders are defined by excess worry, hyperarousal and fear which is both counterproductive and debilitating [52]. Its most extreme form is generalised anxiety disorder (GAD), which is characterised by persistently heightened tension and excessive worry about a range of events, that contributes to impaired functioning [53]. Depression is characterised by a persistently low mood, and loss of interest or pleasure in most activities. Depression may be associated with symptoms including an altered appetite, poor sleep, fatigue, lack of concentration and suicidal thoughts. The degree of depression is determined by the number and severity of associated symptoms, and any related functional impairment [54].

Prevalence in RA

Approximately 38% of patients with RA suffer from depression [55]. The prevalence of anxiety is approximately half that of depression, and estimated to lie between 13 and 20% [56, 57]. When this is compared to the prevalence of depression and anxiety in the general population (with the 2014 Adult Psychiatric Morbidity Survey reporting that 5.9% and 3.3% of the adult English population suffered from generalised anxiety disorder and a depressive disorder, respectively) [58], it is clear that patients with RA have a significantly increased mental health burden.

Aetiology in RA

Margaretten et al. have previously provided a summary of the multifactorial nature of reduced mental health in RA [59]. It is likely that different factors contribute to the initiation and perpetuation of depression in different individuals. Characteristics that have been associated with depression include low socioeconomic status [60], co-morbidities [61, 62], pain [23], and disability [63, 64]. Systemic inflammation has also been linked with depression, leading to the proposal of the "cytokine hypothesis of depression", in which pro-inflammatory cytokines are considered to be important mediators of this disorder [65]. It remains to be determined, however, as to whether such cytokines are causally involved in depression aetiology, or if they represent immunological reactions to depressive disorders [65]. Additionally, in the context of RA, the link between systemic inflammation and the onset of depression is uncertain [23, 66].

The factors underlying the excess anxiety observed in RA have received less attention than those of depression. However, a recent review by Sturgeon et al. highlighted the key issues [67]. Anxiety in RA is driven in part by personal factors including social context combined with the impact of ongoing pain and disability and the inflammatory process. The factors causing depression and anxiety in RA are very similar and often occur together in individual patients.

Impacts

Comorbid mental health problems in RA are associated with worse patient outcomes. Several studies have reported that poorer mental health associates with higher levels of DAS28-defined disease activity, although this appears to be driven by its relationship with the "subjective" components of the DAS28 (the tender joint count (TJC) and patient global assessment of disease activity (PtGA)). Matcham et al.. performed a secondary analysis of the CARDERA trial, reporting that the presence of persistent depression and anxiety associated with higher DAS28 scores over time; exploring relationships with the individual DAS28-components revealed the association was restricted to the TJC and PtGA, with no significant association seen between depression and anxiety and the swollen joint count (SJC) and erythrocyte sedimentation rate (ESR) [68]. Similarly, Cordingley et al. reported a significant association between the PtGA and the Hospital Anxiety and Depression Scale (HADS) depression score in 322 RA patients awaiting biologic therapy, but not the other DAS28 components [69].

Depression has also been linked with increased mortality in RA, with Ang et al.. reporting that amongst 1290 patients with RA observed over 18 years, the presence of clinical depression in the first 4 years of entry into their clinical cohort provided a hazards ratio (HR) on mortality of 2.2 (95% CI 1.2–3.9, $P = 0.01$) [70]. Depression also increases healthcare costs, with Michaud et al. identifying the presence of depression to be a key predictor of increased medical outpatient costs (outpatient procedures, laboratory tests, and physician visits) amongst 7527 RA patients, followed up over a 2-year period [71].

Identifying anxiety and depression

Despite the detrimental impact of mental health disorders on RA outcomes, rheumatologists and primary care physicians do not routinely screen for the presence of mental health issues in patients with RA. In the National Health Service (NHS) this probably reflects a combination of time constraints within clinic appointments, alongside uncertainties as to who is leading on this aspect of patient care (primary or secondary care clinicians). However, to improve the outcomes and HRQoL of patients, the recognition and management of mood problems in RA should be a healthcare priority. Research from the Institute of Psychiatry in London has both highlighted the relative absence of screening in standard care for long-term conditions and shown it can be readily achieved using simple digital assessment methods [72].

One method to implement the routine screening of mental health disorders in RA would be to incorporate it within an annual review. This process is recommended by the National Institute for Health and Care Excellence (NICE), which advise an RA annual review that incorporates an assessment of mood. There are, however, several problems implementing this recommendation. Firstly, there is uncertainty as to where the annual review should occur, and although the NHS Quality and Outcomes Framework (QOF) – which focusses on improving the care of long-term diseases through financial incentives to attain specific clinical targets [73] – incentivises a primary-care based annual review of patients with RA, 20% of GPs feel that this does not benefit their patients [74]. Secondly, it is unclear how mental health should be assessed within an annual review. Thirdly, there is a lack of a standardised approach to the annual review process, with cardiovascular and osteoporosis risk assessments being undertaken more often than depression screening [74].

NICE guidelines for the identification of depression in adults with chronic physical health problems [75], suggest the most sensitive tools for case-finding are the General Health Questionnaire (GHQ-28) and the two-stem questions of the Patient Health Questionnaire (PHQ-9) [75], with the latter often preferred due to their ease of use. These two-stem questions comprise: [1] during the last month, have you often been bothered by feeling down, depressed or hopeless? and [2] during the last month, have you often been bothered by having little interest or pleasure in doing things?

International guidelines for identifying anxiety and experience from the Institute of Psychiatry in London suggests a similar approach can be taken to find patients with significant anxiety [72, 76]. An abbreviated version of the GAD-7 scale, the GAD-2, has been recommended as a case-finding tool for anxiety. This asks two questions: [1] during the last month, have you often been bothered by feeling nervous, anxious or on edge? and [2] during the last month, have you often been bothered by not being able to stop or control worrying? It has a moderately high balance of sensitivity and specificity for detecting clinically relevant anxiety [77].

Managing anxiety and depression in RA

NICE have produced guidelines for the management of depression and generalised anxiety disorder in adults, and also the management of depression in adults with long-term physical health disorders. These recommend a stepped care approach, outlined in Fig. 2, in order to identify the most effective, and least intrusive intervention [53, 54, 75]. If a person declines, or fails to benefit from a treatment, they are offered an appropriate intervention from the next step in the pathway.

Specific to patients with RA, only a handful of trials have evaluated interventions to treat depression and

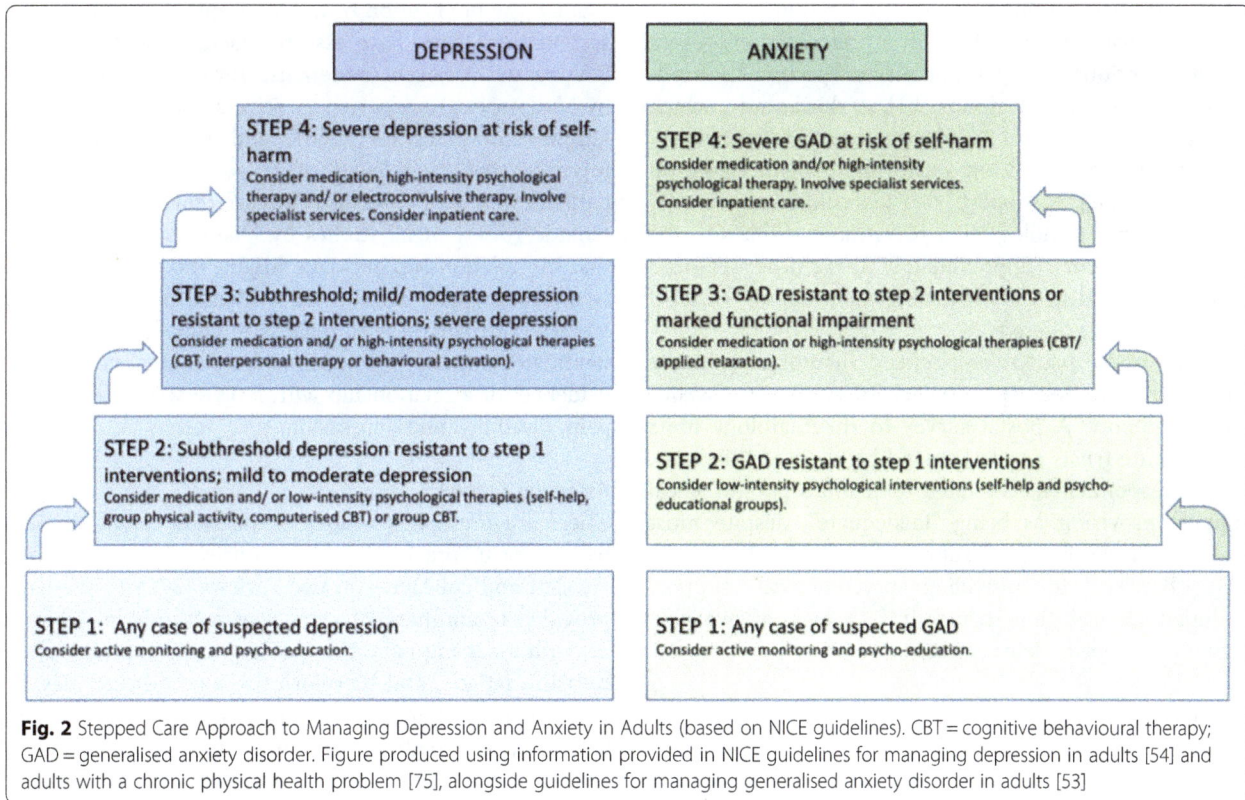

Fig. 2 Stepped Care Approach to Managing Depression and Anxiety in Adults (based on NICE guidelines). CBT = cognitive behavioural therapy; GAD = generalised anxiety disorder. Figure produced using information provided in NICE guidelines for managing depression in adults [54] and adults with a chronic physical health problem [75], alongside guidelines for managing generalised anxiety disorder in adults [53]

anxiety. A recently published systematic literature review has highlighted the paucity of data in this area [78]. This reviewed literature from controlled trials of treatments for depression and anxiety in RA. Only 8 trials were identified, all of which evaluated interventions for depression; no trials evaluated anxiety treatments. Of these, only one trial assessed medications that are often used in contemporary practice (comparing the selective serotonin reuptake inhibitor, paroxetine, with the tricyclic antidepressant, amitriptyline); the remainder used medications that are used infrequently, such as dothiepin and trimipramine, or Chinese herbal remedies. Only 1 trial evaluated non-pharmacological approaches alone, with another assessing a combination of drug and psychological interventions. Overall, a trend towards efficacy was observed with active pharmacological treatments (standardised mean difference – 0.49; 95% CI -1.07 to 0.10), although this was not significant, and significant heterogeneity was observed between study estimates. The one trial of a psychological intervention (randomising 30 patients to cognitive behavioural therapy, and 29 patients to usual care) reported no statistically significant effect on depressive symptoms [79]. Overall, the level of evidence identified by this review was only low-to-moderate, and further research is required before more definitive conclusions can be made regarding pharmacological and non-pharmacological interventions to manage depression and anxiety in RA.

Patient perspectives on management approaches

Qualitative research suggests that patients with RA and comorbid anxiety and depression would favour the use of psychological, over pharmacological interventions. Machin et al. interviewed patients with RA who responded positively to the case-finding questions for anxiety and/or depression (using GAD-2 and/or PHQ-2), to explore their perspectives on this issue [80]. This was conducted in one clinic in England. In the quantitative part of the study 171 patients attending a nurse-led annual review clinic completed the questionnaire; scores in 28% suggested they were anxious or depressed. Fourteen of the patients participated in the qualitative study. They were predominantly white women (68%) reflecting the ethnicity of the local population and the prevalence of RA in females; their average was 63 years and the majority were retired. Patients with mental health problems felt considerable shame and stigma mentioning them to their clinicians. Whereas some participants were open to pharmacological treatments, others feared potential drug interactions, or perceived that medication was offered as a "quick fix". Overall, participants expressed a preference for psychological therapies, although several reported difficulties accessing such care.

This preference for psychological treatments was replicated in a study exploring 46 US Hispanic patients' perspectives of depression associated with RA. Patients often perceived antidepressants to be unnecessary or associated with side-effects, with a preference expressed for interventions incorporating an interpersonal component, such as support groups [81]. A third study, which represented a survey of 2280 patients with inflammatory arthritis that focussed on exploring patient views on their psychological support, also identified a substantial demand for psychological interventions [82]. Of the 1210 respondents, approximately two-thirds reported that they would use a self-management/coping clinic if the service were offered.

Despite these patient preferences, rheumatology units within England self-report a lack of access to psychological support. A postal survey to rheumatology units in 143 acute trusts across England highlighted this issue. Of the respondents, 73% rated their unit's psychological support provision as being "inadequate", despite most feeling that psychological support fell within their remit [83]. Barriers to providing psychological support included clinical time constraints, a lack of available training, alongside delivery costs.

Fatigue

Definition

Fatigue is defined as a state of exhaustion and decreased strength accompanied by a feeling of weariness, sleepiness, and irritability, with a cognitive component [84]. It is unrelated to energy expenditure, and does not improve with rest.

Prevalence in RA

Fatigue is an extremely common symptom in RA. In the Quantitative Standard monitoring of Patients with RA (QUEST-RA) study (evaluating 9874 patients, across 34 countries) high levels of fatigue (defined as a Fatigue VAS of > 6.6 units) were found in almost 1 in 4 patients [85]. A recent systematic review of RA-fatigue aetiology reported that amongst 121 studies (totalling > 100,000 patients with RA) the mean fatigue score (on a normalised scale ranging from 0 (no fatigue) to 1.0 (worst possible fatigue)) was 0.5 units [86].

Aetiology of fatigue in RA

The aetiology of fatigue in RA appears multifactorial. Hewlett et al. proposed a conceptual model for RA-related fatigue, to facilitate research into causal pathways and interventions. This conceptual model has three core, interacting components: [1] the RA disease process (RA), [2] thoughts, feelings and behaviours (cognitive, behavioural) and [3] personal life issues (personal) [87]. An overview of the key proposed factors in each of these components is provided in Fig. 3. This conceptual model highlights the substantial interaction that is considered to occur between fatigue, pain and disability.

Since the publication of this conceptual model, several systematic reviews have assessed factors associated with RA-fatigue. A recent systematic review of 121 studies, by Madsen et al., reported positive associations between fatigue and pain, CRP, ESR and DAS28. They also reported that high levels of fatigue occurred even in patients with well controlled disease [86]. An earlier systematic review of 25 studies by Nikolaus et al, reported that the relationship between fatigue and many variables is uncertain, with conflicting evidence observed across studies (particularly with regards to characteristics of inflammatory activity) [88]. However, the most convincing evidence for a relationship with fatigue was observed for pain, disability, and depression.

Assessing fatigue

There are multiple methods to measure fatigue in RA, which have previously been reviewed in detail by Hewlett and colleagues in two reviews [87, 89]. We have provided a summary of some key methods in Table 2. As with assessing pain, the quickest and simplest way to measure fatigue, and therefore the method that may be preferable to use in routine care, is using a VAS (scoring 0 to 100, with higher scores indicating greater fatigue). As with the pain VAS, as it is a unidimensional measure it cannot fully capture the multidimensional nature of patients' fatigue.

Treatment

Given the multifactorial nature of RA-fatigue, interventions should be multifaceted and directed towards factors which may be exacerbating fatigue, such as pain or mood disturbance, in individual patients.

Although the relationship between disease activity and fatigue is complex, evidence suggests that biologic drugs do reduce fatigue. A systematic review by Almeida et al assessing the impact of biologic agents (20 TNF-inhibitors, and 12 non-TNF-inhibitors) on fatigue reported that biologics in patients with active RA can lead to small-to-moderate improvements in fatigue, with similar magnitudes of effect observed for both TNF-inhibitors and other biologic agents [90]. The authors concluded, however, that "it is unclear whether the improvement results from a direct action of the biologics on fatigue, or indirectly through reduction in inflammation, disease activity or some other mechanism". More recently, similar modest effects on reducing fatigue have been reported with the Janus Kinase inhibitor, baricitinib [91].

A Cochrane systematic review of 24 studies examining non-pharmacological interventions for fatigue by Cramp et al found small but statistically significant benefits of both physical activity interventions and psychosocial interventions [92]. Another systematic review by Kelley et

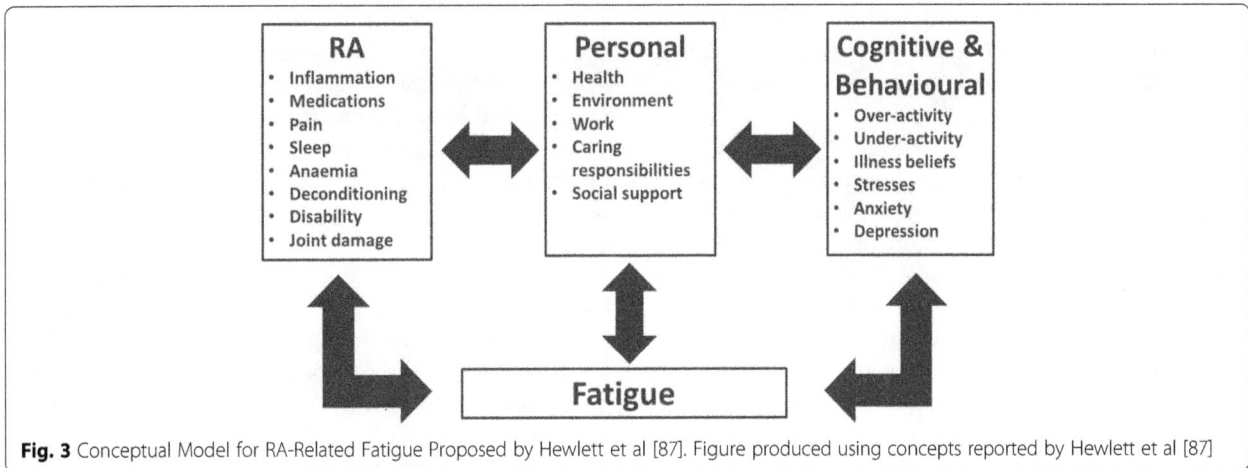

Fig. 3 Conceptual Model for RA-Related Fatigue Proposed by Hewlett et al [87]. Figure produced using concepts reported by Hewlett et al [87]

al of aerobic exercise as a treatment for RA-fatigue, suggested that whilst land-based aerobic exercise is associated with statistically significant reductions in fatigue, it is unlikely that large numbers of people would obtain clinically-relevant reductions [93]. They based their conclusion on changes in relation to the minimal important difference effect size and recommended cut-points. At the same time land-based aerobic exercise did not appear to increase fatigue and is safe; therefore, overall it is likely to be beneficial as part of the overall management of RA.

There is a resource implication in implementing many of these physical or cognitive behavioural approaches, which will limit their uptake within routine clinical care. A simple, more implementable approach to increasing exercise to target fatigue is the use of wearable-technology, such as pedometers. A clinical trial by Katz et al, suggested that this approach is effective in RA. In this trial, 96 patients were randomised to receive either education alone (control group), or a pedometer with step-monitoring diary, with or without step targets. Both intervention groups had significantly higher activity levels and greater reductions in fatigue at 21-weeks compared with the control group [94]. Overall the balance of evidence is strongly in favour of recommending RA patients exercise regularly to limit their fatigue. Although by itself it is unlikely to resolve this feature entirely, it is safe, effective and inexpensive and can be combined with other approaches.

Muscle loss and RA Cachexia
Definition
There are two types of cachexia that can occur in patients with RA. The first is the "classic" low body mass index (BMI) form, in which patients with severe systemic disease lose both muscle mass and fat mass,

Table 2 Key methods to assess fatigue in patients with rheumatoid arthritis

Measure	Population	Content	Completion time (minutes)	Scoring time (minutes)
Bristol RA Fatigue Multi-Dimensional Questionnaire (BRAF MDQ) [125]	Adults with RA	20 items cover domains of physical fatigue, living with fatigue, cognitive fatigue, and emotional fatigue.	5	3
Bristol RA Fatigue Numerical Rating Scales (BRAF NRS) For Severity, Effect, And Coping [125]	Adults with RA	3 single-item numeric rating scales on fatigue severity, effect on patients' lives, and coping with fatigue.	1	1
Fatigue Visual Analogue Scale [89]	Any adult population	Usually one horizontal line, measuring 10 cm, anchored with verbal descriptors such as "not at all tired" and "very tired".	< 1	< 1
Functional Assessment Chronic Illness Therapy (Fatigue) (FACIT-F) [126]	Adults with chronic illness	13 items covering physical fatigue, functional fatigue, emotional fatigue, and social consequences of fatigue.	4	4
Multi-Dimensional Assessment of Fatigue [127]	Adults with RA	15 items covering 4 dimensions of fatigue: severity, distress, interference in activities of daily living, and frequency and change during past week.	8	5
Short-Form 36 Vitality [124]	Any adult population	A 4-item scale covering energy and fatigue.	1	1

leading to an emaciated appearance [95]. The second is "RA cachexia" in which muscle mass is low, but is compensated for by a gain in body fat.

Aetiology

Patients can lose muscle mass for several reasons, including malnutrition, starvation, cachexia and sarcopenia. Malnutrition and starvation are simple concepts related to insufficient food intake. Sarcopenia is predominantly age-related skeletal muscle loss, and is consequently often considered to be a geriatric syndrome [96]. In contrast, cachexia is the consequence of a long-term systemic inflammatory response. The key feature of cachexia is the redistribution of protein content, with skeletal muscle depleted of proteins and an increase in the synthesis of proteins related to the acute-phase response. RA cachexia is considered to be driven by the overproduction of cytokines and inflammation [97], with these metabolic changes of cachexia being cytokine-regulated [98]. RA cachexia has been linked to the metabolic syndrome, with associated abnormalities in lipid levels [99]. Patients with RA cachexia have abnormal energy and protein metabolism and increased inflammatory cytokine production including interleukin-1 and tumour necrosis factor [100].

Prevalence

In RA, there are marked variations in the reported prevalence of cachexia. Some experts suggest it is very common, occurring in as many as two-thirds of patients with RA [101]. Other experts have drawn different conclusions, and suggest it is relatively rare and only occurs in approximately 1% of patients [102]. It is likely that these differences are driven by the use of diverse criteria to define the presence of RA cachexia, with different studies using different definitions, based on varying fat and muscle mass cut-offs [99, 103]. Overall, however, classic cachexia is considered rare, and easily identifiable, and RA cachexia, is considered more common although it is not readily identified by patients and clinicians owing to the presence of a normal, or even increased, BMI [95].

Methods of assessment

Measuring weight and height provide useful information in many settings but are insufficient to assess muscle mass, which is needed to evaluate the presence of RA cachexia. Early studies used a variety of approaches to assess cachexia including energy expenditure profiles and whole body protein turnover [100]. The accurate assessment of cachexia in RA depends upon being able to define the amount of lean body mass, and fat mass that is present. Whole body imaging using computerised tomography and magnetic resonance imaging can

achieve this goal but their use in large numbers of patients is impractical. Dual-energy X-ray absorptiometry, which is widely used to assess bone density in RA, is a reliable and established method for examining the composition of body soft tissue and determining how much is fat and how much is lean mass. It is, therefore, potentially valuable in larger clinical studies of RA cachexia, though it is not currently used for this evaluation in routine practice [104]. A simpler alternative is bioelectrical impedance analysis, which can accurately estimate body composition, particularly the amount of body fat. It determines the electrical impedance, or opposition to the flow of an electric current, through body tissues. This allows an assessment of the total body water, which can be used to estimate fat-free body mass and, by difference with body weight, the amount of body fat. It has been successfully employed in RA patients and is likely to be particularly useful in epidemiological studies [105].

Impact

The loss of lean body mass, a key component of RA cachexia, has been shown across several studies to strongly associate with the presence of disability. Engvall et al. reported that within 60 patients with RA, the correlation coefficient between lean body mass and HAQ scores was -0.42 $(P = 0.001)$ [103]. Other studies have also reported significant associations between loss of lean body mass and disability [106, 107]. The balance of evidence suggests that cachexia causes disability, but there are complex interactions between RA cachexia, sedentary lifestyles and disability in patients with RA. There is a growing body of evidence that sedentary behaviour, which means too much sitting as opposed to movement and exercise, may drive persisting inflammatory disease and elements of cachexia in RA [108].

RA cachexia is often considered to have detrimental impacts on cardiovascular health, although this issue appears controversial. Summers et al [95] have reviewed this relationship in detail, and they identified two studies reporting the association between RA cachexia and cardiovascular disease [99, 109]. The findings of these studies depended on the cut-offs of fat and muscle mass used to define rheumatoid cachexia. Taking a fat free mass index below the 25th percentile and fat mass index above the 50th percentile of a reference population, Elkan et al reported that within 80 patients with RA, 18% of women and 26% of men had "rheumatoid cachexia" and that these individuals had significantly higher total cholesterol and low density lipoprotein, alongside a higher frequency of hypertension and metabolic syndrome [99]. In contrast, using the same definition applied to 400 patients with RA, Metsios et al. reported no significant differences in cardiovascular risk factors, or established cardiovascular disease between patients with and without RA cachexia [109].

Treatment

As cytokines are implicated in the development of RA cachexia there has been considerable interest in evaluating whether cytokine inhibition can improve it. Two small studies evaluated this possibility. One represented a retrospective comparison of 20 RA cases receiving tumour necrosis factor inhibitors and 12 matched controls. Over 12 weeks, biologics improved disease activity and physical function but there were no significant changes in resting energy expenditure and fat-free body mass [110]. The other study was a small 6-month trial of etanercept in 26 patients with early RA; it provided no substantial evidence that this treatment had an important impact on cachexia, though there was some evidence that biologic treatment normalised the anabolic response to overfeeding in a minority of patients [111]. This finding implies that instead of excess food intake resulting in increases in body fat, lean body tissue is preferentially formed in these patients. A larger study of 82 patients subsequently evaluated the impact of tight control using treat-to-target approaches. It also found no evidence that this approach improved RA cachexia [112].The balance of evidence from these small studies is that inhibiting cytokines and controlling synovitis has little impact on RA cachexia, which requires an alternative management strategy.

The impact of exercise appears more positive. An initial small observational study of three months' progressive resistance training as an adjunctive treatment for rheumatoid cachexia in 10 RA patients with matched controls showed it was effective and safe for stimulating muscle growth [113]. A subsequent trial of 28 patients with established, controlled disease showed six months' weekly progressive resistance training was both safe and effective in restoring lean mass and function in these patients [114]. Follow-up of some of these patients at three years showed that stopping the resistance training and resuming normal activity resulted in loss of the benefits of progressive resistance training on lean mass and strength-related function. However, there was substantial retention of the benefits of reduced fat mass and walking ability [115]. Recent research has shown that a short six-week treatment using progressive resistance training can be readily achieved within routine care settings and that this approach is beneficial for patients [116]. The balance of current evidence favours this approach to treat RA cachexia.

Assessing these extra-articular impacts in routine care

Pain, depression and anxiety, fatigue, and rheumatoid cachexia are important issues that would benefit from assessment and management in a routine clinic setting. Delivering this will be challenging, as there are already extensive time pressures in delivering the standard T2T approach. However, the growing use of electronic medical records, and digital technologies to capture PROs (reports of patients' health that come directly from the patient and are measured using standardised, validated questionnaires [117]) that "feed forward" into these, may make this achievable within current medical resources. Although such PROs would not be able to directly identify patients with rheumatoid cachexia, they would identify patients with functional impairment likely to benefit from exercise therapy, which in turn would help improve any co-existing cachexia.

Such an approach, in a rheumatology context, has been pioneered by the Swedish Rheumatology Quality Registry [118]. Patients with rheumatic diseases (including RA) attending a number of clinics across Sweden are able to complete a self-administered health survey prior to their clinic review. This can be undertaken at their routine clinic review using a touch-screen computer in the waiting room area, or at home/work via a secure internet web portal. Patients enter data on a range of PROs, covering general well-being, pain, activities of daily living, quality of life, and ability to work. These patient reported data are then "fed-forward" into their electronic medical records, and summarised in a summary overview "dashboard", which trends their PROs and clinician-reported outcomes over time. During their clinic appointment, the clinician and patient review the co-produced dashboard information together, decide on the next treatment steps, and print an updated summary overview for the patient to bring home. A questionnaire and qualitative interviews of a subset of patients and clinicians confirmed this system to be acceptable, and useful, with 96% of patients rating their "overall impression of the system" as "excellent" or "very good" [119]. A similar approach is being undertaken at the University of Manchester, using a mobile phone application (the Remote Monitoring of RA (REMORA) app), which allows patients to log daily symptoms of their RA and its impact between clinic appointments; these data are sent directly to their electronic healthcare records [120]. Positive feedback was gained from patients in preliminary testing, who felt that it made care "more personal to you", and easier to have a "shared conversation" with the clinician [121]. Additionally, a high-level of data completeness was obtained over a 3-month period of testing [122]. Further research in this area is required, with key questions including which PROs should be measured in a routine NHS setting, how the information should be presented to patients and clinicians, and what management should be undertaken for identified problems.

Conclusions

The evidence outlined in this review has demonstrated that pain, anxiety and depression, fatigue, and muscle loss, are highly prevalent problems in patients with RA. Whilst T2T has revolutionised the overall health and outcomes of patients with RA, it does not directly address these important extra-articular impacts, which can persist despite attaining remission. This suggests that these symptoms are likely to benefit from a more targeted management approach, which is used alongside T2T. This is in-line with patients' preferences, with addressing pain being a key treatment goal across a broad range of patient surveys.

Research suggests that pain, mental health, and fatigue are inter-related problems, that share overlapping aetiologies. As such, they are likely to benefit from a holistic assessment strategy and treatment approach. As detailed in this review, there is evidence to support the use of non-pharmacological strategies, such as psychological interventions and specific forms of exercise to address these issues, with the latter also benefiting muscle loss. Although these interventions have, on the whole, small-to-modest clinical gains, if they are used in combination, and tailored to individual patients, their efficacy is likely to be optimised.

There are many challenges in delivering such a "holistic care" approach to patients. Key barriers include a lack of access to psychological services (with nearly three-quarters of rheumatology units in England self-rating their access to psychological support as being "inadequate"), time constraints in clinic (with follow-up appointments generally lasting 15 min), financial constraints within the NHS, alongside uncertainty as to who should be undertaking this (primary or secondary care clinicians).

Further research is required to clarify the optimal way to address these extra-articular impacts in routine care. This needs to not only focus on how to manage these issues, but also how they can be assessed within a brief clinic appointment. It is likely that digital technologies will play an important role in this area, enabling PRO data to be collected electronically and populated into patients' electronic health care records. Although there is a risk of overwhelming clinicians with information in the short-term, clinical practice should rapidly adjust to incorporate this additional data. A focus on improving co-ordination of care across the primary-secondary care interface is also needed, to ensure that rheumatologists and community services with expertise in managing mental health, are working together in an optimal manner, for the good of patients.

Abbreviations

BMI: body mass index; BP: bodily pain; BRAF MDQ: Bristol RA Fatigue Multi-Dimensional Questionnaire; BRAF NRS: Bristol RA Fatigue Numerical Rating Scales; CBT: cognitive behavioural therapy; DAS28: disease activity score on a 28-joint count; DMARD: disease-modifying anti-rheumatic drug; ESR: erythrocyte sedimentation rate; GAD: generalised anxiety disorder; GHQ-28: general health questionnaire; HADS: hospital anxiety and depression scale; HAQ: health assessment questionnaire; HR: hazards ratio; HRQoL: health-related quality of life; LDA: low disease activity; MDHAQ: multi-dimensional HAQ; MSK: musculoskeletal; MSK-HQ: musculoskeletal health questionnaire; NHS: national health service; NICE: national institute for health and care excellence; NRS: numeric rating scale; NSAIDs: non-steroidal anti-inflammatory drugs; PHQ-9: patient health questionnaire; PRO: patient reported outcome; PtGA: patient global assessment of disease activity; QOF: quality and outcomes framework; QUEST-RA: quantitative standard monitoring of patients with RA; RA: rheumatoid arthritis; RAPID: routine assessment of patient index data; RAPS: RA pain scale; REMORA: remote monitoring of RA; SF-36: short-form 36; SJC: swollen joint count; T2T: treat-to-target; TJC: tender joint count; VAS: visual analogue scale; VDS: verbal descriptive scale

Acknowledgements
Not applicable.

Funding

This article presents independent research funded by the National Institute for Health Research (NIHR) Research Professorship awarded to CDM (Grant number NIHR-RP-2014-04-026). CDM is also supported by the NIHR Collaborations for Leadership in Applied Health Research and Care West Midlands and the NIHR School for Primary Care Research. The views expressed in this article are those of the authors and not necessarily those of the NHS, the NIHR or the Department of Health and Social Care.

Authors' contributions

Manuscript design/conception: ICS, CMD. Drafting of manuscript: SLH (fatigue), AM (depression and anxiety), ICS (remaining sections). Critical revision: all authors. Approval of manuscript: all authors read and approved the final manuscript.

Competing interests

The authors declare that they have no competing interests.

References

1. Smolen JS, Breedveld FC, Burmester GR, Bykerk V, Dougados M, Emery P, et al. Treating rheumatoid arthritis to target: 2014 update of the recommendations of an international task force. Ann Rheum Dis. 2016;75(1):3–15.

2. Drossaers-Bakker KW, de Buck M, van Zeben D, Zwinderman AH, Breedveld FC, Hazes JM. Long-term course and outcome of functional capacity in rheumatoid arthritis: the effect of disease activity and radiologic damage over time. Arthritis Rheum. 1999;42(9):1854–60.

3. Welsing PM, van Gestel AM, Swinkels HL, Kiemeney LA, van Riel PL. The relationship between disease activity, joint destruction, and functional capacity over the course of rheumatoid arthritis. Arthritis Rheum. 2001;44(9):2009–17.

4. Klarenbeek NB, Koevoets R, van der Heijde DMFM, Gerards AH, Ten Wolde S, Kerstens PJSM, et al. Association with joint damage and physical functioning of nine composite indices and the 2011 ACR/EULAR remission criteria in rheumatoid arthritis. Ann Rheum Dis. 2011;70(10):1815–21.

5. Radner H, Smolen JS, Aletaha D. Remission in rheumatoid arthritis: benefit over low disease activity in patient-reported outcomes and costs. Arthritis Res Ther. 2014;16(1):R56.

6. Versteeg GA, Steunebrink LMM, Vonkeman HE, Ten Klooster PM, van der Bijl AE, van de Laar MAFJ. Long-term disease and patient-reported outcomes of a continuous treat-to-target approach in patients with early rheumatoid arthritis in daily clinical practice. Clin Rheumatol. 2018;37:1189-1197.

7. Scott IC, Ibrahim F, Lewis CM, Scott DL, Strand V. Impact of intensive treatment and remission on health-related quality of life in early and established rheumatoid arthritis. RMD open. 2016;2(2):e000270.

8. Lee YC, Cui J, Lu B, Frits ML, Iannaccone CK, Shadick NA, et al. Pain persists in DAS28 rheumatoid arthritis remission but not in ACR/EULAR remission: a longitudinal observational study. Arthritis Res Ther. 2011;13(3):R83.

9. Ishida M, Kuroiwa Y, Yoshida E, Sato M, Krupa D, Henry N, et al. Residual symptoms and disease burden among patients with rheumatoid arthritis in remission or low disease activity: a systematic literature review. Mod Rheumatol. 2017;18:1–11.

10. Druce K, Bhattacharya Y, Jones G, Macfarlane G, Basu N. Most patients who reach disease remission following anti-TNF therapy continue to report fatigue: results from the British Society for Rheumatology biologics register for rheumatoid arthritis. Rheumatol. 2016;55(10):1786–90.

11. Bonica J. Editorial the need of a taxonomy. Pain. 1979;6(3):247–52.

12. McCaffery M. Nursing practice theories related to cognition, bodily pain, and man-environment interactions. Los Angeles: University of California at LA Students Store; 1968.

13. Burckhardt CS, Jones KD. Adult measures of pain: the McGill pain questionnaire (MPQ), rheumatoid arthritis pain scale (RAPS), short-form McGill pain questionnaire (SF-MPQ), verbal descriptive scale (VDS), visual analog scale (VAS), and west haven-Yale multidisciplinary pain inventory (WHYMPI). Arthritis Care Res (Hoboken). 2003;49(S5):S96–104.

14. KEELE KD. The pain chart. Lancet (London, England). 1948;2(6514):6–8.

15. Burckhardt CS. The use of the McGill pain questionnaire in assessing arthritis pain. Pain. 1984;19(3):305–14.

16. Katz J, Melzack R. The McGill pain questionnaire: development, psychometric properties, and usefulness of the long-form, short-form, and short-form-2. In: Handbook of pain assessment. New York: Guilford Press; 2011. p. 45–66.

17. Anderson DL. Development of an instrument to measure pain in rheumatoid arthritis: rheumatoid arthritis pain scale (RAPS). Arthritis Rheum. 2001;45(4):317–23.

18. Ferraz MB, Quaresma MR, Aquino LR, Atra E, Tugwell P, Goldsmith CH. Reliability of pain scales in the assessment of literate and illiterate patients with rheumatoid arthritis. J Rheumatol. 1990;17(8):1022–4.

19. Wolfe F, Michaud K. Assessment of pain in rheumatoid arthritis: minimal clinically significant difference, predictors, and the effect of anti-tumor necrosis factor therapy. J Rheumatol. 2007;34(8):1674–83.

20. Stack RJ, van Tuyl LHD, Sloots M, van de Stadt LA, Hoogland W, Maat B, et al. Symptom complexes in patients with seropositive arthralgia and in patients newly diagnosed with rheumatoid arthritis: a qualitative exploration of symptom development. Rheumatology (Oxford). 2014;53(9):1646–53.

21. Strand V, Wright GC, Bergman MJ, Tambiah J, Taylor PC. Patient expectations and perceptions of goal-setting strategies for disease Management in Rheumatoid Arthritis. J Rheumatol. 2015;42(11):2046–54.

22. Heiberg T, Kvien TK. Preferences for improved health examined in 1,024 patients with rheumatoid arthritis: pain has highest priority. Arthritis Rheum. 2002;47(4):391–7.

23. KOJIMA M, KOJIMA T, SUZUKI S, OGUCHI T, OBA M, TSUCHIYA H, et al. Depression, inflammation, and pain in patients with rheumatoid arthritis. Arthritis Rheum. 2009;61(8):1018–24.

24. Sarzi-Puttini P, Fiorini T, Panni B, Turiel M, Cazzola M, Atzeni F. Correlation of the score for subjective pain with physical disability, clinical and radiographic scores in recent onset rheumatoid arthritis. BMC Musculoskelet Disord. 2002;3:18.

25. Schaible H-G, Ebersberger A, Von Banchet GS. Mechanisms of pain in arthritis. Ann N Y Acad Sci. 2002;966:343–54.

26. Scott DL, Ibrahim F, Farewell V, O'Keeffe AG, Ma M, Walker D, et al. Randomised controlled trial of tumour necrosis factor inhibitors against combination intensive therapy with conventional disease-modifying antirheumatic drugs in established rheumatoid arthritis: the TACIT trial and associated systematic reviews. Health Technol Assess. 2014 Oct;18(66):i-164.

27. Wolfe F, Cathey MA, Kleinheksel SM. Fibrositis (fibromyalgia) in rheumatoid arthritis. J Rheumatol. 1984;11(6):814–8.

28. Wolfe F, Michaud K. Severe rheumatoid arthritis (RA), worse outcomes, comorbid illness, and sociodemographic disadvantage characterize ra patients with fibromyalgia. J Rheumatol. 2004;31(4):695–700.

29. Nieto FR, Clark AK, Grist J, Chapman V, Malcangio M. Calcitonin Gene-Related Peptide–Expressing Sensory Neurons and Spinal Microglial Reactivity Contribute to Pain States in Collagen-Induced Arthritis. Arthritis Rheumatol (Hoboken, N.j). 2015;67(6):1668–77.

30. Nieto FR, Clark AK, Grist J, Hathway GJ, Chapman V, Malcangio M. Neuron-immune mechanisms contribute to pain in early stages of arthritis. J Neuroinflammation. 2016;13(1):96.

31. Ginhoux F, Greter M, Leboeuf M, Nandi S, See P, Gokhan S, et al. Fate mapping analysis reveals that adult microglia derive from primitive macrophages. Science. 2010;330(6005):841–5.

32. Ji R-R, Berta T, Nedergaard M. Glia and pain: is chronic pain a gliopathy? Pain. 2013;154(Suppl):S10–28.

33. Berta T, Park C-K, Xu Z-Z, Xie R-G, Liu T, Lu N, et al. Extracellular caspase-6 drives murine inflammatory pain via microglial TNF-alpha secretion. J Clin Invest. 2014;124(3):1173–86.

34. Miyoshi K, Obata K, Kondo T, Okamura H, Noguchi K. Interleukin-18-mediated microglia/astrocyte interaction in the spinal cord enhances neuropathic pain processing after nerve injury. J Neurosci. 2008;28(48):12775–87.

35. Sokka T, Kankainen A, Hannonen P. Scores for functional disability in patients with rheumatoid arthritis are correlated at higher levels with pain scores than with radiographic scores. Arthritis Rheum. 2000;43(2):386–9.

36. Hazlewood G, van der Heijde DM, Bombardier C. Paracetamol for the management of pain in inflammatory arthritis: a systematic literature review. J Rheumatol Suppl. 2012;90:11–6.

37. Huskisson EC. Simple analgesics for arthritis. Br Med J. 1974;4(5938):196–200.

38. Deeks JJ, Smith LA, Bradley MD. Efficacy, tolerability, and upper gastrointestinal safety of celecoxib for treatment of osteoarthritis and rheumatoid arthritis: systematic review of randomised controlled trials. BMJ. 2002;325(7365):619.

39. Chen Y-F, Jobanputra P, Barton P, Bryan S, Fry-Smith A, Harris G, et al. Cyclooxygenase-2 selective non-steroidal anti-inflammatory drugs (etodolac, meloxicam, celecoxib, rofecoxib, etoricoxib, valdecoxib and lumiracoxib) for osteoarthritis and rheumatoid arthritis: a systematic review and economic evaluation. Health Technol Assess. 2008;12(11):1–iii.

40. Wienecke T, Gotzsche PC. Paracetamol versus nonsteroidal anti-inflammatory drugs for rheumatoid arthritis. Cochrane Database Syst Rev. 2004;1:CD003789.

41. Zamora-Legoff JA, Achenbach SJ, Crowson CS, Krause ML, Davis JM 3rd, Matteson EL. Opioid use in patients with rheumatoid arthritis 2005-2014: a population-based comparative study. Clin Rheumatol. 2016;35(5):1137–44.

42. Whittle SL, Richards BL, van der Heijde DM, Buchbinder R. The efficacy and safety of opioids in inflammatory arthritis: a Cochrane systematic review. J Rheumatol Suppl. 2012;90:40–6.

43. Richards BL, Whittle SL, Buchbinder R. Neuromodulators for pain management in rheumatoid arthritis. Cochrane Database Syst Rev. 2012;1:CD008921.

44. Richards BL, Whittle SL, van der Heijde DM, Buchbinder R. The efficacy and safety of antidepressants in inflammatory arthritis: a Cochrane systematic review. J Rheumatol Suppl. 2012;90:21–7.

45. Bally M, Dendukuri N, Rich B, Nadeau L, Helin-Salmivaara A, Garbe E, et al. Risk of acute myocardial infarction with NSAIDs in real world use: bayesian meta-analysis of individual patient data. BMJ. 2017;357:j1909.

46. Sostres C, Carrera-Lasfuentes P, Lanas A. Non-steroidal anti-inflammatory drug related upper gastrointestinal bleeding: types of drug use and patient profiles in real clinical practice. Curr Med Res Opin. 2017;33(10):1815–20.

47. Roberts E, Delgado Nunes V, Buckner S, Latchem S, Constanti M, Miller P, et al. Paracetamol: not as safe as we thought? A systematic literature review of observational studies. Ann Rheum Dis. 2016;75(3):552–9.

48. Hurkmans E, van der Giesen FJ, Vliet Vlieland TP, Schoones J, den Ende ECHM V. Dynamic exercise programs (aerobic capacity and/or muscle strength training) in patients with rheumatoid arthritis. Cochrane Database Syst Rev. 2009;4:CD006853.

49. Strand V, Boers M, Idzerda L, Kirwan JR, Kvien TK, Tugwell PS, et al. It's good to feel better but it's better to feel good and even better to feel good as soon as possible for as long as possible. Response criteria and the importance of change at OMERACT 10. J Rheumatol. 2011;38(8):1720–7.

50. Knittle K, Maes S, de Gucht V. Psychological interventions for rheumatoid arthritis: examining the role of self-regulation with a systematic review and meta-analysis of randomized controlled trials. Arthritis Care Res (Hoboken). 2010;62(10):1460–72.

51. Astin JA, Beckner W, Soeken K, Hochberg MC, Berman B. Psychological interventions for rheumatoid arthritis: a meta-analysis of randomized controlled trials. Arthritis Rheum. 2002;47(3):291–302.

52. Simpson HB, Neria Y, Lewis-Fernandez RSF. Anxiety disorders – theory, research and clinical perspectives. 2010; 1st ed. Cambridge: Cambridge University Press; 2010.

53. National Institute for Health and Care Excellence (NICE). Generalised anxiety disorder and panic disorder in adults: management. CG113 [Internet]. 2011 [cited 2018 May 9]. Available: https://www.nice.org.uk/guidance/cg113.

54. National Institute for Health and Care Excellence (NICE). Depression in adults: recognition and management. CG90 [Internet]. 2009 [cited 2018 May 9]. Available: https://www.nice.org.uk/guidance/cg90.

55. Matcham F, Rayner L, Steer S, Hotopf M. The prevalence of depression in rheumatoid arthritis: a systematic review and meta-analysis. Rheumatology (Oxford). 2013;52(12):2136–48.

56. Covic T, Cumming SR, Pallant JF, Manolios N, Emery P, Conaghan PG, et al. Depression and anxiety in patients with rheumatoid arthritis: prevalence rates based on a comparison of the depression, anxiety and stress scale (DASS) and the hospital, anxiety and depression scale (HADS). BMC Psychiatry. 2012;12:6.

57. VanDyke MM, Parker JC, Smarr KL, Hewett JE, Johnson GE, Slaughter JR, et al. Anxiety in rheumatoid arthritis. Arthritis Rheum. 2004;51(3):408–12.

58. NatCen Social Research. Adult Psychiatric Morbidity Survey: Survey of Mental Health and Wellbeing, England, 2014 [Internet]. 2016 [cited 2018 May 9]. Available: http://content.digital.nhs.uk/catalogue/PUB21748.

59. Margaretten M, Julian L, Katz P, Yelin E. Depression in patients with rheumatoid arthritis: description, causes and mechanisms. Int J Clin Rheumtol. 2011;6(6):617–23.

60. Berkanovic E, Oster P, Wong WK, Bulpitt K, Clements P, Sterz M, et al. The relationship between socioeconomic status and recently diagnosed rheumatoid arthritis. Arthritis Care Res. 1996;9(6):257–62.

61. Nakajima A, Kamitsuji S, Saito A, Tanaka E, Nishimura K, Horikawa N, et al. Disability and patient's appraisal of general health contribute to depressed mood in rheumatoid arthritis in a large clinical study in Japan. Mod Rheumatol. 2006;16(3):151–7.

62. Wolfe F, Michaud K. Predicting depression in rheumatoid arthritis: the signal importance of pain extent and fatigue, and comorbidity. Arthritis Rheum. 2009;61(5):667–73.

63. Katz PP, Yelin EH. Activity loss and the onset of depressive symptoms: do some activities matter more than others? Arthritis Rheum. 2001;44(5):1194–202.

64. Smedstad LM, Vaglum P, Moum T, Kvien TK. The relationship between psychological distress and traditional clinical variables: a 2 year prospective study of 216 patients with early rheumatoid arthritis. Br J Rheumatol. 1997;36(12):1304–11.

65. Schiepers O, Wichers M, Maes M. Cytokines and major depression. Prog Neuro-Psychopharmacol Biol Psychiatry. 2005;29(2):201–17.

66. Low CA, Cunningham AL, Kao AH, Krishnaswami S, Kuller LH, Wasko MCM. Association between C-reactive protein and depressive symptoms in women with rheumatoid arthritis. Biol Psychol. 2009;81(2):131–4.

67. Sturgeon JA, Finan PH, Zautra AJ. Affective disturbance in rheumatoid arthritis: psychological and disease-related pathways. Nat Rev Rheumatol. 2016;12(9):532–42.

68. Matcham F, Norton S, Scott DL, Steer S, Hotopf M. Symptoms of depression and anxiety predict treatment response and long-term physical health outcomes in rheumatoid arthritis: secondary analysis of a randomized controlled trial. Rheumatology (Oxford). 2016;55(2):268–78.

69. Cordingley L, Prajapati R, Plant D, Maskell D, Morgan C, Ali FR, et al. Impact of psychological factors on subjective disease activity assessments in patients with severe rheumatoid arthritis. Arthritis Care Res (Hoboken). 2014;66(6):861–8.

70. Ang DC, Choi H, Kroenke K, Wolfe F. Comorbid depression is an independent risk factor for mortality in patients with rheumatoid arthritis. J Rheumatol. 2005;32(6):1013–9.

71. Michaud K, Messer J, Choi HK, Wolfe F. Direct medical costs and their predictors in patients with rheumatoid arthritis: a three-year study of 7,527 patients. Arthritis Rheum. 2003;48(10):2750–62.

72. Rayner L, Matcham F, Hutton J, Stringer C, Dobson J, Steer S, et al. Embedding integrated mental health assessment and management in general hospital settings: feasibility, acceptability and the prevalence of common mental disorder. Gen Hosp Psychiatry. 2014;36(3):318–24.

73. Roland M, Guthrie B. Quality and outcomes framework: what have we learnt? BMJ. 2016;354:i4060.

74. Hider SL, Blagojevic-Bucknall M, Whittle R, Clarkson K, Mangat N, Stack R, et al. What does a primary care annual review for RA include? A national GP survey. Clin Rheumatol. 2016;35(8):2137–8.

75. National Institute for Health and Care Excellence (NICE). Depression in adults with a chronic physical health problem: recognition and management, CG91 [Internet]. 2009 [cited 2018 May 9]. Available: https://www.nice.org.uk/guidance/cg91.

76. Ballenger JC, Davidson JR, Lecrubier Y, Nutt DJ, Borkovec TD, Rickels K, et al. Consensus statement on generalized anxiety disorder from the international consensus group on depression and anxiety. J Clin Psychiatry. 2001;62(Suppl 1):53–8.

77. Plummer F, Manea L, Trepel D, McMillan D. Screening for anxiety disorders with the GAD-7 and GAD-2: a systematic review and diagnostic metaanalysis. Gen Hosp Psychiatry. 2016;39:24–31.

78. Fiest KM, Hitchon CA, Bernstein CN, Peschken CA, Walker JR, Graff LA, et al. Systematic review and meta-analysis of interventions for depression and anxiety in persons with rheumatoid arthritis. J Clin Rheumatol. 2017;23(8):425–34.

79. Evers AWM, Kraaimaat FW, van PLCM R, de AJL J. Tailored cognitive-behavioral therapy in early rheumatoid arthritis for patients at risk: a randomized controlled trial. Pain. 2002;100(1–2):141–53.

80. Machin A, Hider S, Dale N, Chew-Graham C. Improving recognition of anxiety and depression in rheumatoid arthritis: a qualitative study in a community clinic. Br J Gen Pract. 2017;67(661):e531–7.

81. Withers M, Moran R, Nicassio P, Weisman MH, Karpouzas GA. Perspectives of vulnerable U.S Hispanics with rheumatoid arthritis on depression: awareness, barriers to disclosure, and treatment options. Arthritis Care Res (Hoboken). 2015;67(4):484–92.

82. Dures E, Almeida C, Caesley J, Peterson A, Ambler N, Morris M, et al. Patient preferences for psychological support in inflammatory arthritis: a multicentre survey. Ann Rheum Dis. 2016;75(1):142–7.

83. Dures E, Almeida C, Caesley J, Peterson A, Ambler N, Morris M, et al. A survey of psychological support provision for people with inflammatory arthritis in secondary care in England. Musculoskeletal Care. 2014;12(3):173–81.

84. Stebbings S, Treharne GJ. Fatigue in rheumatic disease: an overview. Int J Clin Rheumatol. 2010;5:487–502.

85. Gron KL, Ornbjerg LM, Hetland ML, Aslam F, Khan NA, Jacobs JWG, et al. The association of fatigue, comorbidity burden, disease activity, disability and gross domestic product in patients with rheumatoid arthritis. Results from 34 countries participating in the Quest-RA program. Clin Exp Rheumatol. 2014;32(6):869–77.

86. Madsen SG, Danneskiold-Samsoe B, Stockmarr A, Bartels EM. Correlations between fatigue and disease duration, disease activity, and pain in patients with rheumatoid arthritis: a systematic review. Scand J Rheumatol. 2016;45(4):255–61.

87. Hewlett S, Chalder T, Choy E, Cramp F, Davis B, Dures E, et al. Fatigue in rheumatoid arthritis: time for a conceptual model. Rheumatology (Oxford). 2011;50(6):1004–6.

88. Nikolaus S, Bode C, Taal E, van de Laar MAFJ. Fatigue and factors related to fatigue in rheumatoid arthritis: a systematic review. Arthritis Care Res (Hoboken). 2013;65(7):1128–46.

89. Hewlett S, Dures E, Almeida C. Measures of fatigue: Bristol rheumatoid arthritis fatigue multi-dimensional questionnaire (BRAF MDQ), Bristol rheumatoid arthritis fatigue numerical rating scales (BRAF NRS) for severity, effect, and coping, Chalder fatigue questionnaire (CFQ), checklist Individual Strength (CIS20R and CIS8R), Fatigue Severity Scale (FSS), Functional Assessment Chronic Illness Therapy (Fatigue) (FACIT-F), Multi-Dimensional Assessment of Fatigue (MAF), Multi-Dimensional Fatigue Inventory (MFI), Pediatric Quality Of Life (PedsQL) Multi-Dimensional Fatigue Scale, Profile of Fatigue (ProF), Short Form 36 Vitality Subscale (SF-36 VT), and Visual Analog Scales (VAS). Arthritis Care Res (Hoboken). 2011;63(Suppl 11):S263–86.

90. Almeida C, Choy EH, Hewlett S, Kirwan JR, Cramp F, Chalder T, et al. Biologic interventions for fatigue in rheumatoid arthritis. Cochrane database Syst rev. 2016; [cited 2018 Jun 7].

91. Emery P, Blanco R, Maldonado Cocco J, Chen Y-C, Gaich CL, DeLozier AM, et al. Patient-reported outcomes from a phase III study of baricitinib in patients with conventional synthetic DMARD-refractory rheumatoid arthritis. RMD Open. 2017;3(1):e000410.

92. Cramp F, Hewlett S, Almeida C, Kirwan JR, Choy EH, Chalder T, et al. Non-pharmacological interventions for fatigue in rheumatoid arthritis. Cochrane database Syst rev. 2013; [cited 2018 Jun 7].

93. Kelley GA, Kelley KS, Callahan LF. Aerobic exercise and fatigue in rheumatoid arthritis participants: a meta-analysis using the minimal important difference approach. Arthritis Care Res (Hoboken). 2018. [Epub ahead of print]

94. Patricia K, Mary M, Steven G, Laura T. Physical activity to reduce fatigue in rheumatoid arthritis: a randomized controlled trial. Arthritis Care Res (Hoboken). 2017;70(1):1–10.

95. Summers GD, Metsios GS, Stavropoulos-Kalinoglou A, Kitas GD. Rheumatoid cachexia and cardiovascular disease. Nat Rev Rheumatol. 2010;6(8):445–51.

96. Cruz-Jentoft AJ, Landi F, Topinkova E, Michel J-P. Understanding sarcopenia as a geriatric syndrome. Curr Opin Clin Nutr Metab Care. 2010;13(1):1–7.

97. Lemmey AB. Rheumatoid cachexia: the undiagnosed, untreated key to restoring physical function in rheumatoid arthritis patients? Rheumatology (Oxford). 2016;55(7):1149–50.

98. Kotler DP. Cachexia. Ann Intern Med. 2000;133(8):622–34.

99. Elkan A-C, Hakansson N, Frostegard J, Cederholm T, Hafstrom I. Rheumatoid cachexia is associated with dyslipidemia and low levels of atheroprotective natural antibodies against phosphorylcholine but not with dietary fat in patients with rheumatoid arthritis: a cross-sectional study. Arthritis Res Ther. 2009;11(2):R37.

100. Rall LC, Roubenoff R. Rheumatoid cachexia: metabolic abnormalities, mechanisms and interventions. Rheumatology (Oxford). 2004;43(10):1219–23.

101. Lemmey AB, Jones J, Maddison PJ. Rheumatoid cachexia: what is it and why is it important? J Rheumatol. 2011;38(9):2074–5.

102. van Bokhorst-de van der Schueren MAE, Konijn NPC, Bultink IEM, Lems WF, Earthman CP, van Tuyl LHD. Relevance of the new pre-cachexia and cachexia definitions for patients with rheumatoid arthritis. Clin Nutr 2012; 31(6):1008–1010.

103. Engvall I-L, Elkan A-C, Tengstrand B, Cederholm T, Brismar K, Hafstrom I. Cachexia in rheumatoid arthritis is associated with inflammatory activity, physical disability, and low bioavailable insulin-like growth factor. Scand J Rheumatol. 2008;37(5):321–8.

104. Tanner SB, Moore CFJ. A review of the use of dual-energy X-ray absorptiometry (DXA) in rheumatology. Open access Rheumatol Res Rev. 2012;4:99–107.

105. Santillan-Diaz C, Ramirez-Sanchez N, Espinosa-Morales R, Orea-Tejeda A, Llorente L, Rodriguez-Guevara G, et al. Prevalence of rheumatoid cachexia assessed by bioelectrical impedance vector analysis and its relation with physical function. Clin Rheumatol. 2018;37(3):607–14.

106. Hernandez-Beriain JA, Segura-Garcia C, Rodriguez-Lozano B, Bustabad S, Gantes M, Gonzalez T. Undernutrition in rheumatoid arthritis patients with disability. Scand J Rheumatol. 1996;25(6):383–7.

107. Arshad A, Rashid R, Benjamin K. The effect of disease activity on fat-free mass and resting energy expenditure in patients with rheumatoid arthritis versus noninflammatory arthropathies/soft tissue rheumatism. Mod Rheumatol. 2007;17(6):470–5.

108. Fenton SAM, Veldhuijzen van Zanten JJCS, Duda JL, Metsios GS, Kitas GD. Sedentary behaviour in rheumatoid arthritis: definition, measurement and implications for health. Rheumatology (Oxford). 2018;57(2):213–26.

109. Metsios GS, Stavropoulos-Kalinoglou A, Panoulas VF, Sandoo A, Toms TE, Nevill AM, et al. Rheumatoid cachexia and cardiovascular disease. Clin Exp Rheumatol. 2009;27(6):985–8.

110. Metsios GS, Stavropoulos-Kalinoglou A, Douglas KMJ, Koutedakis Y, Nevill AM, Panoulas VF, et al. Blockade of tumour necrosis factor-alpha in rheumatoid arthritis: effects on components of rheumatoid cachexia. Rheumatology (Oxford). 2007;46(12):1824–7.

111. Marcora SM, Chester KR, Mittal G, Lemmey AB, Maddison PJ. Randomized phase 2 trial of anti-tumor necrosis factor therapy for cachexia in patients with early rheumatoid arthritis. Am J Clin Nutr. 2006;84(6):1463–72.

112. Lemmey AB, Wilkinson TJ, Clayton RJ, Sheikh F, Whale J, Jones HS, et al. Tight control of disease activity fails to improve body composition or physical function in rheumatoid arthritis patients. Rheumatology (Oxford). 2016;55(10):1736–45.

113. Marcora SM, Lemmey AB, Maddison PJ. Can progressive resistance training reverse cachexia in patients with rheumatoid arthritis? Results of a pilot study. J Rheumatol. 2005;32(6):1031–9.

114. Lemmey AB, Marcora SM, Chester K, Wilson S, Casanova F, Maddison PJ. Effects of high-intensity resistance training in patients with rheumatoid arthritis: a randomized controlled trial. Arthritis Rheum. 2009;61(12):1726–34.

115. Lemmey AB, Williams SL, Marcora SM, Jones J, Maddison PJ. Are the benefits of a high-intensity progressive resistance training program sustained in rheumatoid arthritis patients? A 3-year followup study. Arthritis Care Res (Hoboken). 2012;64(1):71–5.

116. Morsley K, Berntzen B, Erwood L, Bellerby T, Williamson L. Progressive resistance training (PRT) improves rheumatoid arthritis outcomes: a district general hospital (DGH) model. Musculoskeletal Care. 2018;16(1):13–7.

117. The Kings Fund. The Point of Care Measures of patients' experience in hospital: purpose, methods and uses [Internet]. 2009 [cited 2018 Jun 14]. https://www.kingsfund.org.uk/sites/default/files/Point-of-Care-Measures-of-patients-experience-in-hospital-Kings-Fund-July-2009_0.pdf

118. Nelson EC, Hvitfeldt H, Reid R, Grossman D, Lindblad S, Mastanduno MP, et al. Using patient-reported information to improve health outcomes and health care value: case studies from Dartmouth, Karolinska and Group Health. Lebanon, New Hampshire: The Dartmouth Institute for Health Policy and Clinical Practice. Accessed: 27th August 2018. Available: https ://kiedi t. ki.se/sites /defau lt/files/using patie ntrep orted infor matio n_to_impro ve_ healt h_outcomes_and_healt h_care_value .pdf.

119. Hvitfeldt H, Carli C, Nelson EC, Mortenson DM, Ruppert BA, Lindblad S. Feed forward systems for patient participation and provider support: adoption results from the original US context to Sweden and beyond. Qual Manag Health Care. 2009;18(4):247–56.

120. Dixon W. REmote MOnitoring of Rheumatoid Arthritis (REMORA) [Internet]. 2014 [cited 2018 Jun 14]. Available: http://www.cfe.manchester.ac.uk/research/projects/remora/.

121. Austin L, Sanders C, Dixon WG. Patients' Experiences of Using a Smartphone App for Remote Monitoring of Rheumatoid Arthritis, Integrated into the Electronic Medical Record, and Its Impact on Consultations [abstract]. Arthritis Rheumatol. 2016; 68 (suppl 10). https://acrabstracts.org/abstract/patients-experiences-of-using-a-smartphone-app-for-remote-monitoring-of-rheumatoid-arthritis-integrated-into-the-electronic-medical-record-and-its-impact-on-consultations/. Accessed 11 Oct 2018.

122. Veer S, Van Der AL, Sanders C, Dixon W. FRI0175 Using smartphones to improve remote monitoring of rheumatoid arthritis: completeness of patients' symptom reports. Ann Rheum Dis. 2017;76(Suppl 2):547 LP–547.

123. Farrar JT, Young JPJ, LaMoreaux L, Werth JL, Poole RM. Clinical importance of changes in chronic pain intensity measured on an 11-point numerical pain rating scale. Pain. 2001;94(2):149–58.

124. Ware JE, Kosinski M, Keller S. SF-36 physical and mental health summary scales: a user's manual. Boston: The Health Institute; 1994.

125. Joanna N, Fiona C, John K, Rosemary G, Marie U, Sarah H. Measuring fatigue in rheumatoid arthritis: a cross-sectional study to evaluate the Bristol rheumatoid arthritis fatigue multi-dimensional questionnaire, visual analog scales, and numerical rating scales. Arthritis Care Res (Hoboken). 2010 Jun 25;62(11):1559–68.

126. Cella D, Yount S, Sorensen M, Chartash E, Sengupta N, Grober J. Validation of the functional assessment of chronic illness therapy fatigue scale relative to other instrumentation in patients with rheumatoid arthritis. J Rheumatol. 2005;32(5):811–9.

127. Belza BL. Comparison of self-reported fatigue in rheumatoid arthritis and controls. J Rheumatol. 1995;22(4):639–43.

2

Antibody response to 13-valent pneumococcal conjugate vaccine is not impaired in patients with rheumatoid arthritis or primary Sjögren's syndrome without disease modifying treatment

Per Nived[1,2]* (iD), Tore Saxne[1], Pierre Geborek[1], Thomas Mandl[3], Lillemor Skattum[4,5] and Meliha C. Kapetanovic[1]

Abstract

Background: Pneumococcal vaccination is recommended to patients with rheumatoid arthritis (RA) and primary Sjögren's syndrome (pSS). However, little is known whether the diseases influence pneumococcal vaccine response. This study aimed to investigate antibody response and functionality of antibodies following immunization with 13-valent pneumococcal conjugate vaccine (PCV13) in RA patients or pSS patients without disease modifying anti-rheumatic drugs (DMARD), compared to patients with RA treated with DMARD or to healthy controls.

Methods: Sixty RA patients (50 without DMARD and 10 with MTX), 15 patients with pSS and 49 controls received one dose of PCV13. Serotype-specific antibody concentrations for pneumococcal polysaccharides 6B and 23F and functionality of antibodies (23F) were determined in serum taken before and 4–6 weeks after vaccination using ELISA and opsonophagocytic activity assay (OPA), respectively. Proportions of individuals with positive antibody response (i.e. ≥ 2-fold increase from prevaccination concentrations; antibody response ratio; ARR ≥ 2), percentage of individuals reaching putative protective antibody level (i.e. ≥1.3 μg/mL) for both serotypes, and difference in OPA were calculated.

Results: After vaccination, antibody concentrations for both serotypes increased in RA without DMARD ($p < 0.001$), pSS ($p ≤ 0.05$ and < 0.01) and controls ($p < 0.001$). Antibody responses to 6B and 23F were comparable in RA without DMARD (64% and 74%), pSS (67% and 53%) and controls (65% and 67%), but lower in the small group RA with MTX (both 20%, $p < 0.01$). Similarly, significant increases of patients reaching protective antibody levels were seen in RA without DMARD ($p ≤ 0.001$) and controls ($p < 0.001$). After vaccination, OPA increased significantly in controls, RA and pSS without DMARD ($p < 0.001$ to 0.03), but not in RA with MTX.

Conclusions: Pneumococcal conjugate vaccine is immunogenic in RA and pSS patients without DMARD and in line with previous studies we support the recommendation that vaccination of RA patients should be performed before the initiation of MTX.

Keywords: Rheumatoid arthritis, Sjögren's syndrome, Pneumococcal vaccination, Pneumococcal conjugate vaccine

* Correspondence: per.nived@med.lu.se
[1]Department of Clinical Sciences Lund, Section of Rheumatology, Lund University, Skåne University Hospital, SE-221 85 Lund, Sweden
[2]Department of Infectious Diseases, Central Hospital Kristianstad, J A Hedlunds väg 5, SE-291 85 Kristianstad, Sweden
Full list of author information is available at the end of the article

Background

Infection, in particular pneumonia, is an important cause of the excess mortality in patients with rheumatoid arthritis (RA) [1] and recurrent pulmonary infections are reported in 10–35% of Sjögren's syndrome patients [2]. Doran et al. found an 80% increased risk of infection in a retrospective cohort of RA patients, compared to age- and sex-matched subjects without RA [3]. In addition, the authors reported that older age, presence of extra-articular manifestations, leukopenia, comorbid conditions (e.g. diabetes mellitus), and use of corticosteroids, but not traditional disease modifying anti-rheumatic drugs (DMARDs), were strong predictors of infection [4]. More recently, a systematic review and meta-analysis by Singh et al. showed that in comparison to traditional DMARDs, standard-dose biological drugs and high-dose biological drugs were associated with an increased risk of serious infections, (Odds ratios 1.31 and 1.90, respectively) [5].

Invasive pneumococcal disease (IPD), caused by *Streptococcus pneumoniae*, is a vaccine-preventable life-threatening condition. Retrospective cohort studies have demonstrated increased risks of IPD in patients with autoimmune inflammatory rheumatic diseases, i.e. RA (Rate ratio [RR] 2.47, 95% confidence interval [CI] 2.41–2.52) and primary Sjögren's syndrome (pSS) (RR 3.2, 95% CI 2.9–3.5) [6].

Two pneumococcal vaccine types are currently available for adults, the 23-valent pneumococcal polysaccharide (PPV23) and the 13-valent conjugate vaccine (PCV13). The advantage with the conjugate vaccine is the T cell-dependent (TD) immune response, resulting in the production of memory B-cells. Our group have previously reported that antibody responses to PPV23 [7] and 7-valent pneumococcal conjugate vaccine (PCV7) [8] are impaired in chronic arthritis patients during treatment with methotrexate (MTX), but not with tumour necrosis factor (TNF) inhibitor monotherapy. The current recommendation for adults with immunocompromising conditions, is to receive immunization with a dose of PCV13, followed in at least 8 weeks by a dose of PPV23 [9]. RA and pSS are systemic autoimmune inflammatory diseases, but little is known whether the immunological disturbance as a part of disease itself influences the immune response to PCV13 vaccination since studies of the vaccine response in untreated RA and pSS patients are scarce or non-existing. The aim of this study was to investigate if antibody response and functionality of antibodies following immunization with PCV13 is impaired in patients with RA and pSS without active anti-rheumatic treatment compared to RA patients treated with methotrexate (MTX), or to healthy controls.

Methods

Patient inclusion

Adult patients with RA and pSS, regularly monitored at the Department of Rheumatology in Lund and Malmö at Skåne University Hospital were eligible for this study. At inclusion in the present study all patients' medical records were scrutinised in order to confirm that patients fulfilled the American College of Rheumatology (ACR)/ European League Against Rheumatism (EULAR) criteria for RA or pSS [10, 11]. Ongoing treatment at the time of vaccination was noted as a basis for later patient stratification. Patients were excluded from the study if anti-rheumatic treatment had been changed within 4 weeks before vaccination, if they had been previously vaccinated with PPV23 within 1 year, had a history of allergic reaction at previous vaccinations, were pregnant, or had an ongoing infection. Healthy control subjects were recruited from the staff and relatives at the department of Rheumatology in Lund. The controls were younger (median 57.2 years) than RA patients (median 66.9 years, $p < 0.001$).

Ethics approval and consent to participate

The study was approved by the Regional Ethical Review Board at Lund University, Sweden (Dnr 2011/341). Consecutive patients fulfilling inclusion criteria were invited to participate in the study. All invited participants were provided with oral and written information, and written consent was obtained before study enrolment.

Vaccination protocol

All participants received a single 0.5 mL dose of PCV13 (Prevenar 13®, Pfizer) administered as an intramuscular injection in the deltoid muscle. At the time of vaccination, a rheumatologist performed a clinical examination and data were collected on disease and treatment characteristics and previous vaccinations using a structured protocol. All participants were encouraged to report any adverse events following vaccination, as well as possible changes in rheumatic disease. Adverse events (AEs) and adverse drug reactions (ADRs) were recorded in line with the Guideline for Good Clinical Practice and Clinical Safety Data Management [12].

Pneumococcal serotype-specific IgG measurement

Serum samples were collected immediately before and 4–6 weeks after vaccination. Serotype-specific IgG antibody concentrations for pneumococcal serotypes 6B and 23F, both included in PCV13, were quantified using enzyme-linked immunosorbent assay (ELISA). The World Health Organization consensus pneumococcal IgG ELISA [13] was performed with minor modifications, described previously [14].

Opsonophagocytic activity (OPA) assay

Flow cytometric OPA assay was performed for pneumococcal serotype 23F. The original method has been described by *Martinez* et al. [15] and it was executed with some modifications [14].

Statistical analysis

Differences between groups were analysed using the Chi-square test and the Mann-Whitney U test when appropriate. Geometric mean Ab concentrations (GMCs) and 95% confidence intervals (95% CI) were calculated from log-transformed values. Pre- and post-PCV13 GMCs for larger groups ($n > 30$) were compared using paired samples t-test. Pre- to postvaccine OPA and antibody changes in smaller groups were compared using Wilcoxon signed rank test. Differences in GMCs between patients ($n > 20$) and controls were analysed using independent samples t-test. A positive antibody response was defined as an antibody response ratio (ARR, i.e., the ratio of post- to prevaccination antibody levels) ≥ 2. Putative protective level for each serotype was defined as a titer ≥ 1.3 μg/mL, as recommended by the American Academy of Allergy, Asthma & Immunology [16]. Predictors of positive antibody response for both serotypes were analysed using logistic regression model, adjusted for age. Correlations between "% changes in OPA" and ELISA difference in each groups were calculated using Spearman's rank correlation test. Statistical calculations were performed using IBM® SPSS® version 23 and diagrams were drawn using Graphpad Prism® version 6.

Results

A total of 60 patients with RA (50 without DMARD and 10 on MTX), 15 patients with pSS without

DMARD and 49 controls were vaccinated. None was lost to follow up. In the RA without DMARD group 58% were treated with prednisolone (median dose 5 mg daily, range 0–15 mg). The demographic details, disease characteristics, pre- and postvaccination geometric mean antibody concentrations of the participants are shown in Table 1. Prevaccination GMCs neither differed significantly between the patient groups nor compared to controls. Pre- to postvaccination increases of serotypes 6B and 23F GMCs were found in patients with RA without DMARD (both $p < 0.001$), pSS ($p = 0.05$ and $p = 0.006$) and controls (both $p < 0.001$). The small patient group RA with MTX only showed increase in serotype 6B GMC ($p = 0.05$).

Antibody response

Proportions of subjects with a positive antibody response (i.e. antibody response ratio; ARR ≥ 2) to serotypes 6B and 23F was decreased in patients with RA on MTX treatment (both $p < 0.01$), but not in RA without DMARD or pSS without DMARD, compared to controls (Fig. 1). Proportions of antibody responders to both serotypes did not differ significantly between groups RA without DMARD (52%), pSS without DMARD (40%) and controls (55%). When a logistic regression analysis was performed, RA on MTX was the only group with a significant lower positive antibody response to both serotypes. Due to limited number of patients in this group and patients with pSS only adjustment for age could be performed (Table 2).

Table 1 Demographic and patient characteristics in treatment groups and controls

	RA without DMARD ($n = 50$)	RA with MTX ($n = 10$)	pSS without DMARD ($n = 15$)	Controls ($n = 49$)
Age, median (range) years	66.9 (35–87)	67.4 (39–79)	62.3 (25–89)	57.2 (17–85)
Sex (% female)	78.0	70.0	87.0	63.3
Disease duration, mean (range) years	5.6 (0–36)	13.1 (2–40)	7.0 (0–23)	–
CRP, median (range) mg/L	7 (0–78)	3 (0–11)	1.7 (0.7–38)	–
ESR, median (range) mm/h	21 (4–71)	16 (5–42)	12 (7–66)	–
RF positive, %	78	80	43	–
ACPA positive, %	69	70	8	–
ANA positive, %	–	–	73	–
Anti-ENA positive, %	–	–	73	–
Anti-SSA (anti-Ro) positive, %	–	–	67	–
Anti-SSB (anti-La) positive, %	–	–	40	–
Prednisolone, %	58	0	13	0
Dose, median (range) mg/day	5 (0–15)	0	0 (0–10)	–
Previous PPV23, *n* (%):	1 (2)	0	0	3 (6)

DMARD Disease modifying anti rheumatic drugs, *RA* Rheumatoid arthritis, *pSS* primary Sjögren's syndrome, *CRP* C-reactive protein, *ESR* Erythrocyte sedimentation rate, *ACPA* Antibodies against citrullinated peptides, *ANA* Antinuclear antibodies, *Anti-ENA* Antibodies against extractable nuclear antigens, *Anti-SSA (anti-Ro)* Anti-Sjögren's-syndrome-related antigen A, *Anti-SSB (anti-La)* Anti-Sjögren's-syndrome-related antigen B, *RF* Rheumatoid factor

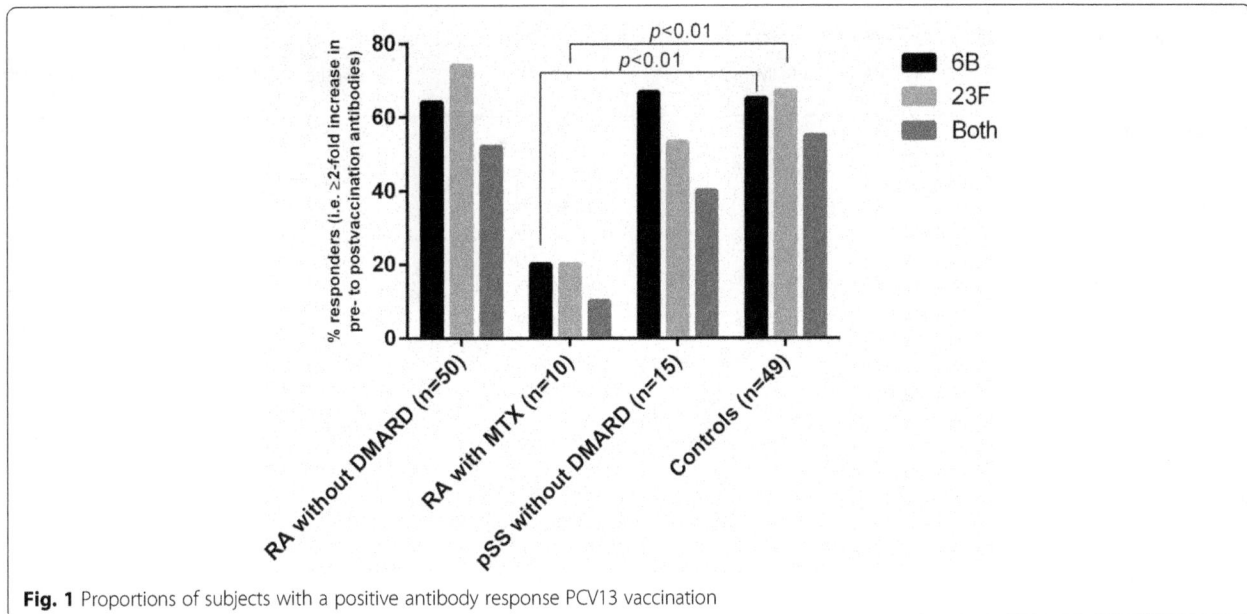

Fig. 1 Proportions of subjects with a positive antibody response PCV13 vaccination

Putative protective levels

The proportions of subjects reaching above protective antibody level (i.e. ≥1.3 µg/mL) for serotype 6B increased after vaccination in RA without DMARD ($p = 0.001$) and controls ($p < 0.001$) but not in RA with MTX and pSS without DMARD (Table 3). For 23F, increases were found in RA without DMARD ($p < 0.001$), pSS without DMARD ($p = 0.05$) and controls ($p < 0.001$) but not in RA with MTX. The pre- to postvaccination percentage increase for serotype 6B and 23F respectively were 24% and 42% in RA without DMARD, 10% and 20% in RA with MTX, 14% and 26% in pSS without DMARD, and 28% and 40% in controls.

Opsonophagocytic activity

After vaccination, OPA increased in groups RA without DMARD ($p < 0.001$), pSS without DMARD ($p = 0.03$) and controls ($p < 0.001$) but did not change significantly in patients with RA on MTX. The mean percentage change in OPA was lower in RA on MTX (1.8%, $p = 0.01$), RA without DMARD (8.9%, $p < 0.01$), but not in pSS without DMARD (10.5%), compared to controls (17.9%). Pre- and postvaccination OPA in patients with RA

Table 2 Predictors of a positive antibody response (i.e. antibody response ratio; ARR ≥ 2) to both 6B and 23F

	p-value	OR	95% CI
RA without DMARD (yes/no)	0.161	1	
RA with MTX (yes/no)	0.037	0.10	0.01–0.87
pSS without DMARDs (yes/no)	0.370	0.58	0.18–1.90
Controls (yes/no)	0.992	0.99	0.42–2.39
Age at vaccination (years)	0.496	0.99	0.97–1.02

and pSS is shown in Fig. 2a and b, respectively. Positive correlations between percentage change in OPA and pre- to postvaccination increase in ELISA were found for patients with RA without DMARD ($ρ = 0.28$, $p = 0.03$) and controls ($ρ = 0.45$, $p = 0.001$).

Effects of age and glucocorticoid treatment

Neither antibody response ratio nor pre- to postvaccination increase in ELISA correlated with age for all patients, subgroups, or controls. A negative correlation was found between percentage change in OPA and age in controls ($ρ = -0.36$, $p = 0.01$) but not in patients. Prednisolone dose did not correlate with antibody response or percentage change in OPA.

Vaccine safety

The vaccine was generally well tolerated, all reported side effects were considered mild-moderate and temporary (duration 1–2 days up to 1–2 weeks). The following side effects were reported in the group RA without DMARD: pain/skin reaction around injection site ($n = 5$), increased arthralgia ($n = 3$), upper respiratory tract symptoms ($n = 2$) and nausea ($n = 1$). In the group RA with MTX, 7 patients had low disease activity and 3 patients no activity (DAS28) at the time of vaccination. None of the patients reported increased disease activity or relapse after vaccination.

Discussion

This study demonstrated that pneumococcal conjugate vaccine was immunogenic in patients with RA and pSS syndrome without DMARD treatment, and the antibody response rates were comparable to those of

Table 3 ELISA IgG geometric mean concentrations and proportions of subjects reaching above putative protective antibody concentration (i.e. ≥1.3 μg/mL) before and after vaccination in treatment groups and controls

	RA without DMARD ($n = 50$)	RA with MTX ($n = 10$)	pSS without DMARD ($n = 15$)	Controls ($n = 49$)
Geometric mean concentrations (μg/mL):				
6B prevaccination (95% CI)	0.6 (0.3–1.0)	1.3 (0.5–2.9)	0.6 (0.2–2.0)	0.8 (0.5–1.3)
6B postvaccination (95% CI)	3.4 (1.8–6.0)	2.1 (0.8–5.6)	2.3 (0.8–6.5)	3.1 (1.9–5.0)
P of increase	< 0.001	0.05	0.05	< 0.001
23F prevaccination (95% CI)	0.5 (0.3–0.8)	1.0 (0.3–3.5)	0.9 (0.4–1.9)	0.6 (0.4–0.9)
23F postvaccination (95% CI)	2.5 (1.5–4.1)	1.7 (0.7–3.9)	3.5 (1.1–11.5)	3.3 (2.0–5.5)
P of increase	< 0.001	0.39	0.006	< 0.001
Proportions of subjects with IgG concentration ≥ 1.3 μg/mL (%):				
6B prevaccination (95% CI)	38 (24–52)	60 (23–97)	33 (6–60)	37 (23–51)
6B postvaccination (95% CI)	62 (48–76)	70 (35–100)	47 (18–75)	65 (51–79)
P of increase	0.001	0.32	0.16	< 0.001
23F prevaccination (95% CI)	26 (13–39)	40 (3–77)	47 (18–75)	29 (15–42)
23F postvaccination (95% CI)	68 (55–81)	60 (23–97)	73 (48–99)	69 (56–83)
P of increase	< 0.001	0.16	0.046	< 0.001

healthy controls. In contrast, a small group of RA patients with MTX treatment had lower antibody responses compared to controls, in accordance with previous findings of our group [8]. These results are in accordance with a meta-analysis of studies investigating immunogenicity of pneumococcal vaccine in RA finding that MTX treated patients with RA had decreased ability to respond to pneumococcal polysaccharide vaccine [17]. Functionality of antibodies after vaccination, measured by an opsonophagocytosis assay, was lower in RA patients without DMARD compared to controls, and a weak positive correlation was found between OPA and ELISA in this group. However, we found a negative correlation between percentage change in OPA and age in controls, and the fact that controls were younger than RA patients could contribute to the difference in functional immune response. To the authors' knowledge, this is the first study of the immune response to pneumococcal conjugate vaccine in patients with RA and pSS without DMARD treatment. The underlying autoimmune pathologies of these diseases are well known to increase the risk of serious infections [3, 6, 18], and pneumococcal vaccination is important to prevent invasive disease. Our findings, i.e. that pneumococcal conjugate vaccine was immunogenic in both RA and pSS without DMARD, support the use of this vaccination in newly diagnosed patients before starting immunosuppressive DMARD treatment.

Among the strengths of this study were the use of both ELISA and a functional antibody assay to evaluate the immune responses. No patients were lost to follow up.

Our study had some limitations. First, we only performed ELISA for two serotypes (6B and 23F). Although the serotypes are among the most common causes of IPD in our part of Sweden [19], we cannot be certain that they are representative of the immune response to PCV13. At the same time, the studies on the immunogenicity of other pneumococcal serotypes prior to the licensure of the conjugate vaccine did not reveal any significant differences between serotypes and probably the impact of the rheumatic diseases or their treatment on antibody response would be similar for the other serotypes [20]. Second, functionality of antibodies was evaluated with a phagocytic OPA assay to only one serotype (i.e. 23F), although validated previously [15], it contrasts to the killing-type OPA assay which is now considered the standard method for vaccine evaluations [21]. Further, small sample sizes may limit the generalizability of our results. Although the group of RA patients with MTX treatment ($n = 10$) arguably is too small for statistical analyses, the purpose of this group was merely to illustrate and confirm what previous studies have shown, i.e. that methotrexate decreases the antibody response to pneumococcal vaccination. The seemingly higher prevaccination antibody level of 6B in this group is probably a result of prior infections and it can explain the lower antibody response to this serotype. The fact that controls were younger than RA patients was considered a minor limitation, and it doesn't contradict our main findings, i.e. that antibody responses in patients with RA without DMARD were comparable to those of healthy controls.

In a recent study, adjuvanted H1N1 influenza vaccination of untreated pSS patients resulted in higher

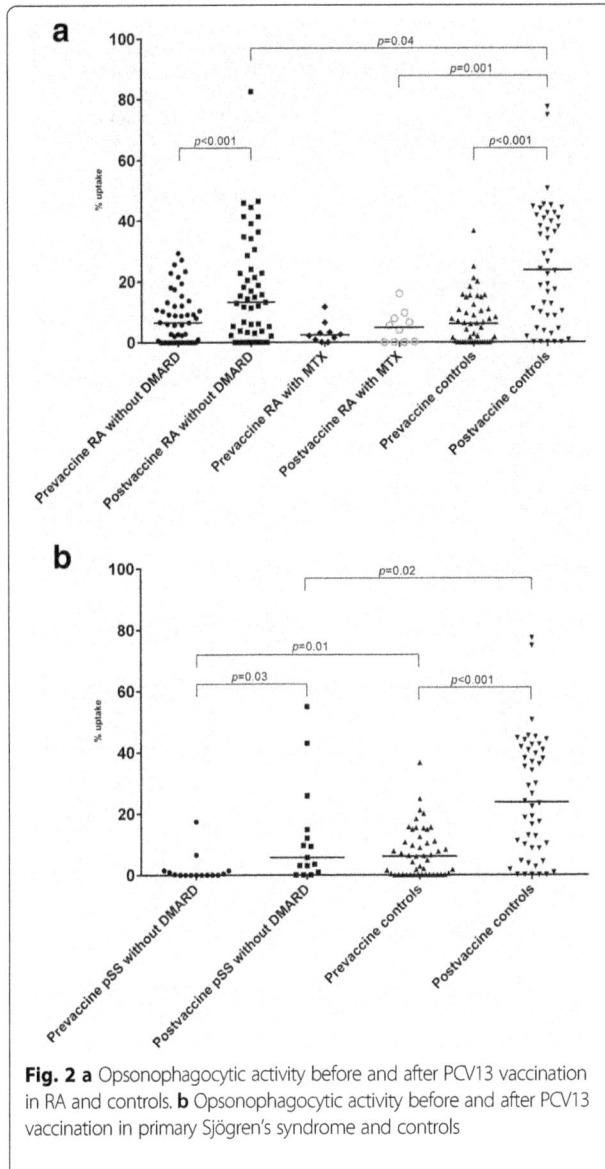

Fig. 2 a Opsonophagocytic activity before and after PCV13 vaccination in RA and controls. **b** Opsonophagocytic activity before and after PCV13 vaccination in primary Sjögren's syndrome and controls

specific IgG titers compared to healthy controls, and autoantibody (Ro/SSA and La/SSB) titers increased. Endosomal toll-like receptor stimulated naïve B-cells in vitro were shown to differentiate and class switch more readily from untreated pSS patients compared with patients receiving hydroxychloroquine and healthy controls [22]. However, in our study with pneumococcal vaccine, this enhanced antibody response could not be reproduced, which could possibly be due to the fact that not all pSS patients in the current study were anti-Ro/SSA and La/SSB seropositives.

Conclusions

Antigen challenge using pneumococcal conjugate vaccine in patients with RA or pSS without active anti-rheumatic treatment resulted in antibody response

comparable to that of healthy controls. Similar to previous findings a decreased response to this vaccine was observed in RA patients treated with methotrexate.

These findings are in line with the previous recommendation that pneumococcal vaccination should be performed before initiation of MTX.

Abbreviations

ARR: Antibody response ratio; DMARD: Disease modifying anti-rheumatic drug; ELISA: Enzyme-linked immunosorbent assay; GMC: Geometric mean antibody concentration; IPD: Invasive pneumococcal disease; MTX: Methotrexate; OPA: Opsonophagocytic activity; PCV13: 13-valent pneumococcal conjugate vaccine; PPV23: 23-valent pneumococcal polysaccharide vaccine; pSS: Primary Sjögren's syndrome; RA: Rheumatoid arthritis

Acknowledgments

This study could not have been conducted without the excellent contributions of the nurses Elna Haglund, Eva-Karin Kristofersson and Nina Svensson in the clinic of Rheumatology at Skåne University Hospital.

Funding

The study was supported by grants from the Swedish Rheumatism Association, the Medical Faculty of Lund University, Alfred Österlund's Foundation, Greta and Johan Kock's foundation, The King Gustaf V Foundation, Lund University Hospital, Inger Bendix Foundation, Apotekare Hedbergs Foundation, Professor Nanna Svartz Foundation, Maggie Stephens Foundation, Åke Wiberg Foundation, the Research and Development Committee at the Central Hospital Kristianstad and Anna-Greta Craford Foundation.

Authors' contributions

The study was conceived by MCK, TS, PG, TM, LS, and PN. PN wrote the manuscript and all authors have revised it critically for important intellectual content. All authors have approved the final version of the manuscript for submission.

Competing interests

The authors declare that they have no competing interests.

Author details

[1]Department of Clinical Sciences Lund, Section of Rheumatology, Lund University, Skåne University Hospital, SE-221 85 Lund, Sweden. [2]Department of Infectious Diseases, Central Hospital Kristianstad, J A Hedlunds väg 5, SE-291 85 Kristianstad, Sweden. [3]Department of Clinical Sciences Malmö, Section of Rheumatology, Lund University, Skåne University Hospital, Malmö, Sweden. [4]Department of Laboratory Medicine, Section of Microbiology, Immunology and Glycobiology, Lund University, Lund, Sweden. [5]Clinical Immunology and Transfusion Medicine, Lund, Region Skåne, Sweden.

References

1. Naz SM, Symmons DPM. Mortality in established rheumatoid arthritis. Best Pract Res Clin Rheumatol. 2007;21:871–83.

2. Flament T, Bigot A, Chaigne B, Henique H, Diot E, Marchand-Adam S. Pulmonary manifestations of Sjögren's syndrome. Eur Respir Rev. 2016; 25:110–23.

3. Doran MF, Crowson CS, Pond GR, O'Fallon WM, Gabriel SE. Frequency of infection in patients with rheumatoid arthritis compared with controls: a population-based study. Arthritis Rheum. 2002;46:2287–93.

4. Doran MF, Crowson CS, Pond GR, O'Fallon WM, Gabriel SE. Predictors of infection in rheumatoid arthritis. Arthritis Rheum. 2002;46:2294–300.

5. Singh JA, Cameron C, Noorbaloochi S, Cullis T, Tucker M, Christensen R, et al. Risk of serious infection in biological treatment of patients with rheumatoid arthritis: a systematic review and meta-analysis. Lancet. 2015; 386:258–65.

6. Wotton CJ, Goldacre MJ. Risk of invasive pneumococcal disease in people admitted to hospital with selected immune-mediated diseases: record linkage cohort analyses. J Epidemiol Community Health. 2012;66:1177–81.

7. Kapetanovic MC, Saxne T, Sjöholm A, Truedsson L, Jönsson G, Geborek P. Influence of methotrexate, TNF blockers and prednisolone on antibody responses to pneumococcal polysaccharide vaccine in patients with rheumatoid arthritis. Rheumatology (Oxford). 2006;45:106–11.

8. Kapetanovic MC, Roseman C, Jönsson G, Truedsson L, Saxne T, Geborek P. Antibody response is reduced following vaccination with 7-valent conjugate pneumococcal vaccine in adult methotrexate-treated patients with established arthritis, but not those treated with tumor necrosis factor inhibitors. Arthritis Rheum. 2011;63:3723–32.

9. Centers for Disease Control and Prevention (CDC). Use of 13-valent pneumococcal conjugate vaccine and 23-valent pneumococcal polysaccharide vaccine for adults with immunocompromising conditions: recommendations of the advisory committee on immunization practices (ACIP). MMWR Morb Mortal Wkly Rep. 2012;61:816–9.

10. Aletaha D, Neogi T, Silman AJ, Funovits J, Felson DT, Bingham CO, et al. 2010 Rheumatoid arthritis classification criteria: an American College of Rheumatology/European league against rheumatism collaborative initiative. Arthritis Rheum. 2010;62:2569–81.

11. Shiboski CH, Shiboski SC, Seror R, Criswell LA, Labetoulle M, Lietman TM, et al. 2016 American College of Rheumatology/European league against rheumatism classification criteria for primary Sjögren's syndrome: a consensus and data-driven methodology involving three international patient cohorts. Ann Rheum Dis. 2017;76:9–16.

12. Online GCP. Guideline for Good Clinical Practice. Available from: http://www.onlinegcp.org. Cited 28 Feb 2017.

13. World Health Organization. The WHO consensus pneumococcal IgG ELISA. Training manual for enzyme-linked immunosorbent assay for the quantitation of Streptococcus pneumonia serotype specific IgG (Pn PS ELISA): a guide to procedures for qualification of materials and analysis of assay performance. Available from: https://www.vaccine.uab.edu/uploads/mdocs/ELISAProtocol(007sp).pdf. Cited 9 May 2017.

14. Nived P, Nagel J, Saxne T, Geborek P, Jönsson G, Skattum L, et al. Immune response to pneumococcal conjugate vaccine in patients with systemic vasculitis receiving standard of care therapy. Vaccine. 2017;35:3639–46.

15. Martinez JE, Romero-Steiner S, Pilishvili T, Barnard S, Schinsky J, Goldblatt D, et al. A flow cytometric opsonophagocytic assay for measurement of functional antibodies elicited after vaccination with the 23-valent pneumococcal polysaccharide vaccine. Clin Diagn Lab Immunol. 1999;6:581–6.

16. Orange JS, Ballow M, Stiehm ER, Ballas ZK, Chinen J, De La Morena M, et al. Use and interpretation of diagnostic vaccination in primary immunodeficiency: a working group report of the basic and clinical immunology interest section of the American Academy of Allergy, Asthma & Immunology. J Allergy Clin Immunol. 2012;130:S1–24.

17. Hua C, Barnetche T, Combe B, Morel J. Effect of methotrexate, anti-tumor necrosis factor α, and rituximab on the immune response to influenza and pneumococcal vaccines in patients with rheumatoid arthritis: a systematic review and meta-analysis. Arthritis Care Res (Hoboken). 2014;66:1016–26.

18. Chang Y-S, Liu C-J, Ou S-M, Hu Y-W, Chen T-J, Lee H-T, et al. Tuberculosis infection in primary Sjögren's syndrome: a nationwide population-based study. Clin Rheumatol. 2014;33:377–83.

19. Nived P, Jørgensen CS, Settergren B. Vaccination status and immune response to 13-valent pneumococcal conjugate vaccine in asplenic individuals. Vaccine. 2015;33:1688–94.

20. European Medicines Agency. Prevenar 13: Summary of product characteristics. Available from: http://www.ema.europa.eu/docs/en_GB/document_library/EPAR_-_Product_Information/human/001104/WC500057247.pdf. Cited 8 May 2017.

21. Romero-Steiner S, Frasch CE, Carlone G, Fleck RA, Goldblatt D, Nahm MH. Use of opsonophagocytosis for serological evaluation of pneumococcal vaccines. Clin Vaccine Immunol. 2006;13:165–9.

22. Brauner S, Folkersen L, Kvarnström M, Meisgen S, Petersen S, Franzén-Malmros M, et al. H1N1 vaccination in Sjögren's syndrome triggers polyclonal B cell activation and promotes autoantibody production. Ann Rheum Dis. 2017;76(10):1755–63. doi:https://doi.org/10.1136/annrheumdis-2016-210509

3

Perioperative medical management for patients with RA, SPA, and SLE undergoing total hip and total knee replacement

Susan M. Goodman*[iD] and Anne R. Bass

Abstract

Total hip (THA) and total knee arthroplasty (TKA) are widely used, successful procedures for symptomatic end stage arthritis of the hips or knees, but patients with rheumatoid arthritis (RA), systemic lupus erythematosus (SLE), and spondyloarthritis (SPA) including ankylosing spondylitis (AS) and psoriatic arthritis (PSA) are at higher risk for adverse events after surgery. Utilization rates of THA and TKA remain high for patients with RA, and rates of arthroplasty have increased for patients with SLE and SPA. However, complications such as infection are increased for patients with SLE, RA, and SPA, most of whom are receiving potent immunosuppressant medications and glucocorticoids at the time of surgery. Patients with SLE and AS are also at increased risk for perioperative cardiac and venous thromboembolism (VTE), while RA patients do not have an increase in perioperative cardiac or VTE risk, despite an overall increase in VTE and cardiac disease. This narrative review will discuss the areas of heightened risk for patients with RA, SLE, and SPA, and the perioperative management strategies currently used to minimize the risks.

Keywords: Total hip arthroplasty, Total knee arthroplasty, Rheumatoid arthritis, Systemic lupus erythematosus, Spondyloarthritis, Perioperative infection, Cardiac risk, Venous-thromboembolism

Background

Total hip (THA) and total knee arthroplasty (TKA) remain valuable options to relieve pain and improve function caused by end-stage arthritis of the hip and knee, including for patients with rheumatoid arthritis (RA), Spondyloarthritis (SPA) including ankylosing spondylitis(AS) and psoriatic arthritis (PSA) and systemic lupus erythematosus (SLE). While rates of THA and TKA for patients with osteoarthritis have increased markedly over the past decade, projections suggest even further increases in utilization by 2015 [1, 2]. Large joint arthroplasty rates for patients with rheumatoid arthritis (RA) have remained stable while rates of arthroplasty for patients with spondyloarthritis (SPA) have increased by 50%, and rates have doubled for patients with systemic lupus erythematosus (SLE) [3–6]. The increased utilization of potent disease

modifying anti-rheumatic drugs (DMARDs) and biologics like the tumor necrosis factor inhibitors (TNFi) has had a clear impact on quality of life for patients with RA, SPA, and SLE, medication use has not been shown to decrease the incidence of large joint arthroplasty for RA, and most RA, PSA, and SLE patients are receiving these immunosuppressant medications at the time of surgery [6–8]. While improvements in pain and function outcomes measured pre and post-operatively are excellent after THA and TKA for patients with RA, SPA, and SLE, adverse events, in particular infection, are increased [9–17]. Ninety day readmission, most commonly for infection, is also increased for patients with RA [18]. Other adverse events increased in patients with SLE include deep venous thrombosis (DVT) and pulmonary embolism (PE), and major acute coronary events (MACE), although patients with RA do not have an increased risk for VTE or MACE after arthroplasty [19, 20]. While the recent literature addressing adverse events in patients with SPA is sparse, increased

* Correspondence: Goodmans@hss.edu
Department of Medicine, Weill Cornell Medical School, Division of Rheumatology Hospital for Special Surgery, 535 E 70th St, New York City, NY 10021, USA

inpatient complications including VTE and cardiac complications have been described using the Agency for Healthcare Research and Quality National Inpatient Sample, a large publically available inpatient database [21], while older studies have demonstrated an increase in infection for patients with PSA undergoing arthroplasty, but have not been repeated since the use of prophylactic perioperative antibiotics became widespread [22, 23]. For patients with RA, the RA specific experience of the surgeon or surgical team decreases the risk of adverse surgical events, but the volume-outcome relationship with SLE or SPA specific volume has not been described [24]. This review will discuss the increased infectious, cardiac, and thromboembolic adverse events seen after THA and TKA in patients with RA, SPA, and SLE, and the perioperative medical evaluation and management options to decrease risk.

Infection

Infection is the most common cause for prosthetic joint failure, and the overall risk of infection is increased in patients with RA, SPA, and SLE [11, 25–29]. The age standardized rate of TKA infection was 1.26% for recipients with RA, compared to 0.84% for recipients with OA, with an adjusted Hazard Ratio (HR) of 1.47, $P = 0.03$, confirmed in a recent meta-analysis demonstrating a relative risk of 1.7 for patients with RA [11, 29]. For patients with SLE whose disease was severe enough to warrant hospitalization within 6 months of surgery, a large study based on Taiwan's National Health Insurance Research Database found the risk of septicaemia to be markedly increased after surgeries including orthopedic procedures (OR = 3.43, 95% CI 2.48 to 4.74) [14]. Immunosuppressant medications including biologics and DMARDs used to treat RA, SPA, and SLE are recognized to increase the risk of infection [30]. Nonetheless, the majority of patients with RA, SPA, and SLE are taking DMARDs, biologics, or other potent immunosuppressant medications at the time of surgery [10, 16, 31, 32]. Medication management, including decisions to continue or withhold medication, is inconsistent, even at high volume centers with experience in arthroplasty for patients with rheumatic diseases [33]. While the increased risk of infection has been attributed to therapy with immunosuppressant medications including DMARDs and biologics, an association with post-operative infection has never been demonstrated directly in randomized controlled trials performed at the time of surgery. The relationship of post-operative infection to anti-rheumatic medication use is unproven, although [32–34] a meta-analysis has demonstrated an increased risk of infection associated with TNFi exposure around the time of surgery when data was pooled [35], a conclusion supported by additional observational studies [15, 34–36]. However, a recent study that used billing data to specify the timing of infliximab infusions in relation to surgery found no clear increase in risk of infection when infliximab was infused within 4 weeks of surgery compared to longer periods of drug withholding [34]. Disease activity and severity may contribute to the risk of peri-operative infection for RA, SPA, and SLE, and might confound the reported association with medication use [14, 37]. Use of glucocorticoids, however, has been consistently associated with an increased risk of infection in multiple settings- including surgery -at dosages above 15 mg./day, yet supraphysiologic doses of glucocorticoids ("stress dose steroids") are routinely administered on the day of surgery out of concern for hemodynamic instability [38, 39]. Synthetic DMARDs including methotrexate, leflunomide, and sulfasalazine have not been demonstrated to increase the risk of perioperative infection, in a randomized controlled trial of perioperative methotrexate use [40].

Using a consensus based process, after analysis of an extensive literature review, The American College of Rheumatology (ACR) and The American Association of Hip and Knee Surgeons (AAHKS) have collaborated on a recently published guideline for the peri-operative management of anti-rheumatic therapy for patients with rheumatic diseases including RA, SPA, and SLE undergoing THA and TKA [41]. The recommendations weighed the risk of infection versus the risk of disease flare when medications were withheld, and were informed by the input of a patient panel that placed far greater importance on the risk of infection, concurring with the panel of experts [42]. The collaborators recommend continuing DMARDs, withholding biologics, based on the dose interval, and withholding tofacitinib for 7 days prior to surgery. Any withheld medications can be re-started after 2 weeks, if there is no evidence of infection either at the surgical site, or elsewhere, and the wound demonstrates good healing. The panel recommends administering the usual daily dose of glucocorticoid (after careful taper when possible to <20 mg. prednisone) rather than supra-physiologic "stress dose steroids" on the day of THA or TKA, specifically for adults receiving glucocorticoids for treatment of their rheumatic condition, excluding patients with juvenile arthritis who may have received glucocorticoids during development or those patients receiving glucocorticoids for adrenal or pituitary insufficiency from this recommendation (Table 1) [41].

Major acute cardiac events

Patients with SLE, SPA, and RA have significantly increased risk of cardiac disease compared to age and sex matched controls. In studies using carotid atherosclerosis as a surrogate for coronary artery disease, patients with RA and SLE had almost 3 times more carotid atherosclerosis (RA 44% versus 15%, $p = .001$; SLE 37.1% vs. 15.2%,

Table 1 Medicatons included in this guideline[a]

DMARDs: CONTINUE these medications through surgery.	Dosing Interval	Continue/Withhold
Methotrexate	Weekly	Continue
Sulfasalazine	Once or twice daily	Continue
Hydroxychloroquine	Once or twice daily	Continue
Leflunomide (Arava)	Daily	Continue
Doxycycline	Daily	Continue
BIOLOGICS: STOP these medications prior to surgery and schedule surgery at the end of the dosing cycle. RESUME medications at minimum 14 days after surgery in the absence wound healing problems, surgical site infection or systemic infection.	Dosing Interval	Schedule Surgery (relative to last biologic dose administered)
Adalimumab (Humira) 40 mg	Every 2 weeks	Week 3
Etanercept (Enbrel) 50 mg or 25 mg	Weekly or twice weekly	Week 2
Golimumab (Simponi)50 mg	Every 4 weeks (SQ)or	Week 5
	Every 8 weeks (IV)	Week 9
Infliximab (Remicade)3 mg/kg	Every 4, 6, or 8 weeks	Week 5, 7, or 9
Abatacept (Orencia) weight-based 500 mg; IV 1000 mg; SQ	Monthly (IV)or	Week 5
125 mg	Weekly (SQ)	Week 2
Rituximab (Rituxan)1000 mg	2 doses 2 weeks apart every 4–6 months	Month 7
Tocilizumab (Actemra) IV 4 mg/kg;	Every week (SQ) or Every 4 weeks	Week 3
SQ 162 mg	(IV)	Week 5
Anakinra (Kineret) SQ 100 mg	Daily	Day 2
Secukinumab (Cosentyx) 150 mg	Every 4 weeks	Week 5
Ustekinumab (Stela) 45 mg	Every 12 weeks	Week 13
Belimumab (Benlysta) 10 mg/kg	Every 4 weeks	Week 5
Tofacitinib (Xeljanz) 5 mg: STOP this medication 7 days prior to surgery.	Daily or twice daily	7 days after last dose
SEVERE SLE-SPECIFIC MEDICATIONS: CONTINUE these medications in the perioperative period.	Dosing Interval	Continue/Withhold
Mycophenolate	Twice daily	Continue
Azathioprine	Daily or twice daily	Continue
Cyclosporine	Twice daily	Continue
Tacrolimus	Twice daily (IV and PO)	Continue
NOT-SEVERE SLE: DISCONTINUE these medications in the perioperative period.	Dosing Interval	Continue/Withhold
Mycophenolate	Twice daily	Withhold
Azathioprine	Daily or twice daily	Withhold
Cyclosporine	Twice daily	Withhold
Tacrolimus	Twice daily (IV and PO)	Continue

Dosing intervals obtained from prescribing information provided online by pharmaceutical companies
[a]2016 American College of Rheumatology/American Association of Hip and Knee Surgeons Guidelines for the Perioperative Management of Anti-rheumatic Medication in Patients with Rheumatic Diseases Undergoing Elective Total Hip or Total Knee Arthroplasty.

$P < 0.001$), even after controlling for traditional cardiac risk factors [43, 44]. For patients with RA, the risk of MI is similar to that seen in patients with diabetes [19, 45, 46]. While cardiac mortality is increased by 50% for patients with RA, they are less likely to report cardiac symptoms such as chest pain [47, 48]. Traditional risk factors such as hypertension and smoking contribute to cardiac risk for patients with RA, and markers of sustained inflammation and disease severity are additional risk factors [49–51]. For patients with SLE, mortality from cardiovascular disease has continued to increase, despite improvements in mortality previously seen for patients with active SLE. The risk of death and cardiac events has doubled, with increases seen even early in the disease [52, 53]. Young women with SLE between the age of 35–44 are 50 times more likely to have an MI than age matched controls [54]. While the extreme increase in relative risk for cardiovascular events is dramatic in young patients with SLE, the absolute risk of cardiovascular events is higher in older women with SLE [55]. In a multicenter Spanish SLE register, 374 (10.9%) of patients had angina, an MI, stroke, or peripheral artery disease. In this cohort, traditional risk factors included smoking and hyperlipidemia, but hypocomplementemia was a risk factor as well, suggesting that for SLE, disease activity contributes to cardiovascular risk [56]. Others have also found that traditional risk factors alone cannot explain the increased risk, and factors such as SLE disease activity and severity contribute to cardiovascular risk [55–58].

Patients with SPA have a higher prevalence of CVD, and have a significant increase in traditional CVD risk factors including hypertension, hyperlipidemia as well as obesity [59–61]. For patients with PSA, the risk of major cardiac events is increased for those not prescribed a DMARD (HR 1.24, 95% CI 1.03 to 1.49), suggesting that either disease severity or activity may also increase cardiac risk in PSA [62].

Perioperative cardiovascular risk is increased in those with known cardiovascular disease. In a large orthopedic hospital, post-operative myocardial infarction (MI) occurred in 0.6% of 8000 inpatient orthopedic procedures, while the risk for those with known ischemic heart disease or risk factors for ischemic heart disease increased to 6.5% [63] suggesting that patients with RA, SPA, and SLE should be at higher risk, given the increase in the prevalence of cardiac disease for these patients and the similarity in risk profile for RA patients when compared to patients with diabetes [45, 54, 57, 64, 65] . However, when a large insurance data-base was queried and patients with RA were compared to patients with DM after surgery, there was a substantially lower rate of cardiac events (RA 0.34% vs. DM 1.07%; p < 0.001) and death (RA 0.30% vs. DM 0.65%; p < 0.001) for patients with RA after intermediate risk procedures including arthroplasty [19]. In addition, there was no increase in in-hospital mortality for RA patients after arthroplasty when compared to controls [66]. However, for patients with SLE, unlike in patients with RA, perioperative risk of cardiac events and death were significantly increased in the US Nationwide Inpatient Sample, with an OR of 4.0 (95% CI 1.9–8.0) for postoperative mortality with hip replacements and an OR of 1.2 (95% CI 0.2–7.5) for mortality with knee replacements [20, 66]. Increased in-hospital mortality for patients with SLE has been confirmed using discharge data from seven states, comprising 8 million discharges, with a higher risk of in-hospital mortality(OR (99% CI) of 1.27 (1.11, 1.47); P < .001), although no increase in in-hospital cardiac events were

reported [67]. Similarly, 30 day post-operative mortality risk is increased in patients with SLE in a report using the Taiwan national insurance database (OR = 2.39, 95% CI 1.28 to 4.45) [14]. For patients with AS, the risk of in-patient cardiac events after THA was significantly higher than in controls [21].

The American Heart Association and American College of Cardiology (AHA/ACC) have formulated guidelines for assessing cardiac risk in preparation for surgery, based on a combination of functional capacity and risk factors including the presence of CAD (angina and/or prior MI), heart failure, stroke or transient ischemic attack, renal insufficiency (serum creatinine [2 mg/dl or creatinine clearance \60 ml/min/1.73 m2), and diabetes requiring insulin therapy [68]. Using this guideline in patients with RA, SPA, and SLE is complicated by the poor functional capacity of many patients prior to THA and TKA, when poor functional capacity is defined as the inability to achieve at least 4 Metabolic Equivalents (METS), achieved by light shoveling, dancing, or gardening, defining "light" as when the activity results in "only minimal perspiration and only a slight increase in breathing above normal" [69]. Moreover, patients with RA with cardiovascular disease may not have symptoms [48, 70, 71]. Using the classic Framingham risk equation (based on age, sex, total cholesterol level, high density lipoprotein cholesterol level, smoking history, and systolic blood pressure), patients with RA, SPA, and SLE may fall into a low risk category, leading some to add the presence of a systemic inflammatory disease such as RA, SPA, and SLE to the list of traditional cardiovascular risk factors, or to add a multiplication factor of 1.4 to the calculation of cardiac risk, recognizing that the current risk assessment tools are unreliable and underestimate cardiac risk in patients with RA, SPA, and SLE [51, 72–76]. Major orthopedic surgery is categorized as an intermediate risk procedure in the ACA/AHA guideline, and carries a 1–5% risk of MI or cardiovascular death [68]. While none of these formulations are entirely satisfactory for estimating perioperative risk in patients with inflammatory diseases, a pragmatic approach has been to include RA, SPA, and SLE as risk factors in the ACA/AHA algorithm; patients with 2 risk factors, one of which could be RA, SPA, and SLE, and poor functional capacity (< 4 METS), would undergo testing for evidence of cardiac ischemia prior to elective intermediate risk surgery.

Venous Thromboembolism

Patients with rheumatic diseases have more than double the risk of VTE compared to the general population, particularly when their disease is active [77–81]. This is not surprising given the association between inflammation and thrombosis [82]. Although RA patients have double the risk of VTE over all [83–85], RA patients undergoing arthroplasty are not at increased VTE risk [11, 32, 85, 86]. For example, in a study of close to a billion hospitalized patients, RA and non-RA patients admitted for surgery on their joints had the same risk of postoperative VTE (0.67%) [85]. In contrast, the RA patients admitted for other reasons had double the risk of VTE compared to their non-RA peers (2.3% vs. 1.15%) [85]. Risk factors for postoperative VTE in RA patients in this study were similar to those in other patients and included advanced age, female gender, and African–American race. It is possible that good disease control in RA patients undergoing arthroplasty explains their relatively low VTE risk. In contrast, a recent retrospective study of patients undergoing spine surgery demonstrated a significantly higher risk of VTE in RA patients than non-RA patients [87]. Although this finding requires validation, it could also reflect the more urgent nature of spine surgery, which may not permit RA disease optimization.

Patients with SPA are at higher risk of VTE than the general population [79]. As with RA patients, however, the risk of VTE after arthroplasty does not appear to be higher in these patients. For example, in a study that looked at complication rates after TKA, there was a higher rate of DVT, but no difference in the rate of PE (or total VTE) in 4575 ankylosing spondylitis patients, and no difference in DVT or PE rates in the 7918 psoriatic arthritis compared to 1,751,938 OA controls [88].

Patients with SLE are also at higher risk for VTE [79–81, 89, 90]. Among lupus patients, VTE risk factors include smoking, obesity, hemolytic anemia and anti-phospholipid antibodies, while Asian race is protective [89, 90]. Lupus patients who have received inpatient care for their lupus in the 6 months prior to surgery are five times more likely to experience postoperative PE [14] reinforcing the concept that it is disease activity that increases thrombotic risk. Lupus patients are also more likely than other individuals to have antiphospholipid antibodies, a well-established risk factor for VTE [89, 91]. Among patients with antiphospholipid antibodies, those with a lupus anticoagulant (LAC) or triple positivity (LAC plus high titer anti-cardiolipin and anti-beta 2 glycoprotein 1 antibodies) are at highest VTE risk [92–94].

Current recommendations for postoperative VTE prophylaxis in patients with the antiphospholipid antibody syndrome (APS) are to minimize the time off anticoagulation, bridge with low molecular weight heparin, and resume warfarin the night of surgery [95, 96]. Although a recent prospective trial demonstrated less thrombin generation in APS patients given rivaroxaban compared to warfarin [97], there are no studies demonstrating the safety and/or efficacy of direct oral anticoagulants in preventing thrombotic events in APS. In patients with APS, surgery can sometimes act as a trigger for catastrophic

antiphospholipid syndrome (CAPS). Patients with CAPS should be managed with parenteral anticoagulation and may require additional treatment with corticosteroids, IVIG and/or rituximab [98] .

It should also be remembered that, in addition to assessing the activity of their rheumatic disease, patients with RA, SPA and SLE should also be assessed for traditional VTE risk factors prior to surgery (Table 2).

Recommended prophylactic anticoagulation for (non-APS) rheumatic disease patients whose disease is quiet is the same as for non-rheumatic disease patients. Patients with active rheumatic disease should, preferably, have their disease controlled prior to undergoing elective orthopedic surgery. Patients with active rheumatic disease who must undergo urgent surgical procedures should be considered at higher than average VTE risk; prophylaxis will depend on their particular procedure.

Conclusion

In summary, while patients with RA, SPA, and SLE continue to utilize THA and TKA, they are at higher risk for complications. Risk of infection is higher in patients with RA, SPA, and SLE, and may be decreased via perioperative medication management strategies that include withholding all biologics prior to surgery, although traditional DMARDs do not appear to increase risk of infection. Perioperative cardiac risk stratification is improved with the recognition that patients with RA, SPA, and SLE are at higher risk of

Table 2 Risk factors for venous thromboembolism in rheumatic disease patients undergoing surgery

Patient-specific risk factors
Active rheumatic disease
History of VTE[a]
Active cancer
Estrogen
Active cancer
Smoking
Advanced age
Black race (Asian race protective)
Obesity
Non-O ABO blood group
Thrombophilia
Surgery-specific risk factors
Orthopedic surgery > other surgery
Hip fracture
Bilateral arthroplasty
Revision arthroplasty
General > Axial/regional anesthesia

[a]VTE = venous thromboembolism

cardiac disease than age matched controls. While patients with SLE are at higher risk of VTE after surgery, VTE risk for patients with RA and SPA is no higher than for others undergoing THA and TKA. Improved outcomes may be achieved with attention to preoperative optimization to minimize perioperative risks.

Acknowledgements
Not applicable

Funding
There are no funding sources associated with this article.

Authors' contributions
SMG and ARB performed the literature search, wrote and revised the manuscript, and gave final approval of the version to be published.

Competing interests
SMG is a member of the Editorial Board of BMC Rheumatology. ARB declares that she has no competing interest.

References
1. Inacio MCS, Paxton EW, Graves SE, Namba RS, Nemes S. Projected increase in total knee arthroplasty in the United States - an alternative projection model. Osteoarthritis Cartilage. 2017; Nov;25(11):1797–803.
2. Kurtz S, Ong K, Lau E, Mowat F, Halpern M. Projections of primary and revision hip and knee arthroplasty in the United States from 2005 to 2030. J Bone Joint Surg Am. 2007; Apr;89(4):780–5.
3. Mertelsmann-Voss C, Lyman S, Pan TJ, Goodman S, Figgie MP, Mandl LA. Arthroplasty rates are increased among US patients with systemic lupus erythematosus: 1991-2005. J Rheumatol. 2014; May;41(5):867–74.
4. Mertelsmann-Voss C, Lyman S, Pan TJ, Goodman SM, Figgie MP, Mandl LA. US trends in rates of arthroplasty for inflammatory arthritis including rheumatoid arthritis, juvenile idiopathic arthritis, and spondyloarthritis. Arthritis Rheumatol. 2014; Jun;66(6):1432–9.
5. Sokka T, Kautiainen H, Hannonen P. Stable occurrence of knee and hip total joint replacement in Central Finland between 1986 and 2003: an indication of improved long-term outcomes of rheumatoid arthritis. Ann Rheum Dis. 2007; Mar;66(3):341–4.
6. Nikiphorou E, Carpenter L, Morris S, Macgregor AJ, Dixey J, Kiely P, et al. Hand and foot surgery rates in rheumatoid arthritis have declined from 1986 to 2011, but large-joint replacement rates remain unchanged: results from two UK inception cohorts. Arthritis Rheumatol. 2014; May;66(5):1081–9.
7. Aaltonen KJ, Virkki LM, Jamsen E, Sokka T, Konttinen YT, Peltomaa R, et al. Do biologic drugs affect the need for and outcome of joint replacements in patients with rheumatoid arthritis? A register-based study. Semin Arthritis Rheum. 2013; Aug;43(1):55–62.
8. Strand V, Sharp V, Koenig AS, Park G, Shi Y, Wang B, et al. Comparison of health-related quality of life in rheumatoid arthritis, psoriatic arthritis and psoriasis and effects of etanercept treatment. Ann Rheum Dis. 2012; Jul; 71(7):1143–50.
9. Shah UH, Mandl LA, Mertelsmann-Voss C, Lee YY, Alexiades MM, Figgie MP, et al. Systemic lupus erythematosus is not a risk factor for poor outcomes after total hip and total knee arthroplasty. Lupus. 2015; Jan 16;24(9):900–8.
10. Goodman SM, Johnson B, Zhang M, Huang WT, Zhu R, Figgie M, et al. Patients with Rheumatoid Arthritis have Similar Excellent Outcomes after Total Knee Replacement Compared with Patients with Osteoarthritis. J Rheumatol. 2016; Jan;43(1):46–53.
11. Ravi B, Croxford R, Hollands S, Paterson JM, Bogoch E, Kreder H, et al. Increased risk of complications following total joint arthroplasty in patients with rheumatoid arthritis. Arthritis Rheumatol. 2014; Feb;66(2):254–63.
12. Ravi B, Croxford R, Hollands S, Paterson MJ, Bogoch E, Kreder H, et al. Patients with rheumatoid arthritis are at increased risk for complications following total joint arthroplasty. Arthritis Rheum. 2013; Nov 19;66(2):254–63.
13. Singh JA, Inacio MC, Namba RS, Paxton EW. Rheumatoid arthritis is associated with higher 90-day hospital readmission rates compared to osteoarthritis after hip or knee arthroplasty: A cohort study. Arthritis Care Res (Hoboken). 2014; Oct 9;67(5):718–24.
14. Lin JA, Liao CC, Lee YJ, Wu CH, Huang WQ, Chen TL. Adverse outcomes after major surgery in patients with systemic lupus erythematosus: a nationwide population-based study. Ann Rheum Dis. 2014; Sep;73(9):1646–51.
15. Salt E, Wiggins AT, Rayens MK, Morris BJ, Mannino D, Hoellein A, et al. Moderating effects of immunosuppressive medications and risk factors for post-operative joint infection following total joint arthroplasty in patients with rheumatoid arthritis or osteoarthritis. Semin Arthritis Rheum. 2017; Feb; 46(4):423–9.
16. Mandl LA, Zhu R, Huang WT, Zhang M, Alexiades MM, Figgie MP, et al. Short Term Total Hip Arthroplasty Outcomes in Patients with Psoriatic Arthritis, Psoriasis Skin Disease, and Osteoarthritis. Arthritis Rheumatol. 2015; Sep 11;68(2):410–7.
17. Goodman SM, Zhu R, Figgie MP, Huang WT, Mandl LA. Short-term total hip replacement outcomes in ankylosing spondylitis. J Clin Rheumatol. 2014; Oct;20(7):363–8.
18. Singh JA, Inacio MC, Namba RS, Paxton EW. Rheumatoid Arthritis is Associated With Higher Ninety-Day Hospital Readmission Rates Compared to Osteoarthritis After Hip or Knee Arthroplasty: A Cohort Study. Arthritis Care Res (Hoboken). 2015; May;67(5):718–24.
19. Yazdanyar A, Wasko MC, Kraemer KL, Ward MM. Perioperative all-cause mortality and cardiovascular events in patients with rheumatoid arthritis: Comparison with unaffected controls and persons with diabetes mellitus. Arthritis Rheum. 2012; Aug;64(8):2429–37.
20. Yazdanyar A, Wasko MC, Scalzi LV, Kraemer KL, Ward MM. Short-term perioperative all-cause mortality and cardiovascular events in women with systemic lupus erythematosus. Arthritis Care Res (Hoboken). 2012; Dec 4;65(6):986–91.
21. Schnaser EA, Browne JA, Padgett DE, Figgie MP, D'Apuzzo MR. Perioperative Complications in Patients With Inflammatory Arthropathy Undergoing Total Hip Arthroplasty. J Arthroplasty. 2016; Oct;31(10):2286–90.
22. Stern SH, Insall JN, Windsor RE, Inglis AE, Dines DM. Total knee arthroplasty in patients with psoriasis. Clin Orthop Relat Res. 1989;248(248):108–10. discussion 111
23. Menon TJ, Wroblewski BM. Charnley low-friction arthroplasty in patients with psoriasis. Clin Orthop Relat Res. 1983; Jun;176(176):127–8.
24. Ravi B, Croxford R, Austin PC, Hollands S, Paterson JM, Bogoch E, et al. Increased surgeon experience with rheumatoid arthritis reduces the risk of complications following total joint arthroplasty. Arthritis Rheumatol. 2014; Mar;66(3):488–96.
25. Mortazavi SM, Molligan J, Austin MS, Purtill JJ, Hozack WJ, Parvizi J. Failure following revision total knee arthroplasty: infection is the major cause. Int Orthop. 2011; Aug;35(8):1157–64.
26. Le DH, Goodman SB, Maloney WJ, Huddleston JI. Current modes of failure in TKA: infection, instability, and stiffness predominate. Clin Orthop Relat Res. 2014; Jul;472(7):2197–200.
27. Thiele K, Perka C, Matziolis G, Mayr HO, Sostheim M, Hube R. Current failure mechanisms after knee arthroplasty have changed: polyethylene wear is less common in revision surgery. J Bone Joint Surg Am. 2015; May 6;97(9):715–20.
28. Jamsen E, Huhtala H, Puolakka T, Moilanen T. Risk factors for infection after knee arthroplasty. A register-based analysis of 43,149 cases. J Bone Joint Surg Am. 2009; Jan;91(1):38–47.
29. Kunutsor SK, Whitehouse MR, Blom AW, Beswick AD, INFORM Team. Patient-Related Risk Factors for Periprosthetic Joint Infection after Total Joint Arthroplasty: A Systematic Review and Meta-Analysis. PLoS One. 2016; Mar 3;11(3):e0150866.
30. Singh JA, Cameron C, Noorbaloochi S, Cullis T, Tucker M, Christensen R, et al. Risk of serious infection in biological treatment of patients with rheumatoid arthritis: a systematic review and meta-analysis. Lancet. 2015; May 11;386(9990):258–65.
31. Shah UH, Mandl LA, Mertelsmann-Voss C, Lee YY, Alexiades MM, Figgie MP, et al. Systemic lupus erythematosus is not a risk factor for poor outcomes after total hip and total knee arthroplasty. Lupus. 2015; Aug;24(9):900–8.
32. ZJ LV, Mandl LA, Johnson BK, Figgie MP, Boettner F, Lee YY, et al. Rheumatoid Arthritis Does Not Increase Risk of Short-term Adverse Events after Total Knee Arthroplasty: A Retrospective Case-control Study. J Rheumatol. 2015; May 1;42(7):1123–30.

33. Johnson BK, Goodman SM, Alexiades MM, Figgie MP, Demmer RT, Mandl LA. Patterns and associated risk of perioperative use of anti-tumor necrosis factor in patients with rheumatoid arthritis undergoing total knee replacement. J Rheumatol. 2013; May;40(5):617–23.

34. George MD, Baker JF, Yenchih Hsu J, Wu Q, Xie F, Chen L, et al. Perioperative timing of infliximab and the risk of serious infection after elective hip and knee arthroplasty. Arthritis Care Res (Hoboken). 2017; Jan 27;69(12):1845–54.

35. Goodman SM, Menon I, Christos PJ, Smethurst R, Bykerk VP. Management of perioperative tumour necrosis factor alpha inhibitors in rheumatoid arthritis patients undergoing arthroplasty: a systematic review and meta-analysis. Rheumatology (Oxford). 2016; Mar;55(3):573–82.

36. Ruyssen-Witrand A, Gossec L, Salliot C, Luc M, Duclos M, Guignard S, et al. Complication rates of 127 surgical procedures performed in rheumatic patients receiving tumor necrosis factor alpha blockers. Clin Exp Rheumatol. 2007; May-Jun;25(3):430–6.

37. Weaver A, Troum O, Hooper M, Koenig AS, Chaudhari S, Feng J, et al. Rheumatoid arthritis disease activity and disability affect the risk of serious infection events in RADIUS 1. J Rheumatol. 2013; Aug;40(8):1275–81.

38. Somayaji R, Barnabe C, Martin L. Risk factors for infection following total joint arthroplasty in rheumatoid arthritis. Open Rheumatol J. 2013; Nov 29;7: 119–24.

39. Harpaz R, Ortega-Sanchez I, Seward J. Prevention of Herpes Zoster: Recommendation of the Advisory Committee on Immunization Practices. MMWR. Morbidity and Mortality Weekly Report. 2008;57(05):1–30.

40. Grennan DM, Gray J, Loudon J, Fear S. Methotrexate and early postoperative complications in patients with rheumatoid arthritis undergoing elective orthopaedic surgery. Ann Rheum Dis. 2001; Mar;60(3):214–7.

41. Goodman SM, Springer B, Guyatt G, Abdel MP, Dasa V, George M, et al. 2017 American College of Rheumatology/American Association of Hip and Knee Surgeons Guideline for the Perioperative Management of Antirheumatic Medication in Patients With Rheumatic Diseases Undergoing Elective Total Hip or Total Knee Arthroplasty. Arthritis Rheumatol. 2017; Jun 16;69(8):1111–24.

42. Goodman SM, Miller AS, Turgunbaev M, Guyatt G, Yates A, Springer B, et al. Clinical Practice Guidelines: Incorporating Input From a Patient Panel. Arthritis Care Res (Hoboken). 2017; Jun 16;69(8):1125–30.

43. Roman MJ, Moeller E, Davis A, Paget SA, Crow MK, Lockshin MD, et al. Preclinical carotid atherosclerosis in patients with rheumatoid arthritis. Ann Intern Med. 2006; Feb 21;144(4):249–56.

44. Roman MJ, Shanker BA, Davis A, Lockshin MD, Sammaritano L, Simantov R, et al. Prevalence and correlates of accelerated atherosclerosis in systemic lupus erythematosus. N Engl J Med. 2003; Dec 18;349(25):2399–406.

45. Lindhardsen J, Ahlehoff O, Gislason GH, Madsen OR, Olesen JB, Torp-Pedersen C, et al. The risk of myocardial infarction in rheumatoid arthritis and diabetes mellitus: a Danish nationwide cohort study. Ann Rheum Dis. 2011; Jun;70(6):929–34.

46. van Halm VP, Peters MJ, Voskuyl AE, Boers M, Lems WF, Visser M, et al. Rheumatoid arthritis versus diabetes as a risk factor for cardiovascular disease: a cross-sectional study, the CARRE Investigation. Ann Rheum Dis. 2009; Sep;68(9):1395–400.

47. Avina-Zubieta JA, Choi HK, Sadatsafavi M, Etminan M, Esdaile JM, Lacaille D. Risk of cardiovascular mortality in patients with rheumatoid arthritis: a meta-analysis of observational studies. Arthritis Rheum. 2008; Dec 15;59(12):1690–7.

48. Maradit-Kremers H, Crowson CS, Nicola PJ, Ballman KV, Roger VL, Jacobsen SJ, et al. Increased unrecognized coronary heart disease and sudden deaths in rheumatoid arthritis: a population-based cohort study. Arthritis Rheum. 2005; Feb;52(2):402–11.

49. Maradit-Kremers H, Nicola PJ, Crowson CS, Ballman KV, Gabriel SE. Cardiovascular death in rheumatoid arthritis: a population-based study. Arthritis Rheum. 2005; Mar;52(3):722–32.

50. Solomon DH, Kremer J, Curtis JR, Hochberg MC, Reed G, Tsao P, et al. Explaining the cardiovascular risk associated with rheumatoid arthritis: traditional risk factors versus markers of rheumatoid arthritis severity. Ann Rheum Dis. 2010; Nov;69(11):1920–5.

51. Alemao E, Cawston H, Bourhis F, Al M, Rutten-van Molken M, Liao KP, et al. Comparison of cardiovascular risk algorithms in patients with vs without rheumatoid arthritis and the role of C-reactive protein in predicting cardiovascular outcomes in rheumatoid arthritis. Rheumatology (Oxford). 2017; May 1;56(5):777–86.

52. Bernatsky S, Boivin JF, Joseph L, Manzi S, Ginzler E, Gladman DD, et al. Mortality in systemic lupus erythematosus. Arthritis Rheum. 2006; Aug;54(8): 2550–7.

53. Bartels CM, Buhr KA, Goldberg JW, Bell CL, Visekruna M, Nekkanti S, et al. Mortality and cardiovascular burden of systemic lupus erythematosus in a US population-based cohort. J Rheumatol. 2014; Apr;41(4):680–7.

54. Manzi S, Meilahn EN, Rairie JE, Conte CG, Medsger TA Jr, Jansen-McWilliams L, et al. Age-specific incidence rates of myocardial infarction and angina in women with systemic lupus erythematosus: comparison with the Framingham Study. Am J Epidemiol. 1997; Mar 1;145(5):408–15.

55. Schoenfeld SR, Kasturi S, Costenbader KH. The epidemiology of atherosclerotic cardiovascular disease among patients with SLE: a systematic review. Semin Arthritis Rheum. 2013; Aug;43(1):77–95.

56. Fernandez-Nebro A, Rua-Figueroa I, Lopez-Longo FJ, Galindo-Izquierdo M, Calvo-Alen J, Olive-Marques A, et al. Cardiovascular Events in Systemic Lupus Erythematosus: A Nationwide Study in Spain From the RELESSER Registry. Medicine (Baltimore). 2015; Jul;94(29):e1183.

57. Esdaile JM, Abrahamowicz M, Grodzicky T, Li Y, Panaritis C, du Berger R, et al. Traditional Framingham risk factors fail to fully account for accelerated atherosclerosis in systemic lupus erythematosus. Arthritis Rheum. 2001; Oct; 44(10):2331–7.

58. Karp I, Abrahamowicz M, Fortin PR, Pilote L, Neville C, Pineau CA, et al. Recent corticosteroid use and recent disease activity: independent determinants of coronary heart disease risk factors in systemic lupus erythematosus? Arthritis Rheum. 2008; Feb 15;59(2):169–75.

59. Wibetoe G, Ikdahl E, Rollefstad S, Olsen IC, Bergsmark K, Kvien TK, et al. Cardiovascular disease risk profiles in inflammatory joint disease entities. Arthritis Res Ther. 2017; Jul 3;19(1):153. 017-1358-1

60. Han C, Robinson DW Jr, Hackett MV, Paramore LC, Fraeman KH, Bala MV. Cardiovascular disease and risk factors in patients with rheumatoid arthritis, psoriatic arthritis, and ankylosing spondylitis. J Rheumatol. 2006; Nov;(11):33, 2167–2172.

61. Haque N, Lories RJ, de Vlam K. Comorbidities Associated with Psoriatic Arthritis Compared with Non-psoriatic Spondyloarthritis: A Cross-sectional Study. J Rheumatol. 2016; Feb;43(2):376–82.

62. Ogdie A, Yu Y, Haynes K, Love TJ, Maliha S, Jiang Y, et al. Risk of major cardiovascular events in patients with psoriatic arthritis, psoriasis and rheumatoid arthritis: a population-based cohort study. Ann Rheum Dis. 2015; Feb;74(2):326–32.

63. Urban MK, Jules-Elysee K, Loughlin C, Kelsey W, Flynn E. The one year incidence of postoperative myocardial infarction in an orthopedic population. HSS J. 2008; Feb;4(1):76–80.

64. Innala L, Moller B, Ljung L, Magnusson S, Smedby T, Sodergren A, et al. Cardiovascular events in early RA are a result of inflammatory burden and traditional risk factors: a five year prospective study. Arthritis Res Ther. 2011; Aug 15;13(4):R131.

65. Peters MJ, van der Horst-Bruinsma IE, Dijkmans BA, Nurmohamed MT. Cardiovascular risk profile of patients with spondylarthropathies, particularly ankylosing spondylitis and psoriatic arthritis. Semin Arthritis Rheum. 2004; Dec;34(3):585–92.

66. Domsic RT, Lingala B, Krishnan E. Systemic lupus erythematosus, rheumatoid arthritis, and postarthroplasty mortality: a cross-sectional analysis from the nationwide inpatient sample. J Rheumatol. 2010; Jul;37(7):1467–72.

67. Babazade R, Yilmaz HO, Leung SM, Zimmerman NM, Turan A. Systemic Lupus Erythematosus Is Associated With Increased Adverse Postoperative Renal Outcomes and Mortality: A Historical Cohort Study Using Administrative Health Data. Anesth Analg. 2017; Apr;124(4):1118–26.

68. Fleisher LA, Fleischmann KE, Auerbach AD, Barnason SA, Beckman JA, Bozkurt B, et al. 2014 ACC/AHA guideline on perioperative cardiovascular evaluation and management of patients undergoing noncardiac surgery: executive summary: a report of the American College of Cardiology/American Heart Association Task Force on practice guidelines. Developed in collaboration with the American College of Surgeons, American Society of Anesthesiologists, American Society of Echocardiography, American Society of Nuclear Cardiology, Heart Rhythm Society, Society for Cardiovascular Angiography and Interventions, Society of Cardiovascular Anesthesiologists, and Society of Vascular Medicine Endorsed by the Society of Hospital Medicine. J Nucl Cardiol. 2015; Feb;22(1):162–215.

69. Jette M, Sidney K, Blumchen G. Metabolic equivalents (METS) in exercise testing, exercise prescription, and evaluation of functional capacity. Clin Cardiol. 1990; Aug;13(8):555–65.

70. Mirfeizi Z, Poorzand H, Javanbakht A, Khajedaluee M. Relationship Between Systemic Lupus Erythematosus Disease Activity Index Scores and Subclinical Cardiac Problems. Iran Red Crescent Med J. 2016; Jul 17;18(8):e38045.

71. Divard G, Abbas R, Chenevier-Gobeaux C, Chanson N, Escoubet B, Chauveheid MP, et al. High-sensitivity cardiac troponin T is a biomarker for atherosclerosis in systemic lupus erythematous patients: a cross-sectional controlled study. Arthritis Res Ther. 2017; Jun 13;19(1):132,017–1352-7.

72. Mosca L, Benjamin EJ, Berra K, Bezanson JL, Dolor RJ, Lloyd-Jones DM, et al. Effectiveness-based guidelines for the prevention of cardiovascular disease in women–2011 update: a guideline from the american heart association. Circulation. 2011; Mar 22;123(11):1243–62.

73. Agca R, Heslinga SC, Rollefstad S, Heslinga M, McInnes IB, Peters MJ, et al. EULAR recommendations for cardiovascular disease risk management in patients with rheumatoid arthritis and other forms of inflammatory joint disorders: 2015/2016 update. Ann Rheum Dis. 2017; Jan;76(1):17–28.

74. Crowson CS, Gabriel SE, Semb AG, van Riel PL, Karpouzas G, Dessein PH, et al. Rheumatoid arthritis-specific cardiovascular risk scores are not superior to general risk scores: a validation analysis of patients from seven countries. Rheumatology (Oxford). 2017; Mar 8;56(7):1102–10.

75. Arts EE, Popa CD, Den Broeder AA, Donders R, Sandoo A, Toms T, et al. Prediction of cardiovascular risk in rheumatoid arthritis: performance of original and adapted SCORE algorithms. Ann Rheum Dis. 2016; Apr;75(4): 674–80.

76. Semb AG, Ikdahl E, Hisdal J, Olsen IC, Rollefstad S. Exploring cardiovascular disease risk evaluation in patients with inflammatory joint diseases. Int J Cardiol. 2016; Nov 15;223:331–6.

77. Johannesdottir SA, Schmidt M, Horvath-Puho E, Sorensen HT. Autoimmune skin and connective tissue diseases and risk of venous thromboembolism: a population-based case-control study. J Thromb Haemost. 2012; May;10(5): 815–21.

78. Kim SC, Schneeweiss S, Liu J, Solomon DH. Risk of venous thromboembolism in patients with rheumatoid arthritis. Arthritis Care Res (Hoboken). 2013; Oct;65(10):1600–7.

79. Zoller B, Li X, Sundquist J, Sundquist K. Risk of pulmonary embolism in patients with autoimmune disorders: a nationwide follow-up study from Sweden. Lancet. 2012; Jan 21;379(9812):244–9.

80. Ramagopalan SV, Wotton CJ, Handel AE, Yeates D, Goldacre MJ. Risk of venous thromboembolism in people admitted to hospital with selected immune-mediated diseases: record-linkage study. BMC Med. 2011; Jan 10; 9(1):7015-9-1.

81. Yusuf HR, Hooper WC, Beckman MG, Zhang QC, Tsai J, Ortel TL. Risk of venous thromboembolism among hospitalizations of adults with selected autoimmune diseases. J Thromb Thrombolysis. 2014; Oct;38(3):306–13.

82. Xu J, Lupu F, Esmon CT. Inflammation, innate immunity and blood coagulation. Hamostaseologie. 2010; Jan;30(1):5,6, 8–9.

83. Bacani AK, Gabriel SE, Crowson CS, Heit JA, Matteson EL. Noncardiac vascular disease in rheumatoid arthritis: increase in venous thromboembolic events? Arthritis Rheum. 2012; Jan;64(1):53–61.

84. Choi HK, Rho YH, Zhu Y, Cea-Soriano L, Avina-Zubieta JA, Zhang Y. The risk of pulmonary embolism and deep vein thrombosis in rheumatoid arthritis: a UK population-based outpatient cohort study. Ann Rheum Dis. 2013; Jul; 72(7):1182–7.

85. Matta F, Singala R, Yaekoub AY, Najjar R, Stein PD. Risk of venous thromboembolism with rheumatoid arthritis. Thromb Haemost. 2009; Jan; 101(1):134–8.

86. Sun Z, Hesler BD, Makarova N, Dalton JE, Doan M, Moraska A, et al. The Association Between Rheumatoid Arthritis and Adverse Postoperative Outcomes: A Retrospective Analysis. Anesth Analg. 2016; Jun;122(6):1887–93.

87. Wei J, Li W, Pei Y, Shen Y, Li J. Clinical analysis of preoperative risk factors for the incidence of deep venous thromboembolism in patients undergoing posterior lumbar interbody fusion. J Orthop Surg Res. 2016; Jun 13;11(1):68,016–0403-0.

88. Cancienne JM, Werner BC, Browne JA. Complications of Primary Total Knee Arthroplasty Among Patients With Rheumatoid Arthritis, Psoriatic Arthritis, Ankylosing Spondylitis, and Osteoarthritis. J Am Acad Orthop Surg. 2016; Aug;24(8):567–74.

89. Mok CC, Tang SS, To CH, Petri M. Incidence and risk factors of thromboembolism in systemic lupus erythematosus: a comparison of three ethnic groups. Arthritis Rheum. 2005; Sep;(9):52, 2774–2782.

90. Calvo-Alen J, Toloza SM, Fernandez M, Bastian HM, Fessler BJ, Roseman JM, et al. Systemic lupus erythematosus in a multiethnic US cohort (LUMINA). XXV. Smoking, older age, disease activity, lupus anticoagulant, and glucocorticoid dose as risk factors for the occurrence of venous thrombosis in lupus patients. Arthritis Rheum. 2005; Jul;52(7):2060–8.

91. Habe K, Wada H, Matsumoto T, Ohishi K, Ikejiri M, Matsubara K, et al. Presence of Antiphospholipid Antibodies as a Risk Factor for Thrombotic Events in Patients with Connective Tissue Diseases and Idiopathic Thrombocytopenic Purpura. Intern Med. 2016;55(6):589–95.

92. Pengo V, Ruffatti A, Legnani C, Gresele P, Barcellona D, Erba N, et al. Clinical course of high-risk patients diagnosed with antiphospholipid syndrome. J Thromb Haemost. 2010; Feb;8(2):237–42.

93. Sciascia S, Cuadrado MJ, Sanna G, Murru V, Roccatello D, Khamashta MA, et al. Thrombotic risk assessment in systemic lupus erythematosus: validation of the global antiphospholipid syndrome score in a prospective cohort. Arthritis Care Res (Hoboken). 2014; Dec;66(12):1915–20.

94. Reynaud Q, Lega JC, Mismetti P, Chapelle C, Wahl D, Cathebras P, et al. Risk of venous and arterial thrombosis according to type of antiphospholipid antibodies in adults without systemic lupus erythematosus: a systematic review and meta-analysis. Autoimmun Rev. 2014; Jun;13(6):595–608.

95. Saunders KH, Erkan D, Lockshin MD. Perioperative management of antiphospholipid antibody-positive patients. Curr Rheumatol Rep. 2014; Jul; 16(7):426. 014-0426-7

96. Raso S, Sciascia S, Kuzenko A, Castagno I, Marozio L, Bertero MT. Bridging therapy in antiphospholipid syndrome and antiphospholipid antibodies carriers: case series and review of the literature. Autoimmun Rev. 2015; Jan; 14(1):36–42.

97. Cohen H, Hunt BJ, Efthymiou M, Arachchillage DR, Mackie IJ, Clawson S, et al. Rivaroxaban versus warfarin to treat patients with thrombotic antiphospholipid syndrome, with or without systemic lupus erythematosus (RAPS): a randomised, controlled, open-label, phase 2/3, non-inferiority trial. Lancet Haematol. 2016; Sep;3(9):e426–36.

98. Cervera R. CAPS Registry Project Group. Catastrophic antiphospholipid syndrome (CAPS): update from the 'CAPS Registry'. Lupus. 2010; Apr;19(4): 412–8.

4

Cardiovascular co-morbidity in patients with rheumatoid arthritis: a narrative review of risk factors, cardiovascular risk assessment and treatment

Aprajita Jagpal[1] and Iris Navarro-Millán[2,3*] (iD)

Abstract

Cardiovascular disease (CVD) is markedly increased in patients with rheumatoid arthritis partly due to accelerated atherosclerosis from chronic inflammation. Traditional cardiovascular risk factors such as hypertension, hyperlipidemia, smoking, diabetes mellitus and physical inactivity are also highly prevalent among patients with rheumatoid arthritis (RA) and contribute to the CVD risk. The impact of traditional risk factors on the CVD risk appears to be different in the RA and non-RA population. However, hyperlipidemia, diabetes mellitus, body mass index and family history of CVD influence the CVD risk in RA patients the same way they do for the non-RA population. Despite that, screening and treatment of these risk factors is suboptimal among patients with RA. Recent guidelines from the European League Against Rheumatism (EULAR) recommend aggressive management of traditional risk factors in addition to RA disease activity control to decrease the CVD risk. Several CVD risk calculators are available for clinical use to stratify a patients' risk of developing a CVD event. Most of these calculators do not account for RA as a risk factor; thus, a multiplication factor of 1.5 is recommended to predict the risk more accurately. In order to reduce CVD in the RA population, national guidelines for the prevention of CVD should be applied to manage traditional risk factors in addition to aggressive control of RA disease activity. While current data suggests a protective effect of non-biologic disease modifying anti-rheumatic drugs (DMARDs) and biologics on cardiovascular events among patients with RA, more data is needed to define this effect more accurately.

Keywords: Cardiovascular disease, Rheumatoid arthritis, Mortality, Myocardial infarction, Cardiovascular risk assessment

Background

Rheumatoid arthritis (RA) is a chronic systemic inflammatory condition which leads to joint damage and physical disability [1]. Compared to the general population, a considerably higher risk of cardiovascular disease (CVD) is seen in patients with RA [2–4]. Hyperlipidemia, diabetes mellitus, family history of CVD, and body mass index are the risk factors associated with CVD risk in these patients [5]. Previous studies indicated that these traditional CVD risk factors do not fully explain the increased CVD risk among RA patients [6]. For example, a prospective cohort study of 114,342 women participating in the Nurses' Health Study found > 2-fold higher risk of myocardial infarction in women with RA compared to non-RA, even after adjusting for cardiovascular risk factors [7]. This data suggests that RA related factors, possibly inflammation, are also associated with the increased CVD risk that exists in this population [8–12]. Thus, adequate control of RA disease activity as well as management of CVD risk factors are needed to mitigate the heightened CVD risk in RA. This is reflected in the recently published treatment guidelines from the European League Against Rheumatism (EULAR), which emphasize the importance of management of traditional CVD risk factors alongside the RA management [13].

* Correspondence: yin9003@med.cornell.edu
[2]Joan and Sanford I Weill Medical College of Cornell University, Division of General Internal Medicine, 525 East 68th Street, F-2019, PO Box #331, New York, NY 10065, USA
[3]Division of Rheumatology, Hospital for Special Surgery, New York, NY, USA
Full list of author information is available at the end of the article

In order to implement preventive measures, CVD risk stratification is the initial step to determine a patients' overall risk for a CVD event. There are several CVD risk prediction models that are used for this purpose. These models were developed in the non-RA population and their accuracy stratifying CVD risk for patients with RA is still a matter of research. Attempts to develop and validate CVD risk prediction models that stratify CVD risk more accurately in patients with RA are on-going [14, 15]. This narrative review summarizes current data about CVD risk in patients with RA, the status of current CVD risk prediction models, and discusses management to reduce this risk. As such, this narrative review does not address risk of bias of the articles included and it may not have taken into consideration all the available data, as a systematic review would have done.

Mortality/morbidity from cardiovascular disease in RA

Rheumatoid arthritis patients suffer from excess mortality from cardiovascular disease [7, 16]. CVD is the leading cause of death even in the general population; however, RA is associated with an increased risk of developing CVD by almost two fold, a risk magnitude comparable to that of diabetes mellitus [17, 18]. RA patients are twice as likely to experience a silent myocardial infarction compared to non-RA subjects [4] and carry a higher burden of coronary plaques even in the absence of clinical history of coronary artery disease [19]. Following a new CVD event, patients with RA have a 17.6% 30-day CVD mortality risk compared to 10.8% in the non-RA population [20]. These patients had an odds ratio (OR) and 95% confidence interval (CI) of 1.6, 1.2-2.2 for increased CVD mortality after 30-days of an myocardial infarction (MI) compared to the non-RA population [20].

Similar findings were observed in a meta-analysis of 111,758 patients with 22,927 cardiovascular events that found a 50% increased risk of CVD death among patients with RA compared to the general population [21]. Another meta-analysis reported a 60% increase in CVD death compared to non-RA subjects [22]. Results from Nurses' health study found that women with RA had 45% increased CVD mortality with a hazard ratio (HR) of 1.5, 95% CI 1.1-1.8, compared to non-RA women [16]. Though the relative risk (RR) and rates of CV mortality may vary among different data sources owing to differences in patient population, duration of follow up, measurement of outcome and missing data on specific cause of death, these studies still considerably support the increase CVD mortality that exists among patients with RA [23].

CVD mortality has been associated with level of inflammation, HLA–DRB1*0404 [10], use of glucocorticoids [24] and presence of RA autoantibodies [25, 26], and can possibly be reduced by effective RA treatments [27, 28].

The time trend studies of overall mortality and CVD specific mortality in RA showed persistently increased CVD mortality except for some recent data suggesting a downward trend. A 2007 study by Gonzalez et al. demonstrated a widening gap between overall mortality in RA compared to general population [29]. A recent (2014) analysis from United Kingdom (U.K.) based cohort, Norfolk Arthritis Register, included 2517 patients with early inflammatory arthritis with 16,485 person-years of follow-up. In this study, CVD mortality decreased with time in the first seven years from recruitment in this register, but was increased among patients who were antibody-positive [25].

In a population-based incident RA cohort from Canada, Lacaille et al. reported improvement in overall mortality and a similar 5-year CV mortality in RA patients with disease onset in 2001-2006 to non-RA patients [30]. Another study showed improved CVD mortality in an RA cohort from 2000 to 07 (2.7%, 95% CI 0.6–4.9%) compared to patients diagnosed in 1990–99 (7.1%, 95% CI 3.9–10.1%) suggesting a decline in CVD mortality in more recent years [31]. It must be noted that results of this particular study were based on only 315 RA patients from a single county in the United States of America (U.S.A) with 8 deaths from CVD, which could be a result of regional differences and may not represent the actual CVD mortality among patients with RA at a population level [31].

Many of the studies that showed a decrease in CVD mortality in the U.S. were not population-based. In order to confirm an actual decrease in CVD mortality, larger population-based studies with longer follow up are needed. Overall, the data thus far remains robust in support of a current and persistent increased CVD mortality among patients with RA [25, 32–36].

Traditional cardiovascular risk factors
Hypertension (HTN)

Hypertension (HTN) is a well-established risk factor for developing cardiovascular disease [37] with a prevalence of 29% in the general population [38]. Prior studies report a wide range of prevalence of hypertension in patients with RA ranging between 3.8%-73% [39–44]. Similar to the general population, hypertension is detrimental for CVD risk among patients with RA and is an independent predictor of CVD events [41, 45]. A meta-analysis of longitudinal studies found an 84% increased risk of myocardial infarction among patients with RA with hypertension compared to non-hypertensive patients with RA (RR 1.8, 95% CI 1.4-2.5) [46].

Multiple factors may impact blood pressure in patients with RA including inflammation, physical inactivity, and drugs [40]. Increased arterial stiffness and reduced elasticity of blood vessels is seen in patients with RA [47, 48]. Studies in animal models suggest an association between ongoing inflammation and hypertension [49]. Although, the exact underlying mechanisms remain to be fully understood. This association can be seen clinically in thedata from the Women's Health Study, an ongoing randomized, double-blind, placebo-controlled trial of low-dose aspirin and vitamin E for the primary prevention of CVD and cancer, that evaluated women with incident hypertension. This study shows that high C-reactive protein (CRP), is associated with increased risk of developing hypertension among healthy women [50, 51]. Finally, medications that are often prescribed to patients with RA, such as non-steroidal anti-inflammatory drugs (NSAIDs) and glucocorticoids, are associated with increased risk for HTN [52, 53].

Despite high prevalence of HTN and associated cardiovascular risk, HTN in rheumatoid arthritis is under-recognized and suboptimally treated [54–56]. Results reported from a U.K. based study showed that among 221 patients with RA and elevated CVD risk, 32% had a systolic blood pressure > 140 mmHg and only 23% were treated with antihypertensive drugs [55]. Among these patients with RA treated with antihypertensive drugs, 50% still had a systolic blood pressure > 140 mmHg [55]. Furthermore, there is a gap in coordinated care for the management of hypertension for patients with RA between rheumatologists and primary care physicians. While rheumatologists routinely screened for hypertension, only 31% of them initiated HTN treatment for these patients [57].

A study from a large academic center used electronic health records to identify patients with hypertension. They identified 14,974 patients with undiagnosed hypertension who were seen regularly in the primary care setting [56]. Among these, 201 patients had RA. When compared to non-RA controls, RA patients had 29% lower hazard of receiving a diagnosis of hypertension at mean follow up of 14 months (HR 0.7, 95%CI 0.6–0.9) even though their number of visits to a primary care physician was equivalent to that of patients without RA [56]. This has significant clinical implications as uncontrolled HTN may lead to a higher number of CVD events. In a study by Singh et al. investigators used cardiovascular risk prediction models from the Framingham Heart Study. This study showed that a 20 mmHg increase in systolic blood pressure in RA patients was associated with 1572 additional ischemic heart disease events yearly [58]. Given the heightened CVD risk imparted by HTN in RA patients, this comorbidity needs more attention for appropriate screening and optimal treatment.

Insulin resistance/metabolic syndrome

Metabolic syndrome has been defined in the general population as having three of five elements including obesity, elevated triglycerides, low high-density lipoproteins (HDL) cholesterol, high systolic and diastolic blood pressure, and elevated fasting glucose [59]. Metabolic syndrome increases CVD risk by 2 fold in general population [60]. Da Cunha et al., in a study conducted in Brazil, found a larger number of patients with RA with metabolic syndrome when compared to healthy non-RA controls (39% vs 19%) [61]. The authors also noted increased prevalence of waist circumference, hypertension, and increased fasting glucose in patients with RA when compared with controls [61].

A recent meta-analysis of prevalence studies of metabolic syndrome in RA patients showed a prevalence of 30.7% (95% CI 27.9-33.4) [62]. Insulin resistance is a key factor for the development of CVD risk in metabolic syndrome [63]. Glucocorticoids (GC), commonly used to treat RA related symptoms, promote insulin resistance; each 5 mg increase of current oral GCs is associated with a 25–30% increased risk of type 2 diabetes mellitus (DM) [64]. Insulin resistance and type 2 DM are linked with elevation of inflammatory markers such as erythrocyte sedimentation rate (ESR), CRP, and RA disease activity [65, 66]. The elevation of these inflammatory markers, in addition to the inflammation caused by RA, further increases the risk for developing atherosclerosis.

Body weight/obesity

Body mass index (BMI), derived from mass and height of an individual (kg/m^2), is a commonly used measure for body composition in RA and non-RA individuals alike. Obese individuals (> 30 kg/m^2) [67] have a two to three times higher mortality than normal weight individuals [68]. Obesity is independently associated with CVD burden as well as other CVD risk factors such as hypertension, dyslipidemia, insulin resistance etc. [69]. It is also associated with endothelial dysfunction and promotion of atherosclerosis [70]. Similar to the general population, obesity contributes to cardiovascular morbidity in patients with RA [71]. In patients with RA, it is independently associated with other CVD risk factors [72]. and also predicts 10-year CVD risk [71, 72]. Adipose tissue is a source of inflammatory factors including interleukin-6, tumor necrosis factor-alpha, and CRP which induce a state of low-grade inflammation that contributes to CVD risk [73].

Paradoxically, a low BMI in RA (< 18.5 kg/m^2) has been associated with high CVD risk in these patients [74]. A possible explanation for this phenomenon of low BMI is rheumatoid cachexia [75]. A chronic inflammatory state such as the one that occurs in RA can cause alterations in body composition. Individuals with RA may lose lean muscle mass and accumulate excess fat. This makes it challenging to use BMI as a marker of body composition because it cannot distinguish the proportion of adipose tissue and muscle. It remains unclear how to best identify those patients with RA who have a disproportionate adipose tissue to muscle ratio. A past study found that, for a given body fat content, patients with RA had a significantly lower BMI by almost $2\,kg/mg^2$ compared to general population. Investigators of this study proposed that the BMI cut off for RA patients should be reduced to 23 kg/m^2 for overweight and 28 kg/m^2 for obesity respectively [66]. While it is an interesting observation, these cut off points have not been used extensively in population-based cohorts to determine whether these are indeed predictive of CVD events in patients with RA. Alternative measures that have been proposed include waist circumference and waist to hip ratio but thus far they have not been proved superior to BMI in assessing obesity-related comorbidity [76]. Further research is needed to identify the optimal way to define obesity in patients with RA.

Smoking

Patients with RA who smoke have aggressive disease and worse clinical outcomes [77]. Despite the associated hazards, a meta-analysis determined that the prevalence of smoking was higher in patients with RA compared with controls (OR 1.6, 95%CI 1.4-1.8) [78]. In the general population, cigarette smoking is associated with CVD [79]. Although among patients with RA its impact on CVD is less clear, some studies in the past showed that there was a weak association between smoking and CVD in patients with RA [5, 80], However, it is possible that this weak association is attributed to under–reporting of smoking status [81] or index event bias (a type of selection bias that occurs when multiple risk factors contribute to the risk of the index outcome (disease) as well as disease sequela) [82].

It is known that cigarette smoking is associated with rheumatoid factor positivity [83], production of anti-citrullinated antibodies (CCP) [84], increased disease severity [77], and poor response to treatment [85], all of which have been associated with CVD morbidity in patients with RA [25, 26, 86, 87]. More recent data have shown that smoking is associated with CVD risk. In a large longitudinal study from the Veterans Health Administration (VHA), (37,568 patients with RA and 896 incident hospitalized myocardial infarction) "current smoking" was associated with an increased risk of myocardial infarction by 42% vs. "never smoker" (HR 1.4, 95% CI 1.1-1.8) [88]. Another study of 5638 patients with RA with no prior CVD who were followed for 5.8 years found that smoking had the highest population attributable risk (PAR) for CVD across different CVD risk factors including RA disease activity (PAR for smoking = 23.7%) [89]. Moreover, a recent meta-analysis of longitudinal studies noted a 50% increased risk of CVD events in smokers compared to non-smoker RA patients (n = 2056, RR 1.5, 95% CI 1.3-1.8) [46]. A significant number of patients with RA continue to smoke

therefore, interventions for smoking cessation should be applied not only to improve RA disease activity but also to ameliorate their overall CVD risk.

Lipids

In the general population, the atherogenic lipid profile is considered to be high total cholesterol (TC), low-density lipoprotein cholesterol (LDL-C) and low high-density lipoprotein cholesterol (HDL-C). Dyslipidemia is commonly seen in patients with RA and is linked to increased cardiovascular disease [90]. A retrospective study of 1078 patients showed that lipid changes (higher TC, lower HDL-C, higher triglycerides) may be present even before the onset of RA [91]. High levels of lipoprotein (a), which is structurally similar to LDL-C and is atherogenic in nature, have also been reported in patients with RA [92, 93].

The relationship of lipids in patients with RA is more complex than in non-RA individuals because of the interplay of cholesterol with inflammation. Cholesterol levels decrease in the presence of active inflammation. The Third National Health and Nutrition Examination Survey (NHANES) compared lipid profiles of 128 patients with RA aged 60 and older to non-RA controls and found that patients with RA who were not on DMARDs or glucocorticoids had significantly low levels of HDL cholesterol [94]. Similarly, low TC and LDL-C levels were seen in patients with active RA while the rate of having a myocardial infarction remained 1.6 times higher than patients without RA [95, 96]. This has been defined as the RA 'lipid paradox' [95]. High CRP among patients with RA representing high level of inflammation correlates with lower TC, LDL-C and HDL-C while at the same time that high CRP is associated with increased CVD risk [97, 98]. While the exact mechanism for the lipid paradox remains unknown, genetic factors, reduced lipid synthesis, increased clearance as well as cholesterol consumption as an essential substrate to develop an inflammatory response have been implicated as causes for the low cholesterol levels [8, 99, 100]. It has also been observed that RA therapies increase the lipid levels while reducing inflammation (See Table 1) [101]. These changes gathered special attention during the clinical trials of tocilizumab (TCZ), an interleukin (IL)-6 receptor blocker. A significant increase in lipid levels was observed in patients who received TCZ [102, 103]. There are ongoing studies to determine whether these changes are detrimental for CVD risk and if so, to what extent. A similar pattern of lipid changes was also seen with other RA therapies such as DMARDs, and tumor necrosis factor (TNF) alpha inhibitors (see Table 1) which suggests that these changes are not only a result of an intrinsic mechanism of action (IL-6 blockade) but also from decreased inflammation.

Table 1 Summary of Changes in Lipid Profiles with Rheumatoid Arthritis Therapies

Study or Author	RA drug	Change in TC (mg/dL)	Change in LDL-C (mg/dL)	Change in HDL-C (mg/dL)	Notes
Yamanaka et al. [171]	TCZ	↑ 12.9	n/a	n/a	Concurrent DMARD use
Yazici et al. [172]	TCZ	↑ 25.9	↑ 17.8	↑ 3.5	Concurrent DMARD use
Genovese et al. [103]	TCZ	↑ 30.9	↑ 3.8	↑ 19.3	Concurrent DMARD use
Gabay et al. [161]	TCZ	↑30.5	↑20.1	↑5.4	Change from baseline to week 8
	Adalimumab	↑6.6	↑2.7	↑2.7	
Tam et al. [173]	Infliximab	↑23.2	↑12.4	↑5.8	Change from baseline to week 14
Kirkham et al. [174]	Golimumab	↑8.0	↑8.0	↑3.0	
Morris et al. [175]	Hydroxychloroquine	↓ 7.7	↓ 7.6	↑ 1.0	
Navarro-Millán et al. [176]	Methotrexate with Etanercept	↑56.8	↑31.4	↑19.3	After 6 months of treatment
	Triple therapy[a]	↑53.0	↑28.7	↑22.3	
	Methotrexate	↑57.3	↑30.0	↑20.6	
Charles-Schoeman et al. [177][b]		↑ week 24	↑ week 24	↑ week 24	Trend of lipids with treatment
		↓week 102	↓week 102	↓week 102	
Novikova et al. [178]	Rituximab	↑19.7	↑4.6	↑12.0	After 6 months of treatment

TC total cholesterol, *LDL-C* low-density lipoprotein cholesterol, *HDL-C* high-density lipoprotein cholesterol, *TCZ* tocilizumab
[a]Triple therapy=methotrexate plus sulfasalazine plus hydroxychloroquine, DMARD = disease modifying anti-rheumatic drugs
[b]Absolute numerical changes not available

Besides the quantitative changes in lipids, inflammation also impacts the qualitative aspect of the cholesterol. The level of inflammation may determine how much impact LDL-C has on CVD risk. For example, LDL-C had more impact on the CVD risk when ESR was more than 30 mm/h [95]. Furthermore, inflammation also affects anti-oxidant capacity of HDL-C. HDL-C under normal circumstances is responsible for inhibiting oxidation of LDL-C and efflux of cholesterol from vessel walls [104]. In a state of inflammation, HDL-C gets altered, losing its ability to remove cholesterol from athero-sclerosis, and indeed becoming pro-atherogenic [105]. HDL-C is also reduced in patients with RA, resulting in a high atherogenic index of totalcholesterol:HDLC ratio [101, 106]. RA treatment, improves HDL-C function as a consequence of decreasing inflammation, which highlights the importance of controlling RA disease activity to improve lipid profiles and decrease overall CVD risk [107].

Physical inactivity and cardiopulmonary fitness
Physical inactivity is associated with higher risk of myocardial infarction in the general population according to the INTERHEART case–control study [108]. Data from 33 large prospective cohorts demonstrated a 35% relative risk reduction in CVD related death associated with being physically active [109]. Unfortunately, several studies indicate that patients with RA are frequently inactive [110–112]. This is partly due to pain

and fatigue [113], lack of motivation [114], and lack of patient understanding of the negative impact of physical inactivity [115].

A recent meta-analysis showed that CVD morbidity was not increased with physical inactivity among RA patients (RR 1, 95%CI 0.7-1.3) [46]. However, the results must be interpreted with caution because this meta-analysis included only two studies, both of which had cross sectional designs. A cross sectional study examined the impact of physical activity on CVD risk profile in RA patients. Levels of physical activity were assessed in 65 patients using a questionnaire. After adjusting for age, weight, sex, smoking status, and RA disease activity, physically active patients with RA had significantly lower systolic blood pressure, cholesterol levels, low density lipoprotein, homocysteine, Apolipoprotein B, von Willebrand Factor, and Type-I plasminogen activator inhibitor antigen [116]. This suggests that CVD risk profile of patients with RA can be improved by implementing increased physical activity. Data from a systematic review of randomized clinical trials of exercise programs among patients with RA showed that exercise improved aerobic and muscle strength among these patients [117]. The benefit on decreasing CVD risk still requires more direct and specific evaluation since none of these trials evaluated this relationship [117].

There is accumulating clinical data that shows improved CVD risk parameters with exercise in RA. Forty patients with RA were divided into an exercise group who received 6 months of tailored aerobic and resistance exercise and a control group who received only information of exercise benefits. Significant improvement in the endothelial function parameters was noted in the exercise group compared to the control group. This suggests that exercise may reduce CVD risk by impacting endothelial dysfunction, though long-term effect of exercise intervention on this parameter needs further evaluation [118]. Other studies show that exercise can reduce CRP levels [119] and also has an anti-atherogenic effect, which further elaborates the impact of exercise on CVD risk [119, 120].

Low levels of cardiopulmonary fitness, measured by the maximal oxygen uptake (VO_2max) test is associated with CVD and all-cause mortality [121–123]. It has been reported that patients with RA have low cardiopulmonary fitness [121]. A recent cross-sectional study evaluated the association of VO_2max with CVD risk in the RA population [124]. Results showed that patients with RA not only had lower VO_2max levels, but also that those with higher levels of VO_2max had better cardiovascular risk profiles. There is evidence that cardiopulmonary fitness in RA can be improved with aerobic and resistance exercise intervention; thus, providing an exercise program to patients with RA is a useful tool to attenuate CVD risk [125]. Based on current evidence, RA patients should be encouraged to exercise not only to improve physical function but also to reduce cardiovascular disease.

RA related factors
Inflammation
Atherosclerosis is no longer thought to be a simple process of lipid accumulation in blood vessels. There is evidence that systemic inflammation plays a pathogenic role in the development of accelerated atherosclerosis. A study found that even in healthy men, inflammation measured by elevated inflammatory markers was associated with increased CVD risk [126]. Atherosclerotic plaque formation begins with endothelial dysfunction, after which pro-inflammatory cytokines and adhesion molecules are released. Inflammatory cells then enter the blood vessel wall along with LDL molecules because of increased endothelial permeability. LDL is oxidized and taken up by the macrophages, which later become foam cells. This is followed by smooth cell proliferation and neovascularization which ultimately cause the thickening of the blood vessel and plaque formation [12].

Past studies have shown that endothelial dysfunction is impaired in RA patients [127] with a magnitude equivalent to that of diabetes, an independent CVD risk factor [18]. Circulating inflammatory substances and autoantibodies, such as anti-CCP and rheumatoid factor, are associated with endothelial dysfunction [128, 129]. A recent systematic review of randomized clinical trials suggested

that endothelial dysfunction in RA can be improved with TNF alpha-blockers, but the conclusion was based on small observational studies and further randomized controlled data is needed to validate these findings [130]. Similarly, inflammatory cytokines such as IL-6, IL-18, and TNF-alpha, which are typically elevated in rheumatoid arthritis, have been associated with cardiovascular disease [131]. Markers of inflammation in patients with RA such as ESR and CRP are associated with intimal media thickness, a surrogate for atherosclerotic disease [132–134]. There is also development of pro-atherogenic HDL in the setting of inflammation from RA [107, 135]. Inflammation thus significantly contributes to CVD risk in patients with RA in addition to traditional CVD risk factors.

NSAIDs and glucocorticoids(GCs)
A broad use of NSAIDs and GCs is common among patients with RA by virtue of their anti-inflammatory properties. However, these drugs have implications pertaining to CVD risk.

GCs are associated with insulin resistance [65], hypertension [53], obesity, hyperlipidemia [136] and DM [64], all of which are associated with development of CVD. They are associated with CVD mortality in a dose dependant fashion [24]. On the contrary, there are studies that suggested that GCs may prove beneficial in reducing CVD risk by controlling inflammation [42]. Robust randomized trials to prove this notion are lacking and EULAR currently recommends keeping GCs at a minimum dosage.

NSAIDs have been associated with CVD risk in the general population, but whether they augment CVD risk in RA needs to be well established. A systematic review and meta-analysis showed that NSAIDs increase risk of CVD events in RA [137]. However, the effect was mainly driven by rofecoxib and not from non-selective NSAIDs or celecoxib, another cyclooxygenase 2 inhibitor. Rofecoxib has now been withdrawn from the market and the recent PRECISION trial found similar CVD safety of celecoxib to ibuprofen and naproxen in patients with arthritis (~ 10% of total population had RA) [138]. In the Danish cohort, investigators found a significantly lower CVD risk associated with NSAIDs in RA compared to non-RA [139]. The evidence as of yet is not strong enough to contraindicate the use of NSAIDs in patients with RA and the recommendation is to use them cautiously in this population [13]. A meta-analysis found naproxen to be least harmful for CVD safety [140]. Nevertheless, further research is needed to understand the impact of NSAIDs in RA patients, particularly in patients with pre-existing CVD risk factors.

Cardiovascular risk assessment
Cardiovascular risk assessment is intended to identify patients who are at high risk of developing CVD in the

future so that preventive strategies could be implemented proactively. Several algorithms that quantify this risk are available to use in the general population, which are also applicable to patients with RA. These models utilize traditional parameters such as age, sex, blood pressure, smoking status, cholesterol levels and presence of diabetes mellitus to compute a risk for CVD in these patients [141]. There are some noteworthy challenges to the use of these algorithms for patients with RA. These models do not account for the increased CVD risk associated with RA inflammation. For instance, the Framingham Score and even the 10-year Pooled Cohort Risk Equation do not take into consideration the effect that RA has on CVD risk as these models do for DM [141, 142]. This is despite the fact that both diseases are independent risk factors for CVD [17]. Therefore it appears that, these instruments can underestimate CVD risk in patients with RA, which has led to multiple studies to determine how more accuraty RA-specific instruments compared to those based on the general population, can predict CVD risk in these patients. Since inflammation and RA disease activity fluctuate over time, the development of a precise CVD prediction model is even more challenging. These changes suggest that CVD risk in patients with RA is more dynamic rather than fixed. Further studies are needed to determine the importance of the changes in RA disease activity and its impact on calculating CVD risk. Nevertheless, using current CVD risk prediction models still provides a valuable starting point to initiate cardiovascular disease primary risk prevention.

Several algorithms are available to stratify CVD risk in a patient. The SCORE (Systematic Coronary Risk Evaluation) CVD death risk score was developed from 12 European cohort studies and is used in European countries [143]. It calculates 10-year risk of any first fatal atherosclerotic event. In the United States, the American College of Cardiology/American Heart Association (ACC/AHA) guildeines on the tratment of blood cholesterol recommends initiation of a lipid-lowering agent and lifestyle modifications if the 10-year CVD risk is => 7.5 [144]. The Reynolds risk score was developed from prospective cohorts of men and women without diabetes [145, 146]. It does account high sensitivity CRP into the equation, so theoretically it can better predict CVD risk in RA. However, CRP is more sensitive for short-term changes in inflammation. A clinical study found that, despite accounting for CRP, the Reynolds risk score substantially underestimated CVD risk in patients with RA (both men and women) [147]. The QRISK-2 calculator is the only calculator that takes RA into account as a CVD risk factor in addition to traditional risk factors [148]. However, studies have shown that QRISK2 may overestimate the CVD risk in patients with RA [149, 150].

Recently, a new cardiovascular risk calculator, called the Expanded Cardiovascular Risk Prediction Score for Rheumatoid Arthritis (ERS-RA) was developed for RA patients using a cohort for 23,605 patients with RA from the Consortium of Rheumatology Researchers of North America (CORRONA) [14, 15]. It includes RA-related variables such as Clinical Disease Activity Index (CDAI) > 10 versus ≤10), disability (modified Health Assessment Questionnaire disability index > 0.5 versus ≤0.5), daily prednisone use and disease duration (≥10 versus < 10 years) in addition to traditional CV risk factors (i.e., age, sex, diabetes mellitus, hypertension, hyperlipidemia, and tobacco use). In this model, actual blood pressure and cholesterol values were not available. Investigators then accounted for these traditional risk factors based on physician reported diagnosis for HTN and hyperlipidemia or the use of medications for either of these conditions. External validation is still needed for this calculator to know whether it could be applied to the general U.S. and non-US populations [14].

A recent study combined data from seven RA cohorts from the U.K., Norway, Netherlands, the United States of America (U.S.A), South Africa, Canada and Mexico and compared the performance of QRISK2, the EULAR multiplier and ERS-RA to risk calculators for the general population: ACC/AHA, Framingham Adult Treatment Panel III, Framingham risk score-Adult Treatment Panel (FRS-ATP) and the Reynolds Risk Score [15]. The study found that RA risk calculators did not perform better than general population risk scores [15]. Hence, it is reasonable to apply these prediction models the same way as they are applied in the general population while specific prediction models for RA are being developed and validated. European League Against Rheumatism (EULAR) 2016 CVD treatment guidelines for RA recommend applying a multiplication factor of 1.5 to the scores that does not account for RA by default [13]. The guidelines also recommend performing CVD risk screening once every 5 years and treating modifiable CVD risk factors in order to decrease the risk. EULAR recommendations is to use national guidelines applicable to the general population to determine which CVD risk prediction model be used. However, if national guidelines are not available, the SCORE model can be used for CVD risk assessment, at least according to the European guidelines.

Management
RA disease activity and the role of RA therapy
Studies have shown that lowering disease activity also decreases CVD events. A 10-point decrease in the clinical disease activity index (CDAI) was associated with a 21% reduction in CVD risk (95% CI 13.0-29.0) [86]. Another study showed that low disease activity measured by the Disease Activity Score-28 joint count DAS28 (≤3.2) was associated with reduced CVD risk compared

to high disease activity (DAS > 3.2) [151]. Recent data from the Brigham and Women's Hospital Rheumatoid Arthritis Sequential Study (BRASS), a prospective observational RA cohort, highlights the improvements in HDL-C efflux capacity with reductions in high sensitivity CRP [152].

Multiple studies have shown that the management of CVD risk should rely on tight RA disease control regardless of type of therapy used. Ljung et al. showed that RA patients on TNF inhibitor therapy who had good EULAR response had 50% lower risk of acute coronary syndrome compared with non-responders [87]. However, EULAR moderate responders had equal risk to that of EULAR non-responders, implying that optimal disease control is needed to reduce CVD risk not just disease control or being on a TNF inhibitor. The number of patients with RA that achieve remission or low disease activity remains low with a prevalence of remission fluctuating between 8 and 20% [153–155]. Given that only a small number of patients achieve clinical remission, it is also important to target traditional modifiable CVD risk factors to ameliorate CVD risk in these patients.

Use of anti-rheumatic therapy is associated with reduced CVD risk. A large meta-analysis of 10 cohort studies showed an 18% to 21% decrease in the risk for CVD related events (myocardial infarction, coronary heart disease, sudden death, and/or stroke) with use of methotrexate (MTX) [156]. MTX may improve HDL-C's anti-inflammatory function [157]. There is an ongoing clinical trial that is evaluating the effect of methotrexate on cardiovascular outcomes in a high CVD risk population without RA [158].

In terms of CVD outcomes, a systematic review and meta-analysis of observational cohorts and randomized controlled trials (RCTs) reporting on cardiovascular events in RA patients showed a decrease in CVD risk with the use of anti-TNF therapy [159], but the results of the meta-analysis were not statistically significant. Del Rincón et al. demonstrated that, even in the presence of a high level of inflammation (represented by ESR), anti-TNF therapy and MTX decreased the progression of intima-media thickness (IMT) [132]. The main limitation of the study was the lack of a non-RA control group.

Interleukin 6 (IL-6) blocker tocilizumab is of particular interest with respect to CVD risk because of their potentially adverse effects on the lipid profile. However, data from a phase 4 clinical trial comparing cardiovascular safety of tocilizumab vs etanercept in patients with RA showed that the rate of major CVD events with tocilizumab was low and comparable to that of etanercept (83 tocilizumab arm versus 78 in etanercept arm, (HR 1.1; 95% CI 0.8, 1.4) [160]. A post hoc analysis from a clinical trial of RA patients that received intravenous tocilizumab or adalimumab noted that LDL-C and

HDL-C increased with both treatments but the magnitude of these changes was higher in the tocilizumab group. While this data suggest that the impact of different therapies on lipid profiles is not equivalent, the observation across studies is that RA treatments increase lipid levels [161]. Further studies are needed to understand the implications of these changes on cardiovascular risk in RA patients, but the data reported to date do not suggest that these changes are detrimental toward CVD risk.

Traditional risk factors:

Several studies showed that primary lipid screening was performed in less than half of patients with RA [162, 163]. It is often questioned which physician (rheumatologist, primary care) should take ownership of performing CVD risk management. In the most recent guidelines, EULAR strongly encouraged rheumatologists to take ownership of the management of this risk factor. National guidelines for the general population should be used to manage traditional risk factors such as hypertension, diabetes and hypercholesterolemia. Lipid management should be carried out similar to the general population. Given that active inflammation in RA can alter the lipid levels, lipid testing should be carried out when a patient's disease activity is stable or in remission [13].

Drugs such as non-steroidal anti-inflammatory drugs and glucocorticoids exert deleterious effects on blood pressure, lipid profile and glucose tolerance and therefore should be kept to minimum [24, 164]. Lifestyle changes should be recommended to all patients with emphasis on a diet without trans fatty acids and high content of fruits and vegetables, regular exercise and smoking cessation. A structured exercise program should be offered as it improves cardiorespiratory fitness and reduces CVD risk [125].

Management of hypertension should be carried out as in the general population. There is no evidence that the treatment thresholds should differ from the general population [37]. Current guidelines for prevention and management of hypertension in adults recommend antihypertensive medication for primary prevention in adults with estimated 10-year atherosclerotic cardiovascular disease => 10% and an average systolic blood pressure => 130 mmHg or diastolic blood pressure => 80mm Hg [165]. Lipid management should be carried out similar to the general population.

Statins are effective at improving lipid profiles [166–168]. Similar to general population, statins reduce CVD risk in RA as well [169]. A multicenter, double blind prospective study of 2986 patients with RA found a 34% reduction in cardiovascular events after treatment with atorvastatin compared to placebo. The results were not statistically significant because the trial was abandoned early because of a lower than anticipated event rate [170]. A recent study examined the impact of lowering LDL-C in two cohorts of RA patients ($n = 1522$ and 1746 respectively) who were matched with a control group comprised of general population and patients with osteoarthritis. All these patients had a hyperlipidemia diagnosis and a statin prescription. It was noted that lower LDL-C levels were associated with reduction of cardiovascular events [169]. Regardless of the "lipid paradox" in RA (low lipid levels but higher incidence of CVD) and the changes in lipid profiles observed with RA treatment, statins should be used in accordance with CVD treatment guidelines for primary prevention in this population. Still, this approach is not regularly used in clinical practice, possibly because of "normal" or "abnormally low" lipid profiles in patients with RA in the presence of high disease activity and the lack of recognition of CVD risk imparted by RA [163]. The practice can be enhanced by a more unanimous agreement of when and how statins should be initiated in patients with RA.

According to the ACC/AHA cholesterol treatment guidelines, statins should be initiated for primary prevention if the calculated 10-year CVD risk ≥7.5% for patients between 40 and 75 years of age in the U.S.A [144]. Once a CVD event has occurred (secondary prevention), every patient with RA should be initiated on a statin. In other countries (such as European countries), statin initiation can be carried out per national guidelines of CVD management for the general population [13].

Conclusion

Cardiovascular burden is significantly increased in rheumatoid arthritis. In addition to RA disease activity control, management of traditional risk factors for CVD is imperative. A multidisciplinary approach should be sought where primary care practitioners, rheumatologists and cardiologists can work together to improve cardiovascular outcomes and reduce mortality among patients with RA.

Abbreviations

ACC/AHA: American College of Cardiology/American Heart Association; BMI: Body mass index; BRASS: Brigham and Women's Hospital Rheumatoid Arthritis Sequential Study; CCP: Cyclic citrullinated peptide; CDAI: Clinical disease activity index; CI: Confidence interval; CORRONA: Consortium of Rheumatology Researchers of North America; CRP: C reactive protein; CVD: Cardiovascular disease; DAS28: Disease Activity Score-28 joint count; DM: Diabetes Mellitus; DMARD: Disease modifying anti-rheumatic drugs; ERS-RA: Expanded Cardiovascular Risk Prediction Score for Rheumatoid Arthritis; ESR: Erythrocyte Sedimentation rate; EULAR: European League Against Rheumatism; FRS-ATP: Framingham risk Score-Adult Treatment Panel; GC: Glucocorticoid; HDL: High density lipoprotein; HDL-C: High density lipoprotein cholesterol; HR: Hazard ratio; HTN: Hypertension; IL: Interleukin; IMT: intima-media thickness; LDL-C: low-density lipoprotein cholesterol; MI: Myocardial infarction; MTX: Methotrexate; NHANES: National Health and Nutrition Examination Survey; NSAIDs: non-steroidal anti-inflammatory drugs; OR: Odds Ratio; PAR: Population attributable risk; RA: Rheumatoid arthritis; RR: Relative risk; SCORE: Systematic Coronary Risk Evaluation; TC: Total cholesterol; TCZ: Tocilizumab; TNF: Tumor necrosis factor; U.S.A: United States of America; VHA: Veterans Health Administration; VO$_2$max: maximal oxygen uptake

Acknowledgments

We would like to thank Anna Cornelius-Schecter and Mary Helen Mays, Ph.D., for editing the manuscript funded by 2U54MD007587 from the National Institute on Minority Health and Health Disparities.

Funding

Dr. Navarro-Millán is funded by National Institute of Arthritis Musculoskeletal and Skin Diseases from the National Institutes of Health Award number K23AR068449.

Authors' contributions

AJ and IN-M performed the literature search, wrote and revised the manuscript, and gave final approval of the version to be published.

Competing interest

The authors declare that they have no competing interests.

Author details

1Division of Clinical Immunology and Rheumatology, University of Alabama at Birmingham, 836 Faculty Office Tower, 510 20th Street South, Birmingham, AL 35294, USA. 2Joan and Sanford I Weill Medical College of Cornell University, Division of General Internal Medicine, 525 East 68th Street, F-2019, PO Box #331, New York, NY 10065, USA. 3Division of Rheumatology, Hospital for Special Surgery, New York, NY, USA.

References

1. Scott DL, Wolfe F, Huizinga TW. Rheumatoid arthritis. Lancet. 2010; 376(9746):1094–108.
2. Radner H, Lesperance T, Accortt NA, Solomon DH. Incidence and prevalence of cardiovascular risk factors among patients with rheumatoid arthritis, psoriasis, or psoriatic arthritis. Arthritis Care Res (Hoboken). 2017; 69(10):1510–8.
3. Pujades-Rodriguez M, Duyx B, Thomas SL, Stogiannis D, Rahman A, Smeeth L, et al. Rheumatoid arthritis and incidence of twelve initial presentations of cardiovascular disease: a population record-linkage cohort study in England. PLoS One. 2016;11(3):e0151245.
4. Maradit-Kremers H, Crowson CS, Nicola PJ, Ballman KV, Roger VL, Jacobsen SJ, et al. Increased unrecognized coronary heart disease and sudden deaths in rheumatoid arthritis: a population-based cohort study. Arthritis Rheum. 2005;52(2):402–11.
5. Gonzalez A, Maradit Kremers H, Crowson CS, Ballman KV, Roger VL, Jacobsen SJ, et al. Do cardiovascular risk factors confer the same risk for cardiovascular outcomes in rheumatoid arthritis patients as in non-rheumatoid arthritis patients? Ann Rheum Dis. 2008;67(1):64–9.
6. del Rincon ID, Williams K, Stern MP, Freeman GL, Escalante A. High incidence of cardiovascular events in a rheumatoid arthritis cohort not explained by traditional cardiac risk factors. Arthritis Rheum. 2001;44(12): 2737–45.
7. Solomon DH, Karlson EW, Rimm EB, Cannuscio CC, Mandl LA, Manson JE, et al. Cardiovascular morbidity and mortality in women diagnosed with rheumatoid arthritis. Circulation. 2003;107(9):1303–7.
8. Zhang J, Chen L, Delzell E, Muntner P, Hillegass WB, Safford MM, et al. The association between inflammatory markers, serum lipids and the risk of cardiovascular events in patients with rheumatoid arthritis. Ann Rheum Dis. 2014;73(7):1301–8.

9.   Arts EE, Fransen J, den Broeder AA, Popa CD, van Riel PL. The effect of disease duration and disease activity on the risk of cardiovascular disease in rheumatoid arthritis patients. Ann Rheum Dis. 2015;74(6):998–1003.

10. Gonzalez-Gay MA, Gonzalez-Juanatey C, Lopez-Diaz MJ, Pineiro A, Garcia-Porrua C, Miranda-Filloy JA, et al. HLA-DRB1 and persistent chronic inflammation contribute to cardiovascular events and cardiovascular mortality in patients with rheumatoid arthritis. Arthritis Rheum. 2007;57(1):125–32.

11. Libby P. Role of inflammation in atherosclerosis associated with rheumatoid arthritis. Am J Med. 2008;121(10 Suppl 1):S21–31.

12. Skeoch S, Bruce IN. Atherosclerosis in rheumatoid arthritis: is it all about inflammation? Nat Rev Rheumatol. 2015;11(7):390–400.

13. Agca R, Heslinga SC, Rollefstad S, Heslinga M, McInnes IB, Peters MJ, et al. EULAR recommendations for cardiovascular disease risk management in patients with rheumatoid arthritis and other forms of inflammatory joint disorders: 2015/2016 update. Ann Rheum Dis. 2017;76(1):17–28.

14. Solomon DH, Greenberg J, Curtis JR, Liu M, Farkouh ME, Tsao P, et al. Derivation and internal validation of an expanded cardiovascular risk prediction score for rheumatoid arthritis: a consortium of rheumatology researchers of North America registry study. Arthritis & rheumatology. 2015;67(8):1995–2003.

15. Crowson CS, Gabriel SE, Semb AG, et al. Rheumatoid arthritis-specific cardiovascular risk scores are not superior to general risk scores: a validation analysis of patients from seven countries. Rheumatology (Oxford). 2017; 56(7):1102–10.

16. Sparks JA, Chang SC, Liao KP, Lu B, Fine AR, Solomon DH, et al. Rheumatoid arthritis and mortality among women during 36 years of prospective follow-up: results from the Nurses' health study. Arthritis Care Res (Hoboken). 2016;68(6):753–62.

17. Peters MJ, van Halm VP, Voskuyl AE, Smulders YM, Boers M, Lems WF, et al. Does rheumatoid arthritis equal diabetes mellitus as an independent risk factor for cardiovascular disease? A prospective study. Arthritis Rheum. 2009;61(11):1571–9.

18. Stamatelopoulos KS, Kitas GD, Papamichael CM, Chryssohoou E, Kyrkou K, Georgiopoulos G, et al. Atherosclerosis in rheumatoid arthritis versus diabetes: a comparative study. Arterioscler Thromb Vasc Biol. 2009;29(10):1702–8.

19. Karpouzas GA, Malpeso J, Choi TY, Li D, Munoz S, Budoff MJ. Prevalence, extent and composition of coronary plaque in patients with rheumatoid arthritis without symptoms or prior diagnosis of coronary artery disease. Ann Rheum Dis. 2014;73(10):1797–804.

20. Van Doornum S, Brand C, King B, Sundararajan V. Increased case fatality rates following a first acute cardiovascular event in patients with rheumatoid arthritis. Arthritis Rheum. 2006;54(7):2061–8.

21. Avina-Zubieta JA, Choi HK, Sadatsafavi M, Etminan M, Esdaile JM, Lacaille D. Risk of cardiovascular mortality in patients with rheumatoid arthritis: a meta-analysis of observational studies. Arthritis Rheum. 2008;59(12):1690–7.

22. Meune C, Touze E, Trinquart L, Allanore Y. Trends in cardiovascular mortality in patients with rheumatoid arthritis over 50 years: a systematic review and meta-analysis of cohort studies. Rheumatology (Oxford). 2009;48(10):1309–13.

23. Michaud K, Berglind N, Franzen S, Frisell T, Garwood C, Greenberg JD, et al. Can rheumatoid arthritis (RA) registries provide contextual safety data for modern RA clinical trials? The case for mortality and cardiovascular disease. Ann Rheum Dis. 2016;75(10):1797–805.

24. del Rincón I, Battafarano DF, Restrepo JF, Erikson JM, Escalante A. Glucocorticoid dose thresholds associated with all-cause and cardiovascular mortality in rheumatoid arthritis. Arthritis Rheumatol. 2014;66(2):264–72.

25. Humphreys JH, Warner A, Chipping J, Marshall T, Lunt M, Symmons DP, et al. Mortality trends in patients with early rheumatoid arthritis over 20 years: results from the Norfolk arthritis register. Arthritis Care Res (Hoboken). 2014;66(9):1296–301.

26. Goodson NJ, Wiles NJ, Lunt M, Barrett EM, Silman AJ, Symmons DP. Mortality in early inflammatory polyarthritis: cardiovascular mortality is increased in seropositive patients. Arthritis Rheum. 2002;46(8):2010–9.

27. Choi HK, Hernán MA, Seeger JD, Robins JM, Wolfe F. Methotrexate and mortality in patients with rheumatoid arthritis: a prospective study. Lancet. 2002;359(9313):1173–7.

28. Kerola AM, Nieminen TV, Virta LJ, Kautiainen H, Kerola T, Pohjolainen T, et al. No increased cardiovascular mortality among early rheumatoid arthritis patients: a nationwide register study in 2000-2008. Clin Exp Rheumatol. 2015;33(3):391–8.

29. Gonzalez A, Maradit Kremers H, Crowson CS, Nicola PJ, Davis JM 3rd, Therneau TM, et al. The widening mortality gap between rheumatoid arthritis patients and the general population. Arthritis Rheum. 2007;56(11):3583–7.

30. Lacaille D, Avina-Zubieta JA, Sayre EC, Abrahamowicz M. Improvement in 5-year mortality in incident rheumatoid arthritis compared with the general population-closing the mortality gap. Ann Rheum Dis. 2017;76(6):1057–63.

31. Myasoedova E, Gabriel SE, Matteson EL, Davis JM, Therneau TM, Crowson CS. Decreased cardiovascular mortality in patients with incident rheumatoid arthritis (RA) in recent years: Dawn of a new era in cardiovascular disease in RA? J Rheumatol. 2017;44(6):732–9.

32. Widdifield J, Bernatsky S, Paterson JM, Tomlinson G, Tu K, Kuriya B, et al. Trends in excess mortality among patients with rheumatoid arthritis in Ontario, Canada. Arthritis care & research. 2015;67(8):1047–53.

33. van den Hoek J, Boshuizen HC, Roorda LD, Tijhuis GJ, Nurmohamed MT, van den Bos GA, et al. Mortality in patients with rheumatoid arthritis: a 15-year prospective cohort study. Rheumatol Int. 2017;37(4):487–93.

34. Dadoun S, Zeboulon-Ktorza N, Combescure C, Elhai M, Rozenberg S, Gossec L, et al. Mortality in rheumatoid arthritis over the last fifty years: systematic review and meta-analysis. Joint Bone Spine. 2013;80(1):29–33.

35. Holmqvist M, Ljung L, Askling J. Mortality following new-onset rheumatoid arthritis: has modern rheumatology had an impact? Ann Rheum Dis. 2018; 77(1):85–91.

36. Holmqvist M, Ljung L, Askling J. Acute coronary syndrome in new-onset rheumatoid arthritis: a population-based nationwide cohort study of time trends in risks and excess risks. Ann Rheum Dis. 2017;76(10):1642–7.

37. James PA, Oparil S, Carter BL, Cushman WC, Dennison-Himmelfarb C, Handler J, et al. 2014 evidence-based guideline for the management of high blood pressure in adults: report from the panel members appointed to the eighth joint National Committee (JNC 8). JAMA. 2014;311(5):507–20.

38. Yoon SS, Carroll MD, Fryar CD. Hypertension prevalence and control among adults: United States, 2011-2014. National Center for Health Statistics data brief. 2015;(220):1–8. https://www.cdc.gov/nchs/data/databriefs/db220.pdf.

39. Dougados M, Soubrier M, Antunez A, Balint P, Balsa A, Buch MH, et al. Prevalence of comorbidities in rheumatoid arthritis and evaluation of their monitoring: results of an international, cross-sectional study (COMORA). Ann Rheum Dis. 2014;73(1):62–8.

40. Panoulas VF, Metsios GS, Pace AV, John H, Treharne GJ, Banks MJ, et al. Hypertension in rheumatoid arthritis. Rheumatology. 2008;47(9):1286–98.

41. Innala L, Moller B, Ljung L, Magnusson S, Smedby T, Sodergren A, et al. Cardiovascular events in early RA are a result of inflammatory burden and traditional risk factors: a five year prospective study. Arthritis Res Ther. 2011;13(4):R131.

42. Naranjo A, Sokka T, Descalzo MA, Calvo-Alén J, Hørslev-Petersen K, Luukkainen RK, et al. Cardiovascular disease in patients with rheumatoid arthritis: results from the QUEST-RA study. Arthritis Res Ther. 2008;10(2):R30.

43. Chung CP, Oeser A, Solus JF, Avalos I, Gebretsadik T, Shintani A, et al. Prevalence of the metabolic syndrome is increased in rheumatoid arthritis and is associated with coronary atherosclerosis. Atherosclerosis. 2008;196(2):756–63.

44. Han C, Robinson DW, Hackett MV, Paramore LC, Fraeman KH, Bala MV. Cardiovascular disease and risk factors in patients with rheumatoid arthritis, psoriatic arthritis, and ankylosing spondylitis. J Rheumatol. 2006;33(11):2167–72.

45. Assous N, Touzé E, Meune C, Kahan A, Allanore Y. Cardiovascular disease in rheumatoid arthritis: single-center hospital-based cohort study in France. Joint Bone Spine. 2007;74(1):66–72.

46. Baghdadi LR, Woodman RJ, Shanahan EM, Mangoni AA. The impact of traditional cardiovascular risk factors on cardiovascular outcomes in patients with rheumatoid arthritis: a systematic review and meta-analysis. PLoS One. 2015;10(2):e0117952.

47. Roman MJ, Devereux RB, Schwartz JE, Lockshin MD, Paget SA, Davis A, et al. Arterial stiffness in chronic inflammatory diseases. Hypertension. 2005;46(1):194–9.

48. Klocke R, Cockcroft JR, Taylor GJ, Hall IR, Blake DR. Arterial stiffness and central blood pressure, as determined by pulse wave analysis, in rheumatoid arthritis. Ann Rheum Dis. 2003;62(5):414–8.

49. Solak Y, Afsar B, Vaziri ND, Aslan G, Yalcin CE, Covic A, et al. Hypertension as an autoimmune and inflammatory disease. Hypertens Res. 2016;39(8):567–73.

50. Sesso HD, Buring JE, Rifai N, Blake GJ, Gaziano JM, Ridker PM. C-reactive protein and the risk of developing hypertension. JAMA. 2003;290(22):2945–51.

51. Rexrode KM, Lee IM, Cook NR, Hennekens CH, Buring JE. Baseline characteristics of participants in the Women's health study. J Womens Health Gend Based Med. 2000;9(1):19–27.

52. Morrison A, Ramey DR, van Adelsberg J, Watson DJ. Systematic review of trials of the effect of continued use of oral non-selective NSAIDs on blood pressure and hypertension. Curr Med Res Opin. 2007;23(10):2395–404.

53. Panoulas VF, Douglas KM, Stavropoulos-Kalinoglou A, Metsios GS, Nightingale P, Kita MD, et al. Long-term exposure to medium-dose glucocorticoid therapy associates with hypertension in patients with rheumatoid arthritis. Rheumatology (Oxford). 2008;47(1):72–5.

54. Panoulas VF, Douglas KM, Milionis HJ, Stavropoulos-Kalinglou A, Nightingale P, Kita MD, et al. Prevalence and associations of hypertension and its control in patients with rheumatoid arthritis. Rheumatology. 2007;46(9):1477–82.

55. van Breukelen-van der Stoep DF, van Zeben D, Klop B, van de Geijn GJ, Janssen HJ, van der Meulen N, et al. Marked underdiagnosis and undertreatment of hypertension and hypercholesterolaemia in rheumatoid arthritis. Rheumatology (Oxford). 2016;55(7):1210–6.

56. Bartels CM, Johnson H, Voelker K, Thorpe C, McBride P, Jacobs EA, et al. Impact of rheumatoid arthritis on receiving a diagnosis of hypertension among patients with regular primary care. Arthritis Care Res (Hoboken). 2014;66(9):1281–8.

57. Nguyen-Oghalai TU, Hunnicutt SE, Smith ST, Maganti R, McNearney TA. Factors that impact decision making among rheumatologists in the initiation of treatment for hypertension in rheumatoid arthritis. Journal of clinical rheumatology : practical reports on rheumatic & musculoskeletal diseases. 2007;13(6):307–12.

58. Singh G, Miller JD, Huse DM, Pettitt D, D'Agostino RB, Russell MW. Consequences of increased systolic blood pressure in patients with osteoarthritis and rheumatoid arthritis. J Rheumatol. 2003;30(4):714–9.

59. National Cholesterol Education Program (NCEP) Expert Panel on Detection Ea, and Treatment of High Blood Cholesterol in Adults (Adult Treatment Panel III). Third Report of the National Cholesterol Education Program (NCEP) Expert Panel on Detection, Evaluation, and Treatment of High Blood Cholesterol in Adults (Adult Treatment Panel III) final report. Circulation. 2002;106(25):3143–421.

60. Mottillo S, Filion KB, Genest J, Joseph L, Pilote L, Poirier P, et al. The metabolic syndrome and cardiovascular risk a systematic review and meta-analysis. J Am Coll Cardiol. 2010;56(14):1113–32.

61. da Cunha VR, Brenol CV, Brenol JC, Fuchs SC, Arlindo EM, Melo IM, et al. Metabolic syndrome prevalence is increased in rheumatoid arthritis patients and is associated with disease activity. Scand J Rheumatol. 2012;41(3):186–91.

62. Hallajzadeh J, Safiri S, Mansournia MA, Khoramdad M, Izadi N, Almasi-Hashiani A, et al. Metabolic syndrome and its components among rheumatoid arthritis patients: a comprehensive updated systematic review and meta-analysis. PLoS One. 2017;12(3):e0170361.

63. Hanley AJ, Williams K, Stern MP, Haffner SM. Homeostasis model assessment of insulin resistance in relation to the incidence of cardiovascular disease: the San Antonio heart study. Diabetes Care. 2002;25(7):1177–84.

64. Movahedi M, Beauchamp ME, Abrahamowicz M, Ray DW, Michaud K, Pedro S, et al. Risk of incident diabetes mellitus associated with the dosage and duration of oral glucocorticoid therapy in patients with rheumatoid arthritis. Arthritis & rheumatology. 2016;68(5):1089–98.

65. Dessein PH, Joffe BI. Insulin resistance and impaired beta cell function in rheumatoid arthritis. Arthritis Rheum. 2006;54(9):2765–75.

66. La Montagna G, Cacciapuoti F, Buono R, Manzella D, Mennillo GA, Arciello A, et al. Insulin resistance is an independent risk factor for atherosclerosis in rheumatoid arthritis. Diab Vasc Dis Res. 2007;4(2):130–5.

67. Obesity: preventing and managing the global epidemic. Report of a WHO consultation. World Health Organ Tech Rep Ser. 2000;894:i-xii, 1-253. http://www.who.int/nutrition/publications/obesity/WHO_TRS_894/en/.

68. Adams KF, Schatzkin A, Harris TB, Kipnis V, Mouw T, Ballard-Barbash R, et al. Overweight, obesity, and mortality in a large prospective cohort of persons 50 to 71 years old. N Engl J Med. 2006;355(8):763–78.

69. Grundy SM, Brewer HB, Cleeman JI, Smith SC, Lenfant C, Association AH, et al. Definition of metabolic syndrome: report of the National Heart, Lung, and Blood Institute/American Heart Association conference on scientific issues related to definition. Circulation. 2004;109(3):433–8.

70. Arcaro G, Zamboni M, Rossi L, Turcato E, Covi G, Armellini F, et al. Body fat distribution predicts the degree of endothelial dysfunction in uncomplicated obesity. Int J Obes Relat Metab Disord. 1999;23(9):936–42.

71. Kremers HM, Crowson CS, Therneau TM, Roger VL, Gabriel SE. High ten-year risk of cardiovascular disease in newly diagnosed rheumatoid arthritis patients: a population-based cohort study. Arthritis Rheum. 2008;58(8):2268–74.

72. Stavropoulos-Kalinoglou A, Metsios GS, Panoulas VF, Douglas KM, Nevill AM, Jamurtas AZ, et al. Associations of obesity with modifiable risk factors for the development of cardiovascular disease in patients with rheumatoid arthritis. Ann Rheum Dis. 2009;68(2):242–5.

73. Hotamisligil GS, Arner P, Caro JF, Atkinson RL, Spiegelman BM. Increased adipose tissue expression of tumor necrosis factor-alpha in human obesity and insulin resistance. J Clin Invest. 1995;95(5):2409–15.

74. Escalante A, Haas RW, del Rincón I. Paradoxical effect of body mass index on survival in rheumatoid arthritis: role of comorbidity and systemic inflammation. Arch Intern Med. 2005;165(14):1624–9.

75. Roubenoff R, Roubenoff RA, Cannon JG, Kehayias JJ, Zhuang H, Dawson-Hughes B, et al. Rheumatoid cachexia: cytokine-driven hypermetabolism accompanying reduced body cell mass in chronic inflammation. J Clin Invest. 1994;93(6):2379–86.

76. Bray GA. Don't throw the baby out with the bath water. Am J Clin Nutr. 2004;79(3):347–9.

77. Saag KG, Cerhan JR, Kolluri S, Ohashi K, Hunninghake GW, Schwartz DA. Cigarette smoking and rheumatoid arthritis severity. Ann Rheum Dis. 1997; 56(8):463–9.

78. Boyer JF, Gourraud PA, Cantagrel A, Davignon JL, Constantin A. Traditional cardiovascular risk factors in rheumatoid arthritis: a meta-analysis. Joint, bone, spine : revue du rhumatisme. 2011;78(2):179–83.

79. Yusuf S, Hawken S, Ounpuu S, Dans T, Avezum A, Lanas F, et al. Effect of potentially modifiable risk factors associated with myocardial infarction in 52 countries (the INTERHEART study): case-control study. Lancet. 2004; 364(9438):937–52.

80. Gabriel SE. Heart disease and rheumatoid arthritis: understanding the risks. Ann Rheum Dis. 2010;69(Suppl 1):i61–4.

81. Connor Gorber S, Schofield-Hurwitz S, Hardt J, Levasseur G, Tremblay M. The accuracy of self-reported smoking: a systematic review of the relationship between self-reported and cotinine-assessed smoking status. Nicotine Tob Res. 2009;11(1):12–24.

82. Choi HK, Nguyen US, Niu J, Danaei G, Zhang Y. Selection bias in rheumatic disease research. Nat Rev Rheumatol. 2014;10(7):403–12.

83. Masdottir B, Jónsson T, Manfredsdottir V, Víkingsson A, Brekkan A, Valdimarsson H. Smoking, rheumatoid factor isotypes and severity of rheumatoid arthritis. Rheumatology. 2000;39(11):1202–5.

84. Linn-Rasker SP, van der Helm-van Mil AH, van Gaalen FA, Kloppenburg M, de Vries RR, le Cessie S, et al. Smoking is a risk factor for anti-CCP antibodies only in rheumatoid arthritis patients who carry HLA-DRB1 shared epitope alleles. Ann Rheum Dis. 2006;65(3):366–71.

85. Mattey DL, Brownfield A, Dawes PT. Relationship between pack-year history of smoking and response to tumor necrosis factor antagonists in patients with rheumatoid arthritis. J Rheumatol. 2009;36(6):1180–7.

86. Solomon DH, Reed GW, Kremer JM, Curtis JR, Farkouh ME, Harrold LR, et al. Disease activity in rheumatoid arthritis and the risk of cardiovascular events. Arthritis & rheumatology. 2015;67(6):1449–55.

87. Ljung L, Rantapää-Dahlqvist S, Jacobsson LT, Askling J. Response to biological treatment and subsequent risk of coronary events in rheumatoid arthritis. Ann Rheum Dis. 2016;75(12):2087–94.

88. Navarro-Millan I, Yang S, DuVall SL, Chen L, Baddley J, Cannon GW, et al. Association of hyperlipidaemia, inflammation and serological status and coronary heart disease among patients with rheumatoid arthritis: data from the National Veterans Health Administration. Ann Rheum Dis. 2016;75(2): 341–7.

89. Crowson CS, Rollefstad S, Ikdahl E, Kitas GD, van Riel PLCM, Gabriel SE, et al. Impact of risk factors associated with cardiovascular outcomes in patients with rheumatoid arthritis. Ann Rheum Dis. 2018;77(1):48–54.

90. Nadkarni A, You M, Resuehr H, Curtis JR. The risk for cardiovascular events associated with hyperlipdemia among patients with and without rheumatoid arthritis. J Arthritis. 2015;4(4):178. https://doi.org/10.4172/2167-7921.1000178.

91. van Halm VP, Nielen MM, Nurmohamed MT, van Schaardenburg D, Reesink HW, Voskuyl AE, et al. Lipids and inflammation: serial measurements of the lipid profile of blood donors who later developed rheumatoid arthritis. Ann Rheum Dis. 2007;66(2):184–8.

92. Boffa MB, Koschinsky ML. Lipoprotein (a): truly a direct prothrombotic factor in cardiovascular disease? J Lipid Res. 2016;57(5):745–57.

93. Zhang C, Li X, Niu D, Zi R, Wang C, Han A, et al. Increased serum levels of β_2-GPI-Lp(a) complexes and their association with premature atherosclerosis in patients with rheumatoid arthritis. Clin Chim Acta. 2011;412(15-16):1332–6.

94. Choi HK, Seeger JD. Lipid profiles among US elderly with untreated rheumatoid arthritis–the third National Health and nutrition examination survey. J Rheumatol. 2005;32(12):2311–6.

95. Myasoedova E, Crowson CS, Kremers HM, Roger VL, Fitz-Gibbon PD, Therneau TM, et al. Lipid paradox in rheumatoid arthritis: the impact of serum lipid measures and systemic inflammation on the risk of cardiovascular disease. Ann Rheum Dis. 2011;70(3):482–7.

96. Semb AG, Kvien TK, Aastveit AH, Jungner I, Pedersen TR, Walldius G, et al. Lipids, myocardial infarction and ischaemic stroke in patients with rheumatoid arthritis in the apolipoprotein-related mortality RISk (AMORIS) study. Ann Rheum Dis. 2010;69(11):1996–2001.

97. Toms TE, Panoulas VF, Douglas KM, Nightingale P, Smith JP, Griffiths H, et al. Are lipid ratios less susceptible to change with systemic inflammation than individual lipid components in patients with rheumatoid arthritis? Angiology. 2011;62(2):167–75.

98. Ridker PM, Danielson E, Fonseca FA, Genest J, Gotto AM Jr, Kastelein JJ, et al. Reduction in C-reactive protein and LDL cholesterol and cardiovascular event rates after initiation of rosuvastatin: a prospective study of the JUPITER trial. Lancet. 2009;373(9670):1175–82.

99. Choy E, Sattar N. Interpreting lipid levels in the context of high-grade inflammatory states with a focus on rheumatoid arthritis: a challenge to conventional cardiovascular risk actions. Ann Rheum Dis. 2009;68(4):460–9.

100. Liao KP, Diogo D, Cui J, Cai T, Okada Y, Gainer VS, et al. Association between low density lipoprotein and rheumatoid arthritis genetic factors with low density lipoprotein levels in rheumatoid arthritis and non-rheumatoid arthritis controls. Ann Rheum Dis. 2014;73(6):1170–5.

101. Robertson J, Peters MJ, McInnes IB, Sattar N. Changes in lipid levels with inflammation and therapy in RA: a maturing paradigm. Nat Rev Rheumatol. 2013;9(9):513–23.

102. Emery P, Keystone E, Tony HP, Cantagrel A, van Vollenhoven R, Sanchez A, et al. IL-6 receptor inhibition with tocilizumab improves treatment outcomes in patients with rheumatoid arthritis refractory to anti-tumour necrosis factor biologicals: results from a 24-week multicentre randomised placebo-controlled trial. Ann Rheum Dis. 2008;67(11):1516–23.

103. Genovese MC, McKay JD, Nasonov EL, Mysler EF, da Silva NA, Alecock E, et al. Interleukin-6 receptor inhibition with tocilizumab reduces disease activity in rheumatoid arthritis with inadequate response to disease-modifying antirheumatic drugs: the tocilizumab in combination with traditional disease-modifying antirheumatic drug therapy study. Arthritis Rheum. 2008;58(10):2968–80.

104. Navab M, Hama SY, Anantharamaiah GM, Hassan K, Hough GP, Watson AD, et al. Normal high density lipoprotein inhibits three steps in the formation of mildly oxidized low density lipoprotein: steps 2 and 3. J Lipid Res. 2000; 41(9):1495–508.

105. Van Lenten BJ, Reddy ST, Navab M, Fogelman AM. Understanding changes in high density lipoproteins during the acute phase response. Arterioscler Thromb Vasc Biol. 2006;26(8):1687–8.

106. Georgiadis AN, Papavasiliou EC, Lourida ES, Alamanos Y, Kostara C, Tselepis AD, et al. Atherogenic lipid profile is a feature characteristic of patients with early rheumatoid arthritis: effect of early treatment–a prospective, controlled study. Arthritis Res Ther. 2006;8(3):R82.

107. Charles-Schoeman C, Yin Lee Y, Shahbazian A, Wang X, Elashoff D, Curtis JR, et al. Improvement of high-density lipoprotein function in patients with early rheumatoid arthritis treated with methotrexate monotherapy or combination therapies in a randomized controlled trial. Arthritis & rheumatology. 2017;69(1):46–57.

108. Anand SS, Islam S, Rosengren A, Franzosi MG, Steyn K, Yusufali AH, et al. Risk factors for myocardial infarction in women and men: insights from the INTERHEART study. Eur Heart J. 2008;29(7):932–40.

109. Nocon M, Hiemann T, Müller-Riemenschneider F, Thalau F, Roll S, Willich SN. Association of physical activity with all-cause and cardiovascular mortality: a systematic review and meta-analysis. European journal of cardiovascular prevention and rehabilitation : official journal of the European Society of Cardiology, Working Groups on Epidemiology & Prevention and Cardiac Rehabilitation and Exercise Physiology. 2008;15(3):239–46.

110. Sokka T, Häkkinen A, Kautiainen H, Maillefert JF, Toloza S, Mørk Hansen T, et al. Physical inactivity in patients with rheumatoid arthritis: data from twenty-one countries in a cross-sectional, international study. Arthritis Rheum. 2008;59(1):42–50.

111. Henchoz Y, Bastardot F, Guessous I, Theler JM, Dudler J, Vollenweider P, et al. Physical activity and energy expenditure in rheumatoid arthritis patients and matched controls. Rheumatology. 2012;51(8):1500–7.

112. Mancuso CA, Rincon M, Sayles W, Paget SA. Comparison of energy expenditure from lifestyle physical activities between patients with rheumatoid arthritis and healthy controls. Arthritis Rheum. 2007;57(4):672–8.

113. Veldhuijzen van Zanten JJ, Rouse PC, Hale ED, Ntoumanis N, Metsios GS, Duda JL, et al. Perceived Barriers, Facilitators and Benefits for Regular Physical Activity and Exercise in Patients with Rheumatoid Arthritis: A Review of the Literature. Sports medicine. 2015;45(10):1401–12.

114. Hurkmans EJ, Maes S, de Gucht V, Knittle K, Peeters AJ, Ronday HK, et al. Motivation as a determinant of physical activity in patients with rheumatoid arthritis. Arthritis care & research. 2010;62(3):371–7.

115. Boo S, Oh H, Froelicher ES, Suh CH. Knowledge and perception of cardiovascular disease risk among patients with rheumatoid arthritis. PLoS One. 2017;12(4):e0176291.

116. Metsios GS, Stavropoulos-Kalinoglou A, Panoulas VF, Wilson M, Nevill AM, Koutedakis Y, et al. Association of physical inactivity with increased cardiovascular risk in patients with rheumatoid arthritis. Eur J Cardiovasc Prev Rehabil. 2009;16(2):188–94.

117. Hurkmans E, van der Giesen FJ, Vliet Vlieland TP, Schoones J, Van den Ende EC. Dynamic exercise programs (aerobic capacity and/or muscle strength training) in patients with rheumatoid arthritis. Cochrane Database Syst Rev. 2009;4:CD006853.

118. Metsios GS, Stavropoulos-Kalinoglou A. Veldhuijzen van Zanten JJ, nightingale P, Sandoo a, Dimitroulas T et al: individualised exercise improves endothelial function in patients with rheumatoid arthritis. Ann Rheum Dis. 2014;73(4):748–51.

119. Albert MA, Glynn RJ, Ridker PM. Effect of physical activity on serum C-reactive protein. Am J Cardiol. 2004;93(2):221–5.

120. Metsios GS, Stavropoulos-Kalinoglou A. Veldhuijzen van Zanten JJ, Treharne GJ, Panoulas VF, Douglas KM et al: rheumatoid arthritis, cardiovascular disease and physical exercise: a systematic review. Rheumatology. 2008;47(3):239–48.

121. Ekdahl C, Broman G. Muscle strength, endurance, and aerobic capacity in rheumatoid arthritis: a comparative study with healthy subjects. Ann Rheum Dis. 1992;51(1):35–40.

122. Sui X, LaMonte MJ, Laditka JN, Hardin JW, Chase N, Hooker SP, et al. Cardiorespiratory fitness and adiposity as mortality predictors in older adults. JAMA. 2007;298(21):2507–16.

123. Ross R, Blair SN, Arena R, Church TS, Després JP, Franklin BA, et al. Importance of assessing cardiorespiratory fitness in clinical practice: a case for fitness as a clinical vital sign: a scientific statement from the American Heart Association. Circulation. 2016;134(24):e653–99.

124. Metsios GS, Koutedakis Y. Veldhuijzen van Zanten JJ, Stavropoulos-Kalinoglou a, Vitalis P, Duda JL et al: cardiorespiratory fitness levels and their association with cardiovascular profile in patients with rheumatoid arthritis: a cross-sectional study. Rheumatology. 2015;54(12):2215–20.

125. Stavropoulos-Kalinoglou A, Metsios GS. Veldhuijzen van Zanten JJ, nightingale P, Kitas GD, Koutedakis Y: individualised aerobic and resistance exercise training improves cardiorespiratory fitness and reduces cardiovascular risk in patients with rheumatoid arthritis. Ann Rheum Dis. 2013;72(11):1819–25.

126. Ridker PM, Cushman M, Stampfer MJ, Tracy RP, Hennekens CH. Inflammation, aspirin, and the risk of cardiovascular disease in apparently healthy men. N Engl J Med. 1997;336(14):973–9.

127. Kerekes G, Szekanecz Z, Dér H, Sándor Z, Lakos G, Muszbek L, et al. Endothelial dysfunction and atherosclerosis in rheumatoid arthritis: a multiparametric analysis using imaging techniques and laboratory markers of inflammation and autoimmunity. J Rheumatol. 2008;35(3):398–406.

128. Zhang C. The role of inflammatory cytokines in endothelial dysfunction. Basic Res Cardiol. 2008;103(5):398–406.

129. Hjeltnes G, Hollan I, Førre O, Wiik A, Mikkelsen K, Agewall S. Anti-CCP and RF IgM: predictors of impaired endothelial function in rheumatoid arthritis patients. Scand J Rheumatol. 2011;40(6):422–7.

130. Ursini F, Leporini C, Bene F, D'Angelo S, Mauro D, Russo E, et al. Anti-TNF-alpha agents and endothelial function in rheumatoid arthritis: a systematic review and meta-analysis. Sci Rep. 2017;7(1):5346.

131. Kaptoge S, Seshasai SR, Gao P, Freitag DF, Butterworth AS, Borglykke A, et al. Inflammatory cytokines and risk of coronary heart disease: new prospective study and updated meta-analysis. Eur Heart J. 2014;35(9):578–89.

132. del Rincon I, Polak JF, O'Leary DH, Battafarano DF, Erikson JM, Restrepo JF, et al. Systemic inflammation and cardiovascular risk factors predict rapid progression of atherosclerosis in rheumatoid arthritis. Ann Rheum Dis. 2015; 74(6):1118–23.

133. Gonzalez-Gay MA, Gonzalez-Juanatey C, Pineiro A, Garcia-Porrua C, Testa A, Llorca J. High-grade C-reactive protein elevation correlates with accelerated atherogenesis in patients with rheumatoid arthritis. J Rheumatol. 2005;32(7): 1219–23.

134. Ambrosino P, Lupoli R, Di Minno A, Tasso M, Peluso R, Di Minno MN. Subclinical atherosclerosis in patients with rheumatoid arthritis. A meta-analysis of literature studies. Thromb Haemost. 2015;113(5):916–30.

135. Arts E, Fransen J, Lemmers H, Stalenhoef A, Joosten L, van Riel P, et al. High-density lipoprotein cholesterol subfractions HDL2 and HDL3 are reduced in women with rheumatoid arthritis and may augment the

cardiovascular risk of women with RA: a cross-sectional study. Arthritis research & therapy. 2012;14(3):R116.

136. Hafström I, Rohani M, Deneberg S, Wörnert M, Jogestrand T, Frostegård J. Effects of low-dose prednisolone on endothelial function, atherosclerosis, and traditional risk factors for atherosclerosis in patients with rheumatoid arthritis–a randomized study. J Rheumatol. 2007;34(9):1810–6.

137. Roubille C, Richer V, Starnino T, McCourt C, McFarlane A, Fleming P, et al. The effects of tumour necrosis factor inhibitors, methotrexate, non-steroidal anti-inflammatory drugs and corticosteroids on cardiovascular events in rheumatoid arthritis, psoriasis and psoriatic arthritis: a systematic review and meta-analysis. Ann Rheum Dis. 2015;74(3):480–9.

138. Nissen SE, Yeomans ND, Solomon DH, Lüscher TF, Libby P, Husni ME, et al. Cardiovascular safety of celecoxib, naproxen, or ibuprofen for arthritis. N Engl J Med. 2016;375(26):2519–29.

139. Lindhardsen J, Gislason GH, Jacobsen S, Ahlehoff O, Olsen AM, Madsen OR, et al. Non-steroidal anti-inflammatory drugs and risk of cardiovascular disease in patients with rheumatoid arthritis: a nationwide cohort study. Ann Rheum Dis. 2014;73(8):1515–21.

140. Trelle S, Reichenbach S, Wandel S, Hildebrand P, Tschannen B, Villiger PM, et al. Cardiovascular safety of non-steroidal anti-inflammatory drugs: network meta-analysis. BMJ. 2011;342:c7086.

141. Goff DC, Lloyd-Jones DM, Bennett G, Coady S, D'Agostino RB, Gibbons R, et al. 2013 ACC/AHA guideline on the assessment of cardiovascular risk: a report of the American College of Cardiology/American Heart Association task force on practice guidelines. J Am Coll Cardiol. 2014;63(25 Pt B):2935–59.

142. D'Agostino RB, Vasan RS, Pencina MJ, Wolf PA, Cobain M, Massaro JM, et al. General cardiovascular risk profile for use in primary care: the Framingham heart study. Circulation. 2008;117(6):743–53.

143. Conroy RM, Pyörälä K, Fitzgerald AP, Sans S, Menotti A, De Backer G, et al. Estimation of ten-year risk of fatal cardiovascular disease in Europe: the SCORE project. Eur Heart J. 2003;24(11):987–1003.

144. Stone NJ, Robinson JG, Lichtenstein AH, Bairey Merz CN, Blum CB, Eckel RH, et al. 2013 ACC/AHA guideline on the treatment of blood cholesterol to reduce atherosclerotic cardiovascular risk in adults: a report of the American College of Cardiology/American Heart Association task force on practice guidelines. Circulation. 2014;129(25 Suppl 2):S1–45.

145. Ridker PM, Buring JE, Rifai N, Cook NR. Development and validation of improved algorithms for the assessment of global cardiovascular risk in women: the Reynolds risk score. JAMA. 2007;297(6):611–9.

146. Ridker PM, Paynter NP, Rifai N, Gaziano JM, Cook NR. C-reactive protein and parental history improve global cardiovascular risk prediction: the Reynolds Risk Score for men. Circulation. 2008;118(22):2243–51. 2244p following 2251

147. Crowson CS, Matteson EL, Roger VL, Therneau TM, Gabriel SE. Usefulness of risk scores to estimate the risk of cardiovascular disease in patients with rheumatoid arthritis. Am J Cardiol. 2012;110(3):420–4.

148. Hippisley-Cox J, Coupland C, Vinogradova Y, Robson J, Minhas R, Sheikh A, et al. Predicting cardiovascular risk in England and Wales: prospective derivation and validation of QRISK2. BMJ. 2008;336(7659):1475–82.

149. Young LE. QRISK underestimated risk of cardiovascular disease in general practice patients; Framingham score overestimated risk. Evid Based Nurs. 2008;11(3):91.

150. Arts EE, Popa C, Den Broeder AA, Semb AG, Toms T, Kitas GD, et al. Performance of four current risk algorithms in predicting cardiovascular events in patients with early rheumatoid arthritis. Ann Rheum Dis. 2015; 74(4):668–74.

151. Arts EE, Fransen J, Den Broeder AA, van PLCM R, Popa CD. Low disease activity (DAS28≤3.2) reduces the risk of first cardiovascular event in rheumatoid arthritis: a time-dependent Cox regression analysis in a large cohort study. Ann Rheum Dis. 2017;76(10):1693–9.

152. Liao KP, Playford MP, Frits M, Coblyn JS, Iannaccone C, Weinblatt ME, et al. The association between reduction in inflammation and changes in lipoprotein levels and HDL cholesterol efflux capacity in rheumatoid arthritis. J Am Heart Assoc. 2015;4:e001588. https://doi.org/10.1161/JAHA. 114.001588.

153. Navarro-Millán I, Chen L, Greenberg JD, Pappas DA, Curtis JR. Predictors and persistence of new-onset clinical remission in rheumatoid arthritis patients. Semin Arthritis Rheum. 2013;43(2):137–43.

154. Shahouri SH, Michaud K, Mikuls TR, Caplan L, Shaver TS, Anderson JD, et al. Remission of rheumatoid arthritis in clinical practice: application of the American College of Rheumatology/European league against rheumatism 2011 remission criteria. Arthritis Rheum. 2011;63(11):3204–15.

155. Prince FH, Bykerk VP, Shadick NA, Lu B, Cui J, Frits M, et al. Sustained rheumatoid arthritis remission is uncommon in clinical practice. Arthritis Res Ther. 2012;14(2):R68.

156. Micha R, Imamura F. Wyler von Ballmoos M, Solomon DH, Hernan MA, Ridker PM et al: systematic review and meta-analysis of methotrexate use and risk of cardiovascular disease. Am J Cardiol. 2011;108(9):1362–70.

157. O'Neill F, Charakida M, Topham E, McLoughlin E, Patel N, Sutill E, et al. Anti-inflammatory treatment improves high-density lipoprotein function in rheumatoid arthritis. Heart. 2017;103(10):766–73.

158. Everett BM, Pradhan AD, Solomon DH, Paynter N, Macfadyen J, Zaharris E, et al. Rationale and design of the Cardiovascular Inflammation Reduction Trial: a test of the inflammatory hypothesis of atherothrombosis. American heart journal. 2013;166(2):199–207. e115

159. Barnabe C, Martin BJ, Ghali WA. Systematic review and meta-analysis: anti-tumor necrosis factor α therapy and cardiovascular events in rheumatoid arthritis. Arthritis Care Res (Hoboken). 2011;63(4):522–9.

160. JT Giles: Comparative Cardiovascular Safety of Tocilizumab Vs Etanercept in Rheumatoid Arthritis: Results of a Randomized, Parallel-Group, Multicenter, Noninferiority, Phase 4 Clinical Trial [abstract]. In. Edited by Sattar N GS, Ridker PM, Gay S, Warne C, Musselman D, Brockwell L, Shittu E, Klearman M, Fleming J, vol. 68 (suppl 10). Arthritis Rheumatol; 2016.

161. Gabay C, McInnes IB, Kavanaugh A, Tuckwell K, Klearman M, Pulley J, et al. Comparison of lipid and lipid-associated cardiovascular risk marker changes after treatment with tocilizumab or adalimumab in patients with rheumatoid arthritis. Ann Rheum Dis. 2016;75(10):1806–12.

162. Bartels CM, Kind AJ, Everett C, Mell M, McBride P, Smith M. Low frequency of primary lipid screening among medicare patients with rheumatoid arthritis. Arthritis Rheum. 2011;63(5):1221–30.

163. Jafri K, Taylor L, Nezamzadeh M, Baker JF, Mehta NN, Bartels C, et al. Management of hyperlipidemia among patients with rheumatoid arthritis in the primary care setting. BMC Musculoskelet Disord. 2015;16:237.

164. Wei L, MacDonald TM, Walker BR. Taking glucocorticoids by prescription is associated with subsequent cardiovascular disease. Ann Intern Med. 2004;141(10):764–70.

165. Whelton PK, Carey RM, Aronow WS, Casey DE, Jr., Collins KJ, Dennison Himmelfarb C et al. 2017 ACC/AHA/AAPA/ABC/ACPM/AGS/APhA/ASH/ ASPC/NMA/PCNA Guideline for the Prevention, Detection, Evaluation, and Management of High Blood Pressure in Adults: A Report of the American College of Cardiology/American Heart Association Task Force on Clinical Practice Guidelines. Hypertension 2017.

166. Ridker PM, Cook NR. Statins: new American guidelines for prevention of cardiovascular disease. Lancet. 2013;382(9907):1762–5.

167. Sever PS, Dahlöf B, Poulter NR, Wedel H, Beevers G, Caulfield M, et al. Prevention of coronary and stroke events with atorvastatin in hypertensive patients who have average or lower-than-average cholesterol concentrations, in the Anglo-Scandinavian cardiac outcomes trial–lipid lowering arm (ASCOT-LLA): a multicentre randomised controlled trial. Drugs. 2004;64(Suppl 2):43–60.

168. Downs JR, Clearfield M, Weis S, Whitney E, Shapiro DR, Beere PA, et al. Primary prevention of acute coronary events with lovastatin in men and women with average cholesterol levels: results of AFCAPS/TexCAPS. Air force/Texas coronary atherosclerosis prevention study. JAMA. 1998;279(20):1615–22.

169. An J, Alemao E, Reynolds K, Kawabata H, Solomon DH, Liao KP, et al. Cardiovascular outcomes associated with lowering low-density lipoprotein cholesterol in rheumatoid arthritis and matched nonrheumatoid arthritis. J Rheumatol. 2016;43(11):1989–96.

170. Kitas G, Nightingale P, Armitage J, et al. SAT0105 Trial of Atorvastatin for the Primary Prevention of Cardiovascular Events in Patients with Rheumatoid Arthritis (TRACE RA). In: Annals of the Rheumatic Diseases, vol. 74; 2015. p. 688.

171. Yamanaka H, Tanaka Y, Inoue E, Hoshi D, Momohara S, Hanami K, et al. Efficacy and tolerability of tocilizumab in rheumatoid arthritis patients seen in daily clinical practice in Japan: results from a retrospective study (REACTION study). Mod Rheumatol. 2011;21(2):122–33.

172. Yazici Y, Curtis JR, Ince A, Baraf H, Malamet RL, Teng LL, et al. Efficacy of tocilizumab in patients with moderate to severe active rheumatoid arthritis and a previous inadequate response to disease-modifying antirheumatic drugs: the ROSE study. Ann Rheum Dis. 2012;71(2):198–205.

173. Tam LS, Tomlinson B, Chu TT, Li TK, Li EK. Impact of TNF inhibition on insulin resistance and lipids levels in patients with rheumatoid arthritis. Clin Rheumatol. 2007;26(9):1495–8.

174. Kirkham BW, Wasko MC, Hsia EC, Fleischmann RM, Genovese MC, Matteson EL, et al. Effects of golimumab, an anti-tumour necrosis factor-alpha human monoclonal antibody, on lipids and markers of inflammation. Ann Rheum Dis. 2014;73(1):161-9.
175. Morris SJ, Wasko MC, Antohe JL, Sartorius JA, Kirchner HL, Dancea S, et al. Hydroxychloroquine use associated with improvement in lipid profiles in rheumatoid arthritis patients. Arthritis Care Res. (Hoboken). 2011;63(4):530-4.
176. Navarro-Millan I, Charles-Schoeman C, Yang S, Bathon JM, Bridges SL Jr, Chen L, et al. Changes in lipoproteins associated with methotrexate or combination therapy in early rheumatoid arthritis: results from the treatment of early rheumatoid arthritis trial. Arthritis Rheum. 2013;65(6):1430-8.
177. Charles-Schoeman C, Wang X, Lee YY, Shahbazian A, Navarro-Millán I, Yang S, et al. Association of triple therapy with improvement in cholesterol profiles over two-year followup in the treatment of early aggressive rheumatoid arthritis trial. Arthritis & rheumatology. 2016;68(3):577-86.
178. Novikova DS, Popkova TV, Lukina GV, Luchikhina EL, Karateev DE, Volkov AV, et al. The effects of rituximab on lipids, arterial stiffness and carotid intima-media thickness in rheumatoid arthritis. J Korean Med Sci. 2016;31(2):202-7.

5

Interpretation of DAS28 and its components in the assessment of inflammatory and non-inflammatory aspects of rheumatoid arthritis

Daniel F. McWilliams[1]* , Patrick D. W. Kiely[2], Adam Young[3], Nalinie Joharatnam[1], Deborah Wilson[4] and David A. Walsh[1,4]

Abstract

Background: DAS28 is interpreted as the inflammatory disease activity of RA. Non-inflammatory pain mechanisms can confound assessment. We aimed to examine the use of DAS28 components or DAS28-derived measures that have been published as indices of non-inflammatory pain mechanisms, to inform interpretation of disease activity.

Methods: Data were used from multiple observational epidemiology studies of people with RA. Statistical characteristics of DAS28 components and derived indices were assessed using baseline and follow up data from British Society for Rheumatology Biologics Registry participants (1) commencing anti-TNF therapy ($n = 10{,}813$), or (2) changing between non-biologic DMARDs ($n = 2992$), (3) Early Rheumatoid Arthritis Network participants ($n = 813$), and (4) participants in a cross-sectional study exploring fibromyalgia and pain thresholds ($n = 45$). Repeatability was tested in 34 patients with active RA. Derived indices were the proportion of DAS28 attributable to patient-reported components (DAS28-P), tender-swollen difference and tender:swollen ratio. Pressure pain detection threshold (PPT) was used as an index of pain sensitisation.

Results: DAS28, tender joint count, visual analogue scale, DAS28-P, tender-swollen difference and tender:swollen ratio were more strongly associated with pain, PPT and fibromyalgia status than were swollen joint count or erythrocyte sedimentation rate. DAS28-P, tender-swollen difference and tender:swollen ratio better predicted pain over 1 year than did DAS28 or its individual components.

Conclusions: DAS28 is strongly associated both with inflammation and with patient-reported outcomes. DAS28-derived indices such as tender-swollen difference are associated with non-inflammatory pain mechanisms, can predict future pain and should inform how DAS28 is interpreted as an index of inflammatory disease activity in RA.

Background

The 28 joint disease activity score incorporating erythrocyte sedimentation rate (DAS28-ESR) is widely used as a measure of inflammatory disease activity in people with RA during clinical decision-making. In the UK, DAS28-ESR is used to determine eligibility for biologic therapies [1]. DAS28-ESR ≥ 3.2 can be used as a threshold for classifying active RA, and DAS28 is often used in clinical trials [2], or as a target for intensive treatment [3]. Current evidence supports these approaches as outcome measures in people with RA [4, 5].

Non-inflammatory mechanisms, through their effects on pain, can confound interpretation of DAS28-ESR ≥ 3.2 as a measure of active inflammation. Swollen joint count (SJC) and ESR are markers of inflammation. However, tender joint counts (TJCs) might be increased in people with centrally augmented pain, and the visual analogue scale for global health (VAS-GH) might be high in people fulfilling fibromyalgia (FM) classification [6, 7]. Persistent

* Correspondence: dan.mcwilliams@nottingham.ac.uk
[1]Arthritis Research UK Pain Centre, NIHR Nottingham Biomedical Research Centre & Division of Rheumatology Orthopaedics and Dermatology, University of Nottingham Clinical Sciences Building, City Hospital, Nottingham NG5 1PB, UK
Full list of author information is available at the end of the article

non-inflammatory pain can result in patients in remission being misclassified as having active inflammatory disease, leading to inappropriate clinical decisions to escalate therapy. Persistent non-inflammatory pain might compromise interpretation of outcomes in clinical trials. Furthermore, clinical tools that identify the subgroup of people with high DAS28 who also have high inflammation (rather than non-inflammatory pain) could help select people for inclusion in clinical trials or for anti-inflammatory treatment.

Several indices have been derived from DAS28-ESR components in an attempt to measure non-inflammatory contributions in people with RA. Pollard et al. have shown an association between tender minus swollen joint count (tender-swollen difference) and concurrent FM status or increased pain sensitivity [8]. We reported DAS28-P, defined as the proportion of DAS28-ESR attributable to patient-reported components (TJC and VAS-GH) [9]. DAS28-P was associated with pain severity, and predicted future pain in early RA [9], and in people commencing or changing biologic or non-biologic disease modifying treatments [10]. DAS28-P was also associated with increased pain sensitivity and concurrent FM in people with RA [7]. Evidence from one national registry suggested that the ratio of tender to swollen joint counts (tender:swollen ratio) might predict less good response of RA to biologic therapy [11], after being trichotomised into three groups. Each of these derived indices attempts to estimate the discordance between patient-reported symptoms and observed or laboratory measured inflammation. Other symptoms such as anxiety, depression and fatigue are strongly associated with chronic pain, and might reflect overlapping mechanisms within the central nervous system in people with RA [12]. We hypothesised that derived indices are associated with non-inflammatory pain and with patient-reported outcome measures of mental health and vitality or fatigue.

We sought to better understand DAS28-ESR, its components and the published derived indices in order to inform interpretation of non-inflammatory mechanisms in RA. To achieve this, we examined:- (1) The statistical properties of each index to show how each may be used in statistical analyses, including distribution (to show their continuum of values) and variability of repeat measurements (higher repeatability between clinicians improves the validity of a measure). (2) Associations of each index with pain and related patient-reported outcomes, and markers of central pain mechanisms, which are the primary objectives of their derivation. (3) Association with inflammatory disease activity (because indices of non-inflammatory mechanisms should not necessarily increase with increasing inflammation). (4) Prediction of future pain (non-inflammatory pain mechanisms might not be responsive to DMARD therapy and their presence might therefore predict poor pain prognosis).

Methods

Datasets from four published studies were used to explore statistical characteristics of DAS28 components and derived indices of inflammatory or non-inflammatory disease activity; baseline data collected from participants in the British Society for Rheumatology Biologics Register (BSRBR) with active, established RA and a valid DAS28-ESR score who were (1) initiating anti-TNF therapy (BSRBR anti-TNF cohort; $n = 10{,}813$) [13], or (2) changing between non-biologic disease modifying anti-rheumatic drugs (DMARDs, BSRBR-Control cohort; $n = 2992$) [14], (3) participants in the Early Rheumatoid Arthritis Network (ERAN cohort; $n = 813$) [15], and (4) participants undergoing routine care in a hospital-based, cross sectional study exploring FM status and pain pressure thresholds (PPT group; $n = 45$) [7]. Written informed consent was obtained from all participants. Data were used only for participants with active disease, as defined by a DAS28-ESR ≥ 3.2. The PPT group included only complete case data available for all variables. Repeatability of the variables was determined from DAS28 assessments performed by multiple assessors in people with RA during training sessions completed during practice standardisation for clinicians in the ERAN study.

The BSRBR anti-TNF cohort is a national register, started in 2002 that tracked biologic naïve people with RA commencing their first anti-TNF agent. The BSRBR control cohort is a multicentre longitudinal study of people with RA who were changing to a new non-biologic treatment at recruitment, and was intended for use as a comparator to biologic cohorts. Both cohorts are coordinated by the University of Manchester. The BSRBR cohorts were approved by NHS North West Multicentre Research Ethics Committee (00/8/53). Baseline data were provided to the authors in de-identified, anonymous formats with no indication of the anti-TNF agent being used, nor the dates of enrolment and treatment. ERAN was a multicentre inception cohort study of newly diagnosed RA spanning the UK and Eire and commenced recruitment in 2002. The study was approved by Trent Research Ethics Committee (01/4/047). Baseline and follow up data up to 1 year were used in the current study. Participants in a hospital-based study of pain pressure thresholds and pain mechanisms in people with RA were recruited through routine annual outpatient appointments for RA management at Sherwood Forest Hospitals NHS Foundation Trust [7]. Ethical approval for this project was obtained from the East Midlands NREC – Nottingham 2 (13/EM/0047).

Participants with RA were eligible for inclusion if their DAS28-ESR ≥ 3.2.

Alterations and rearrangements of the DAS28 formula might possibly increase the variation in the derived scores compared to DAS28-ESR. Repeatability data were derived from DAS28-ESR assessments taken on the same day for each patient by each assessor across four clinical assessment training classes for rheumatology researchers. The total repeatability group contained 34 people with RA across the four sessions. People with RA were assessed in subgroups of 2–4, each individual assessed on two occasions separated by > 1 h by each of 3 to 7 rheumatology healthcare workers. Data were combined with single ESR measurements per individual to give DAS28-ESR or DAS28-P scores. Repeat measures of VAS-GH were available for a subset of 19 people with RA, while the remainder rated VAS-GH once.

The formulae for derived indices were:

$$DAS28\text{-}P = \left(0.56^*\sqrt{TJC} + 0.014^*VAS\text{-}GH\right)/DAS28\text{-}ESR$$
Tender-swollen difference = TJC–SJC
Tender : swollen ratio = TJC/SJC

Participants completed a range of self-report questionnaires addressing symptoms. Bodily Pain, Vitality and Mental Health were assessed in BSR-BR and ERAN groups using Short Form-36 (SF36) and norm-transformed values used for this study (SF36 subscales are negatively oriented, with lower scores reflecting worse quality of life). PPT participants completed the Beck Depression Inventory (BDI) [16]; State-Trait Anxiety Index short form (STAI-SF) [17]; Fatigue Severity Scale (FSS) [18]; Widespread Pain Index (WPI) [19]; Symptom Severity Scale (SSS) [20]. WPI and SSS questionnaires permitted FM classification according to American College of Rheumatology criteria 2010 [20].

PPT testing used an electronic pressure algometer with a laptop recording/display device and a patient switch (Somedic Sensebox). It was carried out by a single, trained observer (NJ) at the anterior tibia [7]. Low PPT (greater sensitivity) distant from affected joints is taken as an index of widespread (possibly central) sensitization.

CRP was included as a covariate marker of concurrent inflammatory disease activity that was not included in any of the derived indices. CRP was measured by clinical laboratories local to recruiting centres. Reported CRP values < 5 mg/ml were imputed with the value of 4 mg/ml. Ln-transformation of CRP was used to adjust for inflammation as a covariate and for regression analyses, because it displayed closer approximation to normality on Q-Q plots than did non-transformed CRP (data not shown).

Statistical analysis

Repeatability was assessed by calculating the inter-observer measures of the same patient volunteer performed on the same day. The average coefficient of variation (CV; calculated as sd/mean) was calculated for each different measurement or index, as recommended as a measure of precision error [21], and is presented as a percentage. Differences between groups were assessed using T-tests

and Cohen's d effect size. Skewness and kurtosis were calculated for each variable [22]. Normality of distributions was assessed by Q-Q plots. For regression analyses, square root transformations of TJC and SJC; and natural logarithms were used for tender:swollen ratio and ESR.

Cross-sectional, baseline-only associations of DAS28-ESR, components or derived indices, transformed where necessary, with other outcomes were determined by linear regression of standardised variables providing B coefficients (95% CI) that could be compared between and across variables. Longitudinal analyses with Generalised Estimating Equations (GEE) used data from baseline to predict 3–6 month and 1 year SF36-Bodily Pain scores. The analyses were controlled for similar variables to other analyses of longitudinal pain performed in ERAN and BSRBR cohorts [9, 23], such as common disease markers for RA severity (disability, serology and disease duration), demographics or lifestyle (age, gender, BMI, smoking) and pain-related factors (mental health and fatigue). The effects of inflammation were adjusted for using CRP measures, as this was the available measure that was the most-independent compared to the other DAS28-ESR components. Analysis was performed using SPSS v22 (IBM, USA) and $p < 0.05$ was taken as statistical significance.

Results

Demographics of each patient group are shown in Table 1. As expected, fewer participants satisfied 1987 ACR RA classification criteria in ERAN at baseline than in those other groups recruited from people with established RA. The BSRBR anti-TNF group displayed highest scores for DAS28 and its components.

Measurement properties of DAS28-ESR, its components and derived indices

Tender:swollen ratio underwent logarithmic transformation to give a closer approximation to a normal distribution (which improves its measurement properties; Additional file 1: Figure S1 and Table S1). Transformed tender:swollen ratio data were therefore used in all analyses. Some measurements displayed prominent floor and ceiling effects. The proportions of cases that displayed either maximum or minimum scores were highest for tender:swollen ratio (≤15% minimum and ≤ 28% maximum depending upon participant group). SJCs were zero in 28% of PPT study, and 7% of ERAN participants, but ≤1% in BSRBR cohorts. Of BSRBR-anti-TNF cohort participants, 6% displayed SJC = 28, and 6% displayed VAS-GH = 100 mm. Other measures all showed ≤3% floor or ceiling prevalence. Inter-observer repeatability was indicated by coefficients of variation; TJC (41%), VAS-GH (16%), SJC (62%),

Table 1 Demographics and clinical features of participant groups at baseline

	ERAN	BSRBR anti-TNF	BSRBR-Control	PPT study	Repeatability
N=	813	10,813	2992	45	34
%female	70%	76%	74%	77%	73%
Age (mean (sd))	57 (14)	56 (12)	60 (12)	60 (11)	60 (13)
Seropositive	59%	65%	58%	90%	79%
DAS28-ESR	5.2 (1.1)	6.6 (1.0)	5.4 (1.1)	4.7 (0.9)	4.8 (1.1)
ESR	34 (24)	46 (29)	37 (25)	21 (13)	39 (29)
SJC	7 (6)	11 (6)	6 (5)	1 (1)	5 (4)
TJC	9 (7)	16 (7)	9 (7)	11 (7)	6 (6)
VAS-GH	50 (24)	73 (20)	57 (23)	53 (23)	39 (20)
CRP	28 (37)	46 (42)	35 (40)	< 5	not collected

Eligible population: proportion (number) of cases from database with DAS28-ESR ≥ 3.2 and therefore included in this study. *TJC* tender joint count, *SJC* swollen joint count, *ESR* erythrocyte sedimentation rate, *VAS-GH* visual analogue scale-general health, *CRP* C-reactive protein (mg per dL)

DAS28-P (17%), tender-swollen difference (188%) and tender:swollen ratio (64%).

Associations with pain and other patient-reported outcomes

DAS28-ESR and its components and each of the derived indices were significantly associated with Bodily Pain scores in each participant group (Additional file 1: Table S2). Cross-sectional associations with Bodily Pain scores were adjusted for CRP to explore possible dependence on non-inflammatory factors (Additional file 1: Table S3). Each study group showed multiple significant associations of worse Bodily Pain scores with DAS28-ESR, and also with the DAS28-ESR components TJC and VAS-GH. Bodily Pain scores were also significantly associated with DAS28-P; tender-swollen difference; and tender:swollen ratio. Less consistent findings were found for ESR and SJC.

Lower PPTs (more sensitive) at the anterior tibia were significantly associated with higher TJC, VAS-GH, DAS28-ESR, and DAS28-P. Lower PPTs were also significantly

associated with tender-swollen difference, but not with SJC, ESR nor tender:swollen ratio (Table 2). DAS28-ESR, TJC, VAS-GH, DAS28-P and tender-swollen difference were higher in participants that satisfied criteria for FM, whereas SJC, ESR and tender:swollen ratio were not (Table 2).

Higher DAS28-ESR was associated with worse mental health, as measured by BDI (depression) or STAI-SF (anxiety), or SF36 Mental Health Score (distress; Table 3A). Higher DAS28-ESR was also associated with worse fatigue/lower vitality in each group (Table 3B). Associations with worse mental health or fatigue were stronger for VAS-GH and TJC than for SJC and ESR, and more consistently significant for DAS28-P and tender-swollen difference than for tender:swollen ratio (Table 3A, B).

Associations between DAS28-related variables, DAS28-ESR and CRP

Indices of non-inflammatory pain might be expected to be independent of inflammation levels. Each individual DAS28-ESR component and derived index displayed the

Table 2 Associations of DAS28-related variables with pressure pain thresholds and fibromyalgia classification

Index	Medial Tibia PPT		Fibromyalgia (FM) classification				
	B (95% CI)	p	RA with FM	RA (no FM)	p	Difference	Effect size
TJC	**− 0.39 (− 0.63 to − 0.15)**	**0.002**	**14 (7)**	**8 (6)**	**0.01**	5.3	0.75
VAS-GH	**− 0.37 (− 0.61 to − 0.13)**	**0.003**	**67 (19)**	**42 (19)**	**< 0.001**	25	1.09
SJC	0.03 (− 0.23 to 0.28)	0.834	1 (1)	1 (2)	0.742	0.15	0.1
ESR	−0.10 (− 0.36 to 0.17)	0.464	23 (16)	20 (11)	0.51	2.7	0.2
DAS28	**− 0.53 (− 0.77 to − 0.29)**	**< 0.001**	**5.2 (0.8)**	**4.4 (0.8)**	**0.001**	0.79	0.93
DAS28-P	**−0.41 (− 0.62 to − 0.13)**	**0.003**	**0.56 (0.11)**	**0.48 (0.09)**	**0.008**	0.09	0.81
Tender-swollen difference	**−0.38 (− 0.62 to − 0.15)**	**0.002**	**12 (8)**	**7 (6)**	**0.011**	5.5	0.76
Tender:swollen ratio	**−0.48 (− 0.79 to − 0.18)**	**0.003**	8.4 (7.0)	6.2 (5.9)	0.363	2.1	0.33

Data from PPT study, n = 45. Linear regression between medal tibial pressure pain thresholds (PPT) and DAS28-related variables (lower values of PPTs indicate greater pain sensitivity). Means (sd); T-Tests and Cohens d effect size for differences between patients with RA ± fibromyalgia (FM). *TJC* tender joint count, *SJC* swollen joint count, *ESR* erythrocyte sedimentation rate, *VAS-GH* visual analogue scale-general health. DAS28-P = proportion of DAS28-ESR attributable to patient-reported components. No corrects were performed for multiple comparisons. Statistically significant findings highlighted in **bold**

Interpretation of DAS28 and its components in the assessment of inflammatory...

49

Table 3 Associations of DAS28-related variables with mental health and vitality or fatigue

A

	BSRBR antiTNF SF36-Mental Health Score		BSRBR-Control SF36-Mental Health Score		ERAN SF36-Mental Health Score		PPT study Beck Depression Index		PPT study State Trait Anxiety Index	
	B (95% CI)	p	B (95% CI)	p	B (95% CI)	p	B (95% CI)	p	B (95% CI)	p
TJC	−0.12 (−0.14 to −0.10)	<0.001	−0.17 (−0.21 to −0.13)	<0.001	−0.19 (−0.26 to −0.11)	<0.001	**0.29 (0.01 to 0.57)**	**0.044**	**0.36 (0.08 to 0.63)**	**0.012**
VAS-GH	−0.19 (−0.21 to −0.17)	<0.001	−0.28 (−0.32 to −0.24)	<0.001	−0.36 (−0.43 to −0.29)	<0.001	**0.47 (0.21 to 0.73)**	**0.001**	**0.45 (0.19 to 0.70)**	**0.001**
SJC	−0.04 (−0.06 to −0.02)	<0.001	−0.05 (−0.09 to −0.01)	0.017	−0.01 (−0.09 to 0.07)	0.735	−0.19 (−0.48 to 0.09)	0.184	−0.22 (−0.50 to 0.06)	0.125
ESR	−0.07 (−0.09 to −0.05)	<0.001	−0.04 (−0.08 to 0.00)	0.078	−0.11 (−0.18 to −0.03)	0.006	0.15 (−0.16 to 0.46)	0.338	0.01 (−0.30 to 0.31)	0.967
DAS28	−0.17 (−0.19 to −0.15)	<0.001	−0.21 (−0.27 to −0.17)	<0.001	−0.25 (−0.32 to −0.18)	<0.001	**0.33 (0.02 to 0.64)**	**0.039**	**0.33 (0.03 to 0.63)**	**0.034**
DAS28-P	−0.10 (−0.12 to −0.08)	<0.001	−0.18 (−0.22 to −0.14)	<0.001	−0.23 (−0.30 to −0.15)	<0.001	**0.37 (0.09 to 0.65)**	**0.012**	**0.41 (0.13 to 0.69)**	**0.005**
Tender-swollen difference	−0.09 (−0.11 to −0.07)	<0.001	−0.14 (−0.18 to −0.10)	<0.001	−0.18 (−0.25 to −0.10)	<0.001	**0.31 (0.04 to 0.59)**	**0.027**	**0.39 (0.12 to 0.66)**	**0.006**
Tender-swollen ratio	−0.06 (−0.08 to −0.04)	<0.001	−0.10 (−0.14 to −0.06)	<0.001	−0.11 (−0.22 to 0.01)	0.060	0.27 (−0.08 to 0.61)	0.128	0.24 (−0.08 to 0.57)	0.135

B

	BSRBR anti-TNF SF36-Vitality		BSRBR control SF36-Vitality		ERAN SF36-Vitality		PPT study Fatigue Severity Scale	
	B (95% CI)	p	B (95% CI)	p	B (95% CI)	p	B (95% CI)	p
TJC	−0.13 (−0.15 to −0.11)	<0.001	−0.17 (−0.21 to −0.13)	<0.001	−0.27 (−0.34 to −0.20)	<0.001	**0.30 (0.01 to 0.58)**	**0.042**
VAS-GH	−0.19 (−0.21 to −0.17)	<0.001	−0.26 (−0.30 to −0.22)	<0.001	−0.36 (−0.43 to −0.29)	<0.001	**0.57 (0.32 to 0.81)**	**<0.001**
SJC	−0.05 (−0.07 to −0.03)	<0.001	−0.06 (−0.10 to −0.02)	0.002	−0.07 (−0.14 to 0.01)	0.100	−0.11 (−0.41 to 0.19)	0.473
ESR	−0.06 (−0.08 to −0.04)	<0.001	−0.09 (−0.13 to −0.05)	0.002	−0.14 (−0.22 to −0.07)	<0.001	0.16 (−0.15 to 0.47)	0.304
DAS28	−0.18 (−0.20 to −0.15)	<0.001	−0.25 (−0.29 to −0.21)	<0.001	−0.33 (−0.40 to −0.26)	<0.001	**0.43 (0.12 to 0.73)**	**0.007**
DAS28-P	−0.11 (−0.13 to −0.09)	<0.001	−0.17 (−0.21 to −0.13)	<0.001	−0.28 (−0.35 to −0.21)	<0.001	**0.38 (0.08 to 0.68)**	**0.013**
Tender-swollen difference	−0.09 (−0.11 to −0.07)	<0.001	−0.13 (−0.17 to −0.09)	<0.001	−0.22 (−0.29 to −0.15)	<0.001	**0.31 (0.03 to 0.60)**	**0.033**
Tender-swollen ratio	−0.07 (−0.09 to −0.05)	<0.001	−0.09 (−0.13 to −0.05)	<0.001	−0.17 (−0.27 to −0.08)	0.001	0.34 (−0.05 to 0.74)	0.087

A: Mental health scores and B: Fatigue scores, with their associations with DAS28-related variables. Standardised linear regression coefficients, 95% confidence intervals and p values. *TJC* tender joint count, *SJC* swollen joint count, *ESR* erythrocyte sedimentation rate, *VAS-GH* visual analogue scale-general health. DAS28-P = proportion of DAS28-ESR attributable to patient-reported components. No corrects were performed for multiple comparisons. Statistically significant findings highlighted in **bold** expected significant positive associations with DAS28-ESR in each participant group (Table 4). Associations of each derived index with DAS28-ESR appeared to have smaller coefficients than those of the individual DAS28-ESR components (Table 4). The weakest association of DAS28-ESR was with tender:swollen ratio. The expected positive associations were found between DAS28-ESR components and serum CRP level. Conversely, none of the derived indices displayed significant positive correlation with serum CRP (Table 4). DAS28-P was significantly negatively associated with serum CRP level in all groups, whereas negative associations with tender-swollen differences and tender:swollen ratios were weaker than with DAS28-P (Table 4).

Longitudinal prediction of pain

The longitudinal prediction of pain was tested for each of the DAS28-ESR components and derived indices using GEE analyses. Baseline DAS28-ESR, derived indices and DAS28-ESR components each predicted worse pain prognosis up to 1 year in univariate analyses (Table 5). Baseline tender-swollen difference and tender:swollen ratio were significantly associated with worse pain prognosis in all longitudinal cohorts using multivariable GEE analysis adjusting for baseline pain, inflammation measured by CRP, and other potential confounders (Table 5). High DAS28-P was significantly associated with worse pain prognosis in ERAN and BSRBR non-biologic cohorts, but not in the BSRBR anti-TNF cohort after multivariable analysis (Table 5). Associations of DAS28-ESR, SJC, TJC or VAS-GH with pain prognosis was significant in only one of the three cohorts for each (Table 5).

Discussion

We have shown that indices derived from DAS28-ESR components can give insight into the non-inflammatory contributions to apparent inflammatory disease activity in people with RA. Tender-swollen difference might have some advantages over other derived indices, although head-to-head statistical comparisons were not made. Derived indices were consistent with being measures of non-inflammatory factors, as they were less strongly associated with DAS28-ESR than were individual DAS28-ESR components; and tender-swollen difference was not consistently associated with CRP. Tender-swollen difference and DAS28-P each was positively associated with FM status, and with PPT evidence of neuronal sensitisation, as found previously [8, 24]. They displayed normal-like distributions and were without notable floor or ceiling effects. Tender-swollen difference more consistently predicted pain outcomes than did DAS28-P. DAS28-derived indices have potential as research tools, to help interpret

DAS28-ESR as a measure of inflammatory disease activity, and to help predict those who might benefit from additional interventions aiming to reduce the long-term burden of pain in people with RA.

DAS28-ESR is an important measure of inflammatory disease activity in RA [25–29]. Our analyses confirm a strong association between DAS28-ESR or its components and self-reported pain, as would be expected where inflammation drives RA symptoms. However, VAS-GH and TJC, and therefore DAS28-ESR, are strongly influenced by non-inflammatory pain mechanisms [7]. Some authors have found benefits from analysing SJC + ESR combined and contrasting to TJC + VAS-GH combined. This may be a way to further examine people in clinical remission with low inflammation, but high pain [30]. Furthermore, as DAS28 shares many components with the Clinical Disease Activity Index [31] and the Simplified Disease Activity Index [32], plus some of the criteria for Boolean Remission [33], there may be scope for cross-validation between different indices.

We have shown that indices derived from DAS28-ESR components are associated with pain, while displaying little dependence on inflammation, as measured by CRP. In cross-sectional analyses, DAS28-ESR and the derived indices were similarly associated with pain and other symptoms. However, each of the derived indices predicted 1 year pain prognosis more strongly than did DAS28-ESR or each of its components. However, examining the exact mechanisms for pain prognosis is a complex task. Modern treatment, including biologic therapies, might counteract the importance of synovitis for pain prognosis. Pain might be more likely to persist where non-inflammatory mechanism make an important contribution and therefore pain outcomes might be best predicted by derived indices that reflect those non-inflammatory mechanisms.

Our data extend previous findings that DAS28-P predicted pain following initiation of biologic or non-biologic DMARDS [9], and that swollen:tender ratio predicted response to biologic treatment [11]. We demonstrate prediction of pain outcomes also by tender-swollen difference, and that pain prediction by derived indices persists after adjusting for other baseline demographic and clinical factors known to influence pain, including measures of inflammatory disease activity, psychological distress, obesity and smoking status.

We found that pain prediction by baseline values of derived indices were weaker in the BSRBR anti-TNF cohort than in the other two studies, consistent with our previous analyses [9, 10]. It is possible that TNF blockade inhibits non-inflammatory as well as inflammatory pain mechanisms [34], or that more effective suppression of an inflammatory drive to central sensitisation might also

Table 4 Associations of DAS28-related variables with DAS28-ESR and CRP

		BSRBR anti-TNF		BSRBR-Control		ERAN	
		B (95% CI)	p	B (95% CI)	p	B (95% CI)	p
DAS28	TJC	**0.72 (0.71 to 0.73)**	**< 0.001**	**0.76 (0.74 to 0.78)**	**< 0.001**	**0.59 (0.55 to 0.62)**	**< 0.001**
	VAS-GH	**0.49 (0.47 to 0.50)**	**< 0.001**	**0.62 (0.59 to 0.65)**	**< 0.001**	**0.46 (0.42 to 0.51)**	**< 0.001**
	SJC	**0.56 (0.55 to 0.58)**	**< 0.001**	**0.60 (0.58 to 0.62)**	**< 0.001**	**0.48 (0.45 to 0.52)**	**< 0.001**
	ESR	**0.49 (0.48 to 0.51)**	**< 0.001**	**0.53 (0.51 to 0.56)**	**< 0.001**	**0.41 (0.37 to 0.45)**	**< 0.001**
	DAS28	Not applicable					
	DAS28-P	**0.19 (0.17 to 0.20)**	**< 0.001**	**0.29 (0.26 to 0.32)**	**< 0.001**	**0.24 (0.19 to 0.29)**	**< 0.001**
	Tender-swollen difference	**0.25 (0.24 to 0.27)**	**< 0.001**	**0.36 (0.32 to 0.39)**	**< 0.001**	**0.15 (0.11 to 0.20)**	**< 0.001**
	Tender:swollen ratio	**0.11 (0.09 to 0.12)**	**< 0.001**	**0.13 (0.10 to 0.16)**	**< 0.001**	**0.07 (0.02 to 0.12)**	**0.011**
CRP	TJC	−0.02 (− 0.05 to 0.01)	0.161	**0.09 (0.02 to 0.16)**	**0.010**	**0.17 (0.07 to 0.26)**	**< 0.001**
	VAS-GH	**0.17 (0.14 to 0.20)**	**< 0.001**	**0.21 (0.13 to 0.28)**	**< 0.001**	**0.17 (0.08 to 0.26)**	**< 0.001**
	SJC	**0.10 (0.07 to 0.13)**	**< 0.001**	**0.11 (0.05 to 0.17)**	**0.001**	**0.23 (0.13 to 0.32)**	**< 0.001**
	ESR	**0.58 (0.55 to 0.60)**	**< 0.001**	**0.56 (0.51 to 0.62)**	**< 0.001**	**0.62 (0.55 to 0.69)**	**< 0.001**
	DAS28	**0.36 (0.33 to 0.39)**	**< 0.001**	**0.47 (0.40 to 0.55)**	**< 0.001**	**0.45 (0.37 to 0.53)**	**< 0.001**
	DAS28-P	**−0.31 (−0.34 to − 0.28)**	**< 0.001**	**−0.28 (− 0.36 to − 0.20)**	**< 0.001**	**−0.20 (− 0.30 to − 0.11)**	**< 0.001**
	Tender-swollen difference	**− 0.10 (− 0.13 to − 0.07)**	**< 0.001**	−0.01 (− 0.08 to 0.06)	0.851	−0.03 (− 0.13 to 0.06)	0.487
	Tender:swollen ratio	**−0.11 (− 0.14 to − 0.08)**	**< 0.001**	**−0.08 (− 0.15 to − 0.01)**	**0.020**	−0.08 (− 0.18 to 0.02)	0.104

Linear regression of z-transformed variables. Regression coefficients (95% CI) and p values for associations with the inflammatory measures, DAS28 and CRP. CRP data were ln-transformed prior to regression analysis. *TJC* tender joint count, *SJC* swollen joint count, *ESR* erythrocyte sedimentation rate, *VAS-GH* visual analogue scale-general health. DAS28-P = proportion of DAS28-ESR attributable to patient-reported components. No corrects were performed for multiple comparisons. Statistically significant findings highlighted in **bold**

Table 5 Longitudinal associations of baseline DAS28-related variables with pain at follow up

| | ERAN | | | | BSRBR anti-TNF | | | | BSRBR-Non-Biologic | | | |
| | Univariate | | Multivariable | | Univariate | | Multivariable | | Univariate | | Multivariable | |
	B (95% CI)	p	B (95% CI)	p	B (95% CI)	p	B (95% CI)	p	B (95% CI)	p	B (95% CI)	p
TJC	**−0.28 (−0.34 to −0.22)**	**< 0.001**	−0.09 (−0.21 to 0.03)	0.131	**−0.10 (−0.12 to −0.08)**	**< 0.001**	−0.02 (−0.05 to 0.01)	0.264	**−0.23 (−0.26 to −0.19)**	**< 0.001**	**−0.10 (−0.16 to −0.05)**	**< 0.001**
SJC	**−0.09 (−0.15 to −0.03)**	**0.004**	0.07 (−0.01 to 0.16)	0.087	−0.02 (−0.04 to 0.00)	0.090	**0.03 (0.00 to 0.06)**	**0.029**	**−0.04 (−0.08 to −0.01)**	**0.019**	−0.02 (−0.07 to 0.03)	0.523
VAS-GH	**−0.36 (−0.44 to −0.29)**	**< 0.001**	−0.10 (−0.23 to 0.02)	0.102	**−0.14 (−0.16 to −0.12)**	**< 0.001**	−0.02 (−0.05 to 0.01)	0.139	**−0.29 (−0.32 to −0.26)**	**< 0.001**	**−0.14 (−0.20 to −0.09)**	**< 0.001**
ESR	**−0.18 (−0.25 to −0.11)**	**< 0.001**	0.07 (−0.07 to 0.20)	0.338	**−0.07 (−0.09 to −0.05)**	**< 0.001**	0.01 (−0.02 to 0.03)	0.695	**−0.09 (−0.13 to −0.05)**	**< 0.001**	−0.04 (−0.11 to 0.04)	0.349
DAS28	**−0.31 (−0.38 to −0.23)**	**< 0.001**	−0.04 (−0.17 to 0.09)	0.564	**−0.14 (−0.16 to −0.12)**	**< 0.001**	−0.02 (−0.04 to 0.01)	0.176	**−0.25 (−0.28 to −0.21)**	**< 0.001**	**−0.13 (−0.19 to −0.07)**	**< 0.001**
DAS28-P	**−0.26 (−0.34 to −0.19)**	**< 0.001**	**−0.15 (−0.27 to −0.04)**	**0.007**	**−0.07 (−0.09 to −0.05)**	**< 0.001**	−0.02 (−0.04 to 0.00)	0.089	**−0.20 (−0.24 to −0.17)**	**< 0.001**	**−0.14 (−0.23 to −0.05)**	**0.002**
Tender-swollen difference	**−0.25 (−0.32 to −0.18)**	**< 0.001**	**−0.14 (−0.24 to −0.04)**	**0.004**	**−0.08 (−0.10 to −0.06)**	**< 0.001**	**−0.03 (−0.05 to −0.00)**	**0.019**	**−0.20 (−0.23 to −0.16)**	**< 0.001**	**−0.11 (−0.17 to −0.05)**	**< 0.001**
Tender-swollen ratio	**−0.17 (−0.23 to −0.10)**	**< 0.001**	**−0.14 (−0.21 to 0.06)**	**< 0.001**	**−0.06 (−0.08 to −0.05)**	**< 0.001**	**−0.03 (−0.05 to −0.01)**	**0.007**	**−0.15 (−0.19 to −0.11)**	**< 0.001**	**−0.08 (−0.14 to −0.02)**	**0.016**

Generalised Estimating Equations for prediction of longitudinal pain (3/6 month and 1 year SF36-Bodily Pain). Univariate analyses show the associations between baseline DAS28-related variables and longitudinal pain with no adjustments. Multivariable analyses were similar, but with adjustments for baseline measures of pain, DAS28, CRP, seropositive, age, gender, BMI, smoking, SF36-physical function, SF36-vitality, SF36-mental health. TJC tender joint count, SJC swollen joint count, ESR erythrocyte sedimentation rate, VAS-GH visual analogue scale-general health. DAS28-P = proportion of DAS28-ESR attributable to patient-reported components. No corrects were performed for multiple comparisons. Statistically significant findings highlighted in **bold** inhibit non-inflammatory pain mechanisms [35]. Confounding by the higher baseline RA severity in the BSRBR biologics cohort might also contribute to differences in pain prediction. DAS28-P did not predict EULAR-defined inflammatory disease responses 3 months after initiation of biologic therapy in another study [36], and factors that predict pain response to treatment might differ from those predicting inflammatory disease suppression.

Low PPTs indicate neuronal sensitisation and, when observed at a distance from affected joints, might reflect central sensitisation [37]. Concurrent classification of FM is common in people with RA [7] and is considered also to reflect central sensitisation. Derived indices displayed significant associations with PPTs and FM classification, suggesting that they might reflect central sensitisation in RA. Central sensitisation might indicate comorbid conditions such as FM or result from sustained nociceptive input from joint inflammation [12] or other co-morbidities, such as osteoarthritis and low back pain. We did not observe significant associations between SJC or ESR and PPTs or FM classification, indicating that ongoing inflammation might not be necessary to sustain sensitisation in RA, although inflammation might yet contribute to the development of sensitisation in earlier disease.

Self-reported fatigue and poor mental health scores are associated with worse pain and greater central sensitisation in people with RA [38, 39]. DAS28-ESR was significantly associated with fatigue and mental health in each study group. However, SJC and ESR were less consistently or less strongly (smaller coefficients) associated with fatigue or mental health than were TJC and VAS-GH, paralleling the various associations seen with bodily pain. Furthermore, we now extend our previous findings on pain [7] to show that derived indices were significantly associated with fatigue and mental health scores in both early and established disease. Fatigue and/or poor mental health might, therefore, be additional centrally mediated non-inflammatory mechanisms that confound inflammatory disease assessment using DAS28-ESR.

Derived indices displayed less positive association with CRP than did DAS28-ESR or its components, and therefore have some external validity as measures of non-inflammatory mechanisms. Testing against additional measures of inflammation, for example using ultrasound or magnetic resonance imaging, might further extend these findings. Tender-swollen difference displayed some advantages over the other derived measures, in being simple to calculate, displaying a normal distribution without important floor and ceiling effects, displaying consistent associations with pain, PPT and FM status, and consistently predicting worse pain outcome across all three cohort studies. The inclusion of

four items in DAS28-P might improve its validity over indices derived from only two items, but the significant negative association of DAS28-P with CRP, possibly due to the inclusion of ESR in its denominator, suggests potential confounding by inflammation. DAS28-P displayed a lower coefficient of variation than did the tender-swollen difference. However, the coefficient of variation statistic tends towards infinity where mean values approach zero, and this might underestimate the repeatability of the tender-swollen difference. It showed similar standardised coefficients and confidence intervals with other indices, and we believe that it has similar validity to DAS28-P when used to analyse these data. Inclusion of a single ESR measurement might also have led us to overestimate the repeatability of DAS28-P. Tender:-swollen ratio had a number of disadvantages including floor and ceiling effects, and skewness that necessitated transformation prior to parametric analysis. When the swollen:tender ratio was derived, it was split into three response levels to deal with the effects of zero values [11], whereas this analysis focussed on comparisons of continuous indices. Tender-swollen difference might be a preferred continuous derived index for studying non-inflammatory contributions to RA pain.

Our study is subject to several limitations, despite the availability of data from several large groups with early or established RA. The consistent pattern of findings for each index is presented across a variety of data sources. As most of the comparisons were complementary, no corrections were made for multiple testing. Derived indices have value in epidemiology or secondary data analyses where more specific measures of non-inflammatory mechanisms such as central sensitisation are unfeasible or not available. However, their interpretation as surrogates for pain sensitivity or central sensitisation should be cautious in the context of other potential confounders such as mental health or fatigue. In the absence of a gold-standard measure of central sensitisation or non-inflammatory pain, we have used PPTs and bodily pain as surrogates. Using other surrogate measures might have altered the study findings. Further research is required to determine which specific non-inflammatory disease mechanisms modulate assessment of inflammation using DAS28-ESR. Our study used CRP as a measure of inflammation, although some patients with RA might have continuing inflammatory disease activity despite normal CRP, in particular since the introduction of interleukin-6 blockade. CRP was selected because it was not included in any of the DAS28-related variables, and so would be the least likely to be a confounder. Other measures of synovitis might reveal possible associations of derived indices with residual synovitis. Lack of formal reliability data is a limitation, and necessitated use of CV values. The repeatability data are limited by their collection from a large number of practitioners with varying experience, and may reflect the "real world" variability, rather than an optimal variability. CV values of VAS-GH might be underestimated because it was not possible to blind participants to previous instructions or responses during repeated assessment by successive practitioners. It should be noted that other definitions of disease activity, treatment response and remission are available [40–42]. Data from observational cohort studies cannot distinguish effects on treatment from those on placebo response or natural history. Future studies should therefore also test the ability of derived measures to predict response to treatments within the context of randomised controlled trials, either targeting synovitis or non-inflammatory disease mechanisms.

Non-inflammatory contributions are of particular clinical importance where DAS28-ESR suggests active inflammatory disease. Overestimation of synovitis might result in inappropriate exposure of patients to potentially toxic or expensive treatments, and underestimation of inflammatory disease suppression might lead to discontinuation of treatments that would otherwise prevent joint damage and subsequent disability. The presence of non-inflammatory pain mechanisms does not, however, exclude concurrent inflammation, and even moderate disease activity is longitudinally associated with both poor function and joint damage [28]. Specific measures of synovitis such as ultrasound assessment might help guide treatment titration to achieve low disease activity or remission in all cases, particularly where non-inflammatory mechanisms might conceal contributions of persistent synovitis to DAS28-ESR. Non-inflammatory mechanisms underlying important symptoms such as pain, fatigue or impaired mental health are important even where DAS28-ESR suggests that inflammation is well controlled. Derived measures are unlikely to be appropriate in people with remission of inflammatory disease, where more experimental measures such as PPT or other forms of quantitative sensory testing might reveal non-inflammatory pain mechanisms. Where DAS28-ESR < 3.1, DAS28-P displays a skewed distribution and high measurement errors are generated by ratios in which denominators are close to zero [9].

Conclusion

In conclusion, we demonstrate the potential of derived indices as measures of non-inflammatory mechanisms in people with apparently active RA (DAS28-ESR ≥ 3.2). Our analyses suggest that tender-swollen difference, DAS28-P and tender:swollen ratio are surrogate indices of non-inflammatory pain mechanisms, and we propose that central sensitisation is a likely candidate. DAS28-ESR remains a valuable measure of active synovitis,

which continues to facilitate the development of disease modifying treatments and helps target treatments those to those who gain most benefit [4, 5, 43, 44]. Derived indices, such as tender-swollen difference, conveniently assist interpretation of DAS28-ESR as a measure of inflammatory disease activity. With further research to establish thresholds, they may have potential to help identify people with RA who might benefit from interventions that target non-inflammatory mechanisms in order to improve their pain prognosis.

Abbreviations

BDI: Beck Depression Inventory; BSRBR: British Society for Rheumatology Biologics Register; CRP: C-reactive protein; DAS28: Disease activity score for 28 joints; ERAN: Early Rheumatoid Arthritis Network; ESR: Erythrocyte sedimentation rate; FM: Fibromyalgia; FSS: Fatigue Severity Scale; PPT: Pressure pain thresholds; SJC: Swollen joint count; SSS: Symptom Severity Scale; STAI-SF: State-Trait Anxiety Index short form; TJC: Tender joint count; VAS-GH: Visual analogue scale; WPI: Widespread Pain Index

Acknowledgements

We would like to acknowledge staff and patients at ERAN and BSRBR collection centres; patient volunteers for training days (repeatability study); patients for PPT study; Drs Kimme Hyrich, Kath Watson, Chris Hiley and Alan Roach (BSRBR studies).

Funding

Funded by Pfizer iCRP grant #WI190792. The funder did not contribute to the design of the study, the data collection, the analysis, the interpretation of the data, the writing of the manuscript nor the decision to submit for publication.
The BSRBR-RA register is funded by restricted income from UK pharmaceutical companies, presently Abbvie, Pfizer, Roche, MSD and UCB Pharma. This income finances a wholly separate contract between the BSR and the Register at the University of Manchester. The principal investigators, their team and other researchers using the data have full academic freedom and are able to work independently of pharmaceutical industry influence. All decisions concerning analyses, interpretation and publication are made autonomously of any industry contribution.

Authors' contributions

DFM was involved in study design, analysis, writing, editing, critical appraisal of the manuscript and its final approval. PDWK was involved in study design, data collection, writing, editing, critical appraisal of the manuscript and its final approval. AY was involved in study design, data collection, writing, editing, critical appraisal of the manuscript and its final approval. NJ was involved in study design, data collection, writing, editing, critical appraisal of the manuscript and its final approval. DW was involved in study design, data collection, writing, editing, critical appraisal of the manuscript and its final approval. DAW was involved in study design, analysis, data collection, writing, editing, critical appraisal of the manuscript and its final approval. All authors read and approved the final manuscript.

Competing interests

DFM and DAW declare grant support from Pfizer Ltd (iCRP scheme; grant #WI190792). DAW has undertaken paid consultancy, outside of this work, for Pfizer Ltd. and GSK Consumer Healthcare.

Author details

[1]Arthritis Research UK Pain Centre, NIHR Nottingham Biomedical Research Centre & Division of Rheumatology Orthopaedics and Dermatology, University of Nottingham Clinical Sciences Building, City Hospital, Nottingham NG5 1PB, UK. [2]Department of Rheumatology, St Georges Healthcare NHS Trust, London, UK. [3]University of West Hertfordshire, Watford, UK. [4]Department of Rheumatology, Sherwood Forest Hospitals NHS Foundation Trust, Sutton-in-Ashfield, UK.

References

1. NICE. NICE guidelines [CG79]: rheumatoid arthritis: the management of rheumatoid arthritis in adults: NICE; 2009. Available from: http://www.nice.org.uk/guidance/cg79. Accessed 12 Mar 2018.

2. Allaart CF, Goekoop-Ruiterman YP, de Vries-Bouwstra JK, Breedveld FC, Dijkmans BA. Aiming at low disease activity in rheumatoid arthritis with initial combination therapy or initial monotherapy strategies: the BeSt study. Clin Exp Rheumatol. 2006;24(6 Suppl 43):S-77-82.

3. Fransen J, van Riel PL. The Disease Activity Score and the EULAR response criteria. Clin Exp Rheumatol. 2005;23(5 Suppl 39):S93-9.

4. Goekoop-Ruiterman YP, de Vries-Bouwstra JK, Allaart CF, van Zeben D, Kerstens PJ, Hazes JM, et al. Clinical and radiographic outcomes of four different treatment strategies in patients with early rheumatoid arthritis (the BeSt study): a randomized, controlled trial. Arthritis Rheum. 2008;58 (2 Suppl):S126-35.

5. Nikiphorou E, Norton S, Young A, Carpenter L, Dixey J, Walsh DA, et al. Association between rheumatoid arthritis disease activity, progression of functional limitation and long-term risk of orthopaedic surgery: combined analysis of two prospective cohorts supports EULAR treat to target DAS thresholds. Ann Rheum Dis. 2016;75(12):2080-6.

6. Wolfe F, Cathey MA, Kleinheksel SM. Fibrositis (Fibromyalgia) in rheumatoid arthritis. J Rheumatol. 1984;11(6):814-8.

7. Joharatnam N, McWilliams DF, Wilson D, Wheeler M, Pande I, Walsh DA. A cross sectional study of pain sensitivity, disease activity assessment, mental health and fibromyalgia status in rheumatoid arthritis. Arthritis Res Ther. 2015;17(1):11.

8. Pollard LC, Kingsley GH, Choy EH, Scott DL. Fibromyalgic rheumatoid arthritis and disease assessment. Rheumatology (Oxford). 2010;49(5):924-8.

9. McWilliams DF, Zhang W, Mansell JS, Kiely PD, Young A, Walsh DA. Predictors of change in bodily pain in early rheumatoid arthritis: an inception cohort study. Arthritis Care Res (Hoboken). 2012;64(10):1505-13.

10. McWilliams DF, Walsh DA. Factors predicting pain and early discontinuation of tumour necrosis factor-α-inhibitors in people with rheumatoid arthritis: results from the British society for Rheumatology biologics register. BMC Musculoskelet Disord. 2016; In Press

11. Kristensen LE, Bliddal H, Christensen R, Karlsson JA, Gulfe A, Saxne T, et al. Is swollen to tender joint count ratio a new and useful clinical marker for biologic drug response in rheumatoid arthritis? Results from a Swedish cohort. Arthritis Care Res (Hoboken). 2014;66(2):173-9.

12. Walsh DA, McWilliams DF. Mechanisms, impact and management of pain in rheumatoid arthritis. Nat Rev Rheumatol. 2014;10(10):581-92.

13. Hyrich KL, Watson KD, Silman AJ, Symmons DP, British Society for Rheumatology Biologics R. Predictors of response to anti-TNF-alpha therapy among patients with rheumatoid arthritis: results from the British Society for Rheumatology Biologics Register. Rheumatology (Oxford). 2006;45(12):1558-65.

14. Hyrich KL, Watson KD, Isenberg DA, Symmons DP, Register BSRB. The British society for rheumatology biologics register: 6 years on. Rheumatology (Oxford). 2008;47(10):1441-3.

15. Kiely P, Williams R, Walsh D, Young A, Early Rheumatoid Arthritis N. Contemporary patterns of care and disease activity outcome in early rheumatoid arthritis: the ERAN cohort. Rheumatology (Oxford). 2009;48(1):57-60.

16. Schwab J, Bialow M, Clemmons R, Martin P, Holzer C. The Beck depression inventory with medical inpatients. Acta Psychiatr Scand. 1967;43(3):255-66.

17. Spielberger CD, Gorssuch RL, Lushene PR, Vagg PR, Jacobs GA. Manual for the state-trait anxiety inventory. Palo Alto: Consulting Psychologists Press, Inc; 1983.

18. Krupp LB, LaRocca NG, Muir-Nash J, Steinberg AD. The fatigue severity scale. Application to patients with multiple sclerosis and systemic lupus erythematosus. Arch Neurol. 1989;46(10):1121-3.

19. Wolfe F. Pain extent and diagnosis: development and validation of the regional pain scale in 12,799 patients with rheumatic disease. J Rheumatol. 2003;30(2):369-78.

20. Wolfe F, Clauw DJ, Fitzcharles MA, Goldenberg DL, Katz RS, Mease P, et al. The American College of Rheumatology preliminary diagnostic criteria for fibromyalgia and measurement of symptom severity. Arthritis Care Res (Hoboken). 2010;62(5):600-10.

21. Gluer CC, Blake G, Lu Y, Blunt BA, Jergas M, Genant HK. Accurate assessment of precision errors: how to measure the reproducibility of bone densitometry techniques. Osteoporos Int. 1995;5(4):262-70.

22. IBM Knowledge Center. Display Statistics: IBM Corporation, USA. Available from: https://www.ibm.com/support/knowledgecenter/SS3RA7_15.0.0/com.ibm.spss.modeler.help/dataaudit_displaystatistics.htm. Accessed 12 Mar 2018.

23. McWilliams DF, Walsh DA. Factors predicting pain and early discontinuation of tumour necrosis factor-alpha-inhibitors in people with rheumatoid arthritis: results from the British society for rheumatology biologics register. BMC Musculoskelet Disord. 2016;17:337.

24. Pollard LC, Ibrahim F, Choy EH, Scott DL. Pain thresholds in rheumatoid arthritis: the effect of tender point counts and disease duration. J Rheumatol. 2012;39(1):28-31.

25. Mandl P, Balint PV, Brault Y, Backhaus M, D'Agostino MA, Grassi W, et al. Clinical and ultrasound-based composite disease activity indices in rheumatoid arthritis: results from a multicenter, randomized study. Arthritis Care Res (Hoboken). 2013;65(6):879-87.

26. Salaffi F, Carotti M, Ciapetti A, Gasparini S, Filippucci E, Grassi W. Relationship between time-integrated disease activity estimated by DAS28-CRP and radiographic progression of anatomical damage in patients with early rheumatoid arthritis. BMC Musculoskelet Disord. 2011;12:120.

27. Aletaha D, Funovits J, Keystone EC, Smolen JS. Disease activity early in the course of treatment predicts response to therapy after one year in rheumatoid arthritis patients. Arthritis Rheum. 2007;56(10):3226-35.

28. Nikiphorou E, Norton S, Young A, Carpenter L, Dixey J, Walsh DA, et al. Association between rheumatoid arthritis disease activity, progression of functional limitation and long-term risk of orthopaedic surgery: combined analysis of two prospective cohorts supports EULAR treat to target DAS thresholds. Ann Rheum Dis. 2016;75(12):2080-2086. https://doi.org/10.1136/annrheumdis-2015-208669.

29. Norton S, Fu B, Scott DL, Deighton C, Symmons DP, Wailoo AJ, et al. Health Assessment Questionnaire disability progression in early rheumatoid arthritis: systematic review and analysis of two inception cohorts. Semin Arthritis Rheum. 2014;44(2):131-44.

30. Druce KL, Jones GT, Macfarlane GJ, Basu N. Examining changes in central and peripheral pain as mediates of fatigue improvement: results from the British Society for Rheumatology Biologics Register for Rheumatoid Arthritis. Arthritis Care Res. 2016;68(7):922-6.

31. Aletaha D, Neogi T, Silman AJ, Funovits J, Felson DT, Bingham CO 3rd, et al. 2010 rheumatoid arthritis classification criteria: an American College of Rheumatology/European League Against Rheumatism collaborative initiative. Ann Rheum Dis. 2010;69(9):1580-8.

32. Smolen JS, Breedveld FC, Schiff MH, Kalden JR, Emery P, Eberl G, et al. A simplified disease activity index for rheumatoid arthritis for use in clinical practice. Rheumatology (Oxford). 2003;42(2):244-57.

33. Felson DT, Smolen JS, Wells G, Zhang B, van Tuyl LH, Funovits J, et al. American College of Rheumatology/European League against Rheumatism provisional definition of remission in rheumatoid arthritis for clinical trials. Ann Rheum Dis. 2011;70(3):404-13.

34. Rech J, Hess A, Finzel S, Kreitz S, Sergeeva M, Englbrecht M, et al. Association of brain functional magnetic resonance activity with response to tumor necrosis factor inhibition in rheumatoid arthritis. Arthritis Rheum. 2013;65(2):325-33.

35. Hess A, Axmann R, Rech J, Finzel S, Heindl C, Kreitz S, et al. Blockade of TNF-alpha rapidly inhibits pain responses in the central nervous system. Proc Natl Acad Sci U S A. 2011;108(9):3731-6.

36. Jurgens MS, Overman CL, Jacobs JW, Geenen R, Cuppen BV, Marijnissen AC, et al. Contribution of the subjective components of the disease activity score to the response to biologic treatment in rheumatoid arthritis. Arthritis Care Res. 2015;67(7):923-8.

37. Suokas AK, Walsh DA, McWilliams DF, Condon L, Moreton B, Wylde V, et al. Quantitative sensory testing in painful osteoarthritis: a systematic review and meta-analysis. Osteoarthr Cartil. 2012;20(10):1075-85.

38. Druce KL, Jones GT, Macfarlane GJ, Basu MN. Determining pathways to improvements in rheumatoid arthritis fatigue: results from the BSRBR-RA. Arthritis Rheumatol. 2015;67(9):2303-10. https://doi.org/10.1002/art.39238.

39. Odegard S, Finset A, Mowinckel P, Kvien TK, Uhlig T. Pain and psychological health status over a 10-year period in patients with recent onset rheumatoid arthritis. Ann Rheum Dis. 2007;66(9):1195-201.

40. Aletaha D, Ward MM, Machold KP, Nell VP, Stamm T, Smolen JS. Remission and active disease in rheumatoid arthritis: defining criteria for disease activity states. Arthritis Rheum. 2005;52(9):2625-36.

41. Chandrashekara S, Priyanka BU. Remission in rheumatoid arthritis by different criteria does not converge over the inflammatory markers. Int J Rheum Dis. 2013;16(3):291-6.

42. Kuriya B, Sun Y, Boire G, Haraoui B, Hitchon C, Pope JE, et al. Remission in early rheumatoid arthritis — a comparison of new ACR/EULAR remission criteria to established criteria. J Rheumatol. 2012;39(6):1155–8.

43. Kiely P, Walsh D, Williams R, Young A, Early Rheumatoid Arthritis N. Outcome in rheumatoid arthritis patients with continued conventional therapy for moderate disease activity—the early RA network (ERAN). Rheumatology (Oxford). 2011;50(5):926–31.

44. Nikiphorou E, Morris S, Dixey J, Williams PL, Kiely P, Walsh DA, et al. The effect of disease severity and comorbidity on length of stay for orthopedic surgery in rheumatoid arthritis: results from 2 UK inception cohorts, 1986–2012. J Rheumatol. 2015;42(5):778–85.

6

The underrated prevalence of depression in Japanese patients with rheumatoid arthritis

Rosarin Sruamsiri[1,2], Yuko Kaneko[3] and Jörg Mahlich[1,4*] (iD)

Abstract

Background: To determine the prevalence of depression among Japanese people with rheumatoid arthritis (RA) and explore the relationships between depression and an array of variables.

Methods: Nation-wide, cross-sectional online survey ($n = 500$) of people with RA including the Patient Health Questionnaire (PHQ-9) to measure the presence and severity of depressive symptoms were performed.

Results: While only 5% of the population studied had been officially diagnosed with depression, 35% had PHQ-9 scores indicating depression was present. People with RA are more likely to experience depression if they are younger, have greater functional impairment, or whose treatment regimen includes pain medications not biologic agents.

Conclusions: It is a potential risk of under-diagnosis and under-reporting of depression in Japanese people with RA. People with RA are more likely to experience depression if they are younger, have greater functional impairment, or whose treatment regimen includes pain medications without biologic drugs.

Keywords: Depression, Rheumatoid arthritis, Prevalence, PHQ-9

Background

Significant evidence in the scholarly literature suggests that depression is a common comorbidity among patients with rheumatoid arthritis (RA) [1–3]. The prevalence of depression varies significantly between different studies, but by some estimates occurs in as many as 42% of RA patients [4]. A meta-analysis of 72 studies involving 13,189 people with RA revealed that from 14.8 to 38.8% of people with RA receive a diagnosis of a major depressive disorder [5].

Depression in RA is a risk factor not only for suicidal ideation [6] but for cardiovascular disease [7], myocardial infarction [8], and mortality [9]. Patients with RA are at greater risk of experiencing anxiety, depression, and low self-esteem, with higher levels of associated mortality and suicide

[10]. It was suggested that nearly 11% of people with RA experience suicidal thoughts, a statistic that rises to an alarming 30% in patients with a co-morbidity of depression [11]. Previous study found that people with comorbid RA and depression may use more health services and are less likely to adhere to their medication regimens [12, 13]. A comorbidity of RA and depression is also associated with higher unemployment, work productivity losses, and increased healthcare costs to both individual patient and society [13, 14].

More often than not comorbid depression with RA is undiagnosed and therefore untreated [15] often because rheumatologists and their patients seldom communicate about depression [13, 16]. In the USA and Europe, the prevalence of depression was high in people with RA and the prevalence was found to be greater in younger patients [5]. Similar findings were found in only one Japanese study that identified factors associated with depression in female people with RA and found that among sociodemographic factors, "a decrease in the frequency of going out socially after having RA" and "a higher education" were significantly

* Correspondence: joerg.mahlich@gmail.com
[1]Health Economics, Janssen Pharmaceutical KK, 5-2, Nishi-kanda 3-chome Chiyoda-ku, Tokyo 101-0065, Japan
[4]Düsseldorf Institute for Competition Economics (DICE), University of Düsseldorf, Düsseldorf, Germany
Full list of author information is available at the end of the article

associated with depression [17]. However, evidence of depression in people with RA is limited in Asia studies and also Japan.

The present study was undertaken to determine the prevalence of depression in Japanese People with RA and explore the relationships between RA patient, depression and an array of demographic variables.

Methods

Patient population and data collection

A nationwide cross-sectional online survey was carried out in Japan during the months of July and August in 2016. The survey was national in its scope, drawing from a pool of more than 2000 people with RA. Figure 1 showed patient flow of this study. The study included 500 people with RA who had been diagnosed with RA for at least 1 year, whose current treatment scheme included at least one RA medication and completed all questionnaires.

The survey instrument contained questions about a variety of patient demographic characteristics such as age, gender, marital status, education, employment, and income. It also included questions covering clinical characteristics such as length of time since diagnosis, functional impairment as assessed using the Japanese version of the Stanford Health Assessment Questionnaire (J-HAQ score) [18], and the participant's current medical treatment scheme including whether biologic agents and conventional synthetic disease modifying anti-rheumatic drugs (conventional synthetic disease-modifying antirheumatic drugs; csDMARDs) are being used.

The Patient Health Questionnaire with 9 items (PHQ-9) was used to measure the presence and severity of depressive symptoms. The study used a Japanese language version of the PHQ-9 shown to be a valid screening tool to detect potential depression patients in Japanese hospitals [19]. In addition, the similar findings have been shown when using the PHQ-9 web-base and paper based survey [20]. The cut-off scores were defined as follows: no depression (0–4), mild (5–9), and moderate-to-severe (≥10) [21].

Statistical analysis

Descriptive statistics were used to quantify baseline characteristics and depression condition while one-way analysis of variance was used to determine differences among relevant patient groupings. Ordered logistic regression was used to identify the determinants of depression conditions among survey respondents. We also reported univariate correlation coefficients between depression conditions and all other variables to assess associations of depression condition with each factor. In the multivariate model, all factors with p values in the univariate analyses of $p < 0.2$ were included (stepwise regression). All analyses were calculated using STATA version 14.0 (College Station, TX, USA). A P value of <0.05 was considered statistically significant.

Results

Patient demographics

Data from a total of 500 patients with RA were included in the analysis. The mean age was 54.3 years old and 67% of the patients were female (Table 1).

Depression prevalence

Table 1 reveals the prevalence of depression among the 500 People with RA analyzed across a number of demographic characteristics. Overall, 176 (35%) had depressive

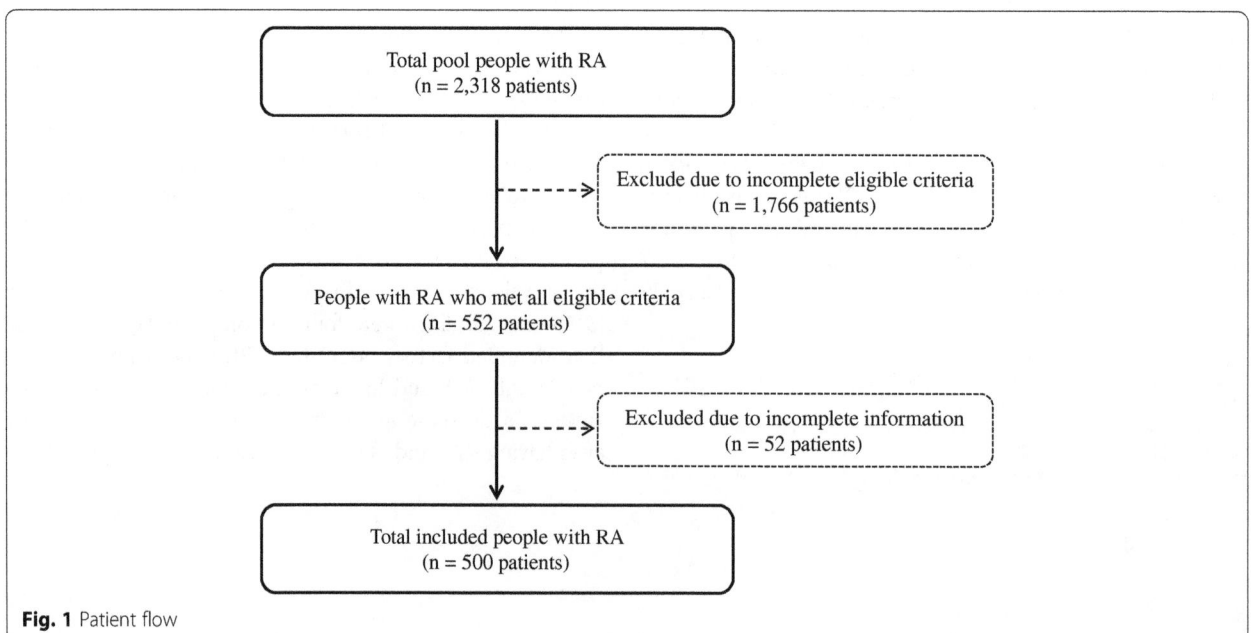

Fig. 1 Patient flow

Table 1 Depression in RA patients analyzed by demographic characteristics

Characteristics	Overall, N (%)	No depression, N (%)	Mild depression, N (%)	Moderate to severe depression, N (%)	P-value
Patients	500	324 (65)	118 (24)	58 (11)	
Age (mean ± SD)	54.28 ± 10.02	56.04 ± 9.91	51.57 ± 10.02	49.93 ± 9.59	<0.001
≤ 50 years	178 (36)	94 (29)	53 (45)	31 (54)	
51–60 years	196 (39)	130 (40)	45 (38)	21 (36)	
> 60 years	126 (25)	100 (31)	20 (17)	6 (10)	
Gender					0.036
Male	163 (33)	118 (37)	28 (24)	17 (29)	
Female	337 (67)	206 (64)	90 (76)	41 (71)	
Marital status					0.004
Single	97 (19)	49 (15)	34 (29)	14 (24)	
Married	403 (81)	275 (85)	84 (71)	44 (76)	
Highest Education					0.109
High school or less	180 (36)	107 (33)	47 (40)	26 (44)	
College	120 (24)	74 (23)	30 (25)	16 (28)	
Bachelor's degree or higher	200 (40)	143 (44)	41 (35)	16 (28)	
Occupation					0.141
Full-time	164 (33)	112 (34)	36 (30)	16 (28)	
Part-time	78 (16)	43 (13)	26 (22)	9 (15)	
Self-employed	37 (7)	28 (9)	6 (5)	3 (5)	
Housewife	141 (28)	89 (27)	33 (28)	19 (33)	
Retired	20 (4)	18 (6)	1 (1)	1 (2)	
Unemployed	57 (11)	32 (10)	16 (14)	9 (15)	
Other	3 (1)	2 (1)	0 (0)	1 (2)	
Region					
Hokkaido	26 (5)	15 (5)	4 (3)	7 (12)	0.038
Tohoku	23 (5)	17 (5)	4 (3)	2 (3)	0.645
Kanto	230 (46)	147 (45)	53 (46)	30 (52)	0.646
Chubu	63 (13)	45 (14)	10 (8)	8 (14)	0.303
Kansai	95 (19)	58 (18)	30 (25)	7 (12)	0.073
Chugoku	21 (4)	14 (4)	7 (6)	0 (0)	0.180
Shikoku	11 (2)	6 (2)	2 (2)	3 (5)	0.259
Kyushu	31 (6)	22 (7)	8 (7)	1 (2)	0.323
Annual individual income					
< 3.7 M Yen	286 (57)	173 (53)	73 (62)	40 (69)	0.272
3.7–7.7 M Yen	105 (21)	74 (23)	22 (19)	9 (15)	
> 7.7 M Yen	45 (9)	34 (11)	7 (6)	4 (7)	
I don't know	64 (13)	43 (13)	16 (13)	5 (9)	
Time since diagnosis (mean ± SD)	10.67 ± 8.63	10.45 ± 8.99	11.07 ± 8.07	11.12 ± 7.63	0.242
≤ 5 years	165 (33)	111 (34)	38 (32)	16 (28)	
6–10 years	146 (29)	101 (31)	27 (23)	18 (31)	
> 10 years	189 (38)	112 (35)	53 (45)	24 (41)	

Table 1 Depression in RA patients analyzed by demographic characteristics (Continued)

Characteristics	Overall, N (%)	No depression, N (%)	Mild depression, N (%)	Moderate to severe depression, N (%)	P-value
Current Medication					
Painkillers (NSAIDs/oral pain medication)	80 (16)	39 (12)	27 (23)	14 (24)	0.005
Steroid	110 (22)	66 (20)	29 (25)	15 (26)	0.481
DMARDs					0.112
csDMARDs	329 (66)	214 (66)	79 (67)	36 (62)	
csDMARDs + biologic agent	113 (23)	65 (20)	30 (25)	18 (31)	
Biologic agent	58 (12)	45 (14)	9 (8)	4 (7)	
Functional impairment					
J-HAQ score (mean ± SD)	0.40 ± 0.81	0.26 ± 0.55	0.52 ± 0.78	0.98 ± 1.50	<0.001
Comorbidity with depression					
Depression	25 (5)	7 (2)	6 (5)	12 (21)	<0.001
Comorbidity other than depression					
Hypertension	79 (16)	52 (16)	16 (14)	11 (19)	0.638
High cholesterol	42 (8)	24 (7)	11 (9)	7 (12)	0.458
Diabetes	26 (5)	15 (5)	10 (9)	1 (2)	0.122
Migraines	11 (2)	0 (0)	5 (4)	6 (10)	<0.001
Heart condition	8 (2)	3 (1)	2 (2)	3 (5)	0.060
Anxiety	8 (2)	3 (1)	2 (2)	3 (5)	0.060

N number, % percentage, SD standard deviation, M Million, NSAID nonsteroidal anti-inflammatory drugs, RA rheumatoid arthritis, DMARDs disease modifying anti-rheumatic drugs, csDMARDs conventional synthetic disease modifying anti-rheumatic drugs, J-HAQ Japanese version of the Stanford Health Assessment Questionnaire

symptoms, whereas only 25 (5%) had been officially diagnosed with depression or visited physicians due to depression, suggesting depression might be under-diagnosed or under-reported in people with RA.

The average age of patients with no depression based on self-report PHQ-9 assessment was 56.04 years. By comparison, the average age of patients with mild depression was 51.57 years, and that of patients with moderate to severe depression was 49.93 years, suggesting that younger people with RA are more susceptible to depression. Among people with RA, the majority of major depression patients were female and married. Comorbidity conditions, except for migraine and heart conditions (for example chronic heart failure and ischemic heart disease), were not different between patients with depression and those without.

Painkillers were taken more in patients with depression than in those without (23% vs 12%, P = 0.005). No difference was found in treatment of steroid, csDMARDs and biologic agents.

Among the 324 patients who showed no signs of depression, the average J-HAQ score was 0.26, whereas the score among those with mild depression was 0.52 and those with moderate to severe depression had an average J-HAQ score of 0.98 (P < 0.001), indicating that the greater physical disability patients experience greater depression.

Determinant of depression among people with RA

Table 2 shows the results of multivariable regression analysis for the determinants of depressive conditions among Japanese people with RA. A negative correlation with the prevalence of depression was found for age, meaning younger patients were more likely to experience depression, with a corresponding odds ratio (ORs) of 0.96 [95% confidence interval (CI); 0.94–0.98]. Higher education was also negatively correlated with depression, meaning more education resulted in less depression (ORs, 0.61 (CI 0.38–1.00) for a bachelor's degree or higher. Another negative correlation was related to the biologic agent monotherapy (ORs, 0.36 (0.17–0.75)). People with RA with high J-HAQ score also had a high probability of developing depression (ORs 1.86: CI 1.40–2.48)). In summary, people with RA more likely to experience depression are those who are younger, less educated, have greater functional impairment, and who are treated with csDMARDs alone.

Discussion

The results of this study reveal that one third of Japanese people with RA might potentially have depression as assessed by PHQ-9 while only 5% are officially diagnosed. Additionally, younger, less educated, more functionally impaired patients, and patients who are being treated with csDMARDs alone are more likely to

Table 2 Determinants of depression among RA patients

Characteristics	Univariate analysis		Multivariate analysis	
	ORs (95%CI)	P-value	ORs (95%CI)	P-value
Age	**0.95 (0.93–0.97)**	**<0.001**	**0.96 (0.94–0.98)**	**0.001**
Gender (Reference: Male)				
Female	**1.59 (1.07–2.38)**	**0.023**	0.86 (0.49–1.51)	0.599
Marital status (Reference: Single)				
Married	**0.52 (0.34–0.80)**	**0.003**	0.68 (0.40–1.17)	0.168
Highest Education (Reference: High school or less)				
College	0.91 (0.51–1.47)	0.690	0.89 (0.53–1.47)	0.639
Bachelor's degree or higher	**0.57 (0.38–0.87)**	**0.010**	**0.61 (0.38–1.00)**	**0.050**
Occupation (Reference: Full-time)				
Part-time	**1.63 (0.96–2.78)**	**0.072**	1.26 (0.68–2.35)	0.459
Self-employed	0.70 (0.31–1.58)	0.396	0.85 (0.35–2.06)	0.725
Housewife	1.28 (0.81–2.05)	0.289	1.09 (0.59–2.00)	0.781
Retired	**0.25 (0.06–1.10)**	**0.067**	0.46 (0.94–2.30)	0.348
Unemployed	**1.69 (0.93–3.08)**	**0.086**	1.14 (0.55–2.37)	0.728
Other	1.60 (0.12–19.85)	0.715	1.48 (0.08–25.86)	0.787
Region				
Hokkaido	1.71 (0.77–3.21)	0.212		
Tohoku	0.64 (0.25–1.65)	0.361		
Kanto	1.10 (0.77–1.59)	0.584		
Chubu	0.75 (0.42–1.34)	0.333		
Kansai	1.09 (0.70–1.71)	0.692		
Chugoku	0.79 (0.32–1.92)	0.600		
Shikoku	1.88 (0.57–6.19)	0.296		
Kyushu	0.68 (0.31–1.48)	0.336		
Annual individual income (Reference <3.7 M Yen)				
3.7–7.7 M Yen	**0.63 (0.39–1.01)**	**0.058**	0.78 (0.46–1.34)	0.058
> 7.7 M Yen	**0.50 (0.24–1.03)**	**0.059**	0.75 (0.31–1.79)	0.059
Time since diagnosis (Reference: ≤5 years)				
6–10 years	0.96 (0.60–1.54)	0.872	0.99 (0.59–1.65)	0.964
> 10 years	**1.40 (0.91–2.13)**	**0.124**	1.13 (0.69–1.87)	0.624
J-HAQ score	**2.01 (1.59–2.53)**	**<0.001**	**1.86 (1.40–2.48)**	**<0.001**
Comorbidity				
Hypertension	0.99 (0.60–1.64)	0.986		
High cholesterol	1.46 (0.78–2.72)	0.233		
Diabetes	1.15 (0.54–2.45)	0.716		
Migraines	**13.23 (4.29–40.81)**	**<0.001**	9.27 (0.99–32.19)	0.087
Heart condition	**3.84 (1.01–14.61)**	**0.048**	4.18 (0.95–18.30)	0.058
Anxiety	**3.84 (1.01–14.61)**	**0.048**	2.20 (0.47–10.27)	0.317
Current medication				
Pain killer (NSAIDs/oral pain medication)	**2.11 (1.34–3.34)**	**0.001**	1.60 (0.94–2.72)	0.084
Steroid	1.30 (0.85–1.98)	0.228		
DMARDs (Reference: csDMARDs)				
csDMARDs + biologic agent	**1.40 (0.92–2.15)**	**0.117**	0.82 (0.49–1.37)	0.459
Biologic agent	**0.54 (0.28–1.05)**	**0.067**	**0.36 (0.17–0.75)**	**0.007**

Bold numbers indicate significance. Univariate analysis: significant p value < 0.2, multivariate analysis (stepwise approach): significant value = 0.05. *ORs* odds ratio, *CI* confidence interval, *RA* rheumatoid arthritis, *M* Million, *NSAID* nonsteroidal anti-inflammatory drugs, *DMARDs* disease modifying anti-rheumatic drugs, *csDMARDs* conventional synthetic disease modifying anti-rheumatic drugs, *J-HAQ* Japanese version of the Stanford Health Assessment Questionnaire have depressive syptoms. These findings are important to increase awareness of rheumatologist regarding depression. Furthermore, the results call for multidisciplinary treatment teams that do not only focus on the treatment of physical symptoms but also take into account a patient's psychological condition. This approach will bring together the skills and knowledge of all team members which may may comprise case managers, pharmacists, physical and occupational therapists, social workers, physiatrists, orthopedists, or other health professionals to assess and manage care for the individual patient's needs [22].

The key finding of this study is that a potential significant under-reporting of depression among Japanese people with RA might exist. The prevalence of depression among people with RA has been reported in previous studies worldwide [5], ranging from 15% up to 39%, and our finding of 35% by PHQ-9 is consistent with those results. Severe depressive symptom (PHQ ≥ 10) was less frequent in this study (11%) than the frequency reported in Asians and Pacific Islanders reported in 2009 (36%), which might be due to the development of treatment along with less physical functional impairment. However, there was still discrepancy in the prevalence between PHQ-9 and the official diagnosis. One explanation of the under-reporting of depression might be related to Asian cultural factors. People in Asian societies such as China and Japan are less likely to speak openly about depression due to the stigma attached to it as well as the need to maintain perceived strength of character [23]. However, differences in prevalence can be found when using different measurement instruments. For example, the point prevalence of major depressive disorders in Japanese people with RA was 6.8% when using the Mini-International Neuropsychiatric Interview [24]. This observation makes it the more important for physicians and all healthcare professional who are members of multidisciplinary team in Asia to be highly attuned to potential depression when treating their people with RA.

In this study, people with comorbid RA and depression tended to be younger than people without depression. This comparison is evident as well in the national Japanese survey conducted by the Ministry of Health, Labor, and Welfare in 2014 [25] and an Japanese employee survey conducted by the Northern-Japan Occupational Health Promotion Centers Collaboration Study for Mental Health [26]. Additionally, the results of the present study showed a positive association between depression and migraine and heart condition comorbidities. Several studies reported the relationship of depression with cardiovascular disease [27, 28], which is well known to be correlated with RA [29, 30].

Several studies show a positive correlation between depression and RA disease activity scores such as disease activity score for 28-joint (DAS28) or clinical disease activity

index (CDAI) [31, 32]. Although the current study did not measure disease severity by such composite measures due to the limitations of online survey, people with RA were asked to rate their functional disability using J-HAQ [18], which closely correlates to both DAS28 and CDAI [33]. The results indicate that a higher J-HAQ score was correlated with depression. J-HAQ can measure a variety of functional limitations caused not only by inflammatory disease activity but also by joint damage and long-term disability. The resulting loss of valued activities has been shown to be a strong predictor of depression in patients with RA [13, 34]. Additionally, systemic inflammation that also causes functional disability is associated with, causes, or contributes to depressive symptoms experienced during the course of disorders that include chronic inflammation [35]. Patients with major depression have increased Interleukin 6 (IL-6) [36]. concentrations and pro-inflammatory tumor necrosis factor-alpha (TNF-α) [37] in serum, plasma, or both. A recent meta-analysis showed raised inflammatory markers such as IL-6 or C-reactive protein (CRP) are significantly associated with the subsequent development of depressive symptoms, which supports the hypothesis that there is an association between the inflammation and depression [38]. Consequently, medications that result in lower IL-6 and TNF-α level might have a direct positive impact on treating depression. Our findings also showed that patients receiving biologic agents had lower probability of developing depression compared to patients treated with csDMARDs alone, which can also be explained by the mechanism of the reduction of cytokine level that might be linked to depression [38–40]. These findings suggest that further research on the connection between biologic treatment and depression is needed.

There were several limitations to the present study. First, the analysis was based on a cross-sectional survey. As this was a single sample, the study was unable to demonstrate a causal relationship or account for changes in perception that might occur over time. Second, the study did not show that the documented depression condition was the direct consequence of the patient's RA condition – other factors in patients' lives could be the cause. Third, the exact disease activity was not completely known because this was an online survey consisting of patients reports. This hampered the analysis for the direct relationship between disease activity and depression. Furthermore, this was an online survey which might not be representative of the overall Japanese RA population. Usually, people that are more familiar with the Internet take part in online surveys which are in turn younger and probably better educated. On the other hand, the average age of our sample (54.28 years) does not differ much from a recent Japanese claims database analysis with more than 16,000 RA patients [41]. In that study the average patient age was 53.96 years which makes us believe that the potential selection bias in our sample is low. Last, there is a possibility of diagnostic over-shadowing if some physical symptoms of RA are misattributed to depression. An example is feeling tired or having little energy which are both symptoms of depression as well as RA. This can potentially lead to an overestimation of depression in RA.

Conclusions

In conclusion, the results of this study suggest that depression among Japanese people with RA is potentially under-reported and under-diagnosed. Rheumatologists should take particular care in assessing the psychological status of people with RA, particularly those susceptible to depression –younger patients, patients with greater functional impairment, and patients with a treatment regimen of csDMARDs alone.

Abbreviations

CDAI: Clinical disease activity index; CI: Confidence interval; CRP: C-reactive protein; csDMARDs: Conventional synthetic disease modifying anti-rheumatic drugs; DAS28: Disease activity score for 28-joint; DMARDs: Disease modifying anti-rheumatic drugs; IL-6: Interleukin 6; J-HAQ: Japanese version of the Stanford Health Assessment Questionnaire; ORs: Odds ratio; PHQ-9: The Patient Health Questionnaire with 9 items; RA: Rheumatoid arthritis; TNF-α: Tumor necrosis factor-alpha

Acknowledgements

We would like to thank Medilead, Inc. to identify patients and also collected all questionnaires.
We wish to thank those who reviewed the manuscript for their constructive comments (Additional file 1).

Funding

We received funding from Janssen pharmaceutical KK to conduct the survey. The study design, data collection, data analysis, data interpretation, and writing of the report, was solely done by the authors. The findings and conclusions in this report do not necessarily reflect the views of Janssen Pharmaceutical KK.

Authors' contributions

JM, YK and RS made substantial contributions to conception and design, and interpretation of data; RS performed the analysis; JM was drafting the manuscript; JM, YK and RS discussed for critical important intellectual content; JM has given final approval of the version to be published. All authors read and approved the final manuscript.

Competing interests

JM and RS are employed at Janssen Pharmaceutical KK, YK has received lecture fees from AbbVie, Eisai Pharmaceutical, Chugai Pharmaceutical, Bristol Myers Squibb, Astellas Pharmaceutical, Mitsubishi Tanabe Pharma Corporation, Pfizer, Janssen, and UCB.

Author details

[1]Health Economics, Janssen Pharmaceutical KK, 5-2, Nishi-kanda 3-chome Chiyoda-ku, Tokyo 101-0065, Japan. [2]Center of Pharmaceutical Outcomes Research, Naresuan University, Phitsanulok, Thailand. [3]Division of Rheumatology, Department of Internal Medicine, Keio University School of Medicine, Tokyo, Japan. [4]Düsseldorf Institute for Competition Economics (DICE), University of Düsseldorf, Düsseldorf, Germany.

References

1. Dickens C, McGowan L, Clark-Carter D, Creed F. Depression in rheumatoid arthritis: a systematic review of the literature with meta-analysis. Psychosom Med. 2002;64(1):52–60.
2. Löwe B, Willand L, Eich W, Zipfel S, Ho AD, Herzog W, Fiehn C. Psychiatric comorbidity and work disability in patients with inflammatory rheumatic diseases. Psychosom Med. 2004;66(3):395–402.
3. Isik A, Koca SS, Ozturk A, Mermi O. Anxiety and depression in patients with rheumatoid arthritis. Clin Rheumatol. 2007;26(6):872–8.
4. Bruce TO. Comorbid depression in rheumatoid arthritis: pathophysiology and clinical implications. Curr Psychiatry Rep. 2008;10(3):258–64.
5. Matcham F, Rayner L, Steer S, Hotopf M. The prevalence of depression in rheumatoid arthritis: a systematic review and meta-analysis. Rheumatology (Oxford). 2013;52(12):2136–48.
6. Tektonidou MG, Dasgupta A, Ward MM. Suicidal ideation among adults with arthritis: prevalence and subgroups at highest risk. Data from the 2007–2008 National Health and nutrition examination survey. Arthritis Care Res. 2011;63(9):1322–33.
7. Treharne GJ, Hale ED, Lyons AC, Booth DA, Banks MJ, Erb N, Douglas KM, Mitton DL, Kitas GD. Cardiovascular disease and psychological morbidity among rheumatoid arthritis patients. Rheumatology (Oxford). 2005;44(2):241–6.
8. Scherrer JF, Virgo KS, Zeringue A, Bucholz KK, Jacob T, Johnson RG, True WR, Carney RM, Freedland KE, Xian H, et al. Depression increases risk of incident myocardial infarction among veterans administration patients with rheumatoid arthritis. Gen Hosp Psychiatry. 2009;31(4):353–9.
9. Ang DC, Choi H, Kroenke K, Wolfe F. Comorbid depression is an independent risk factor for mortality in patients with rheumatoid arthritis. J Rheumatol. 2005;32(6):1013–9.
10. Gettings L. Psychological well-being in rheumatoid arthritis: a review of the literature. Musculoskeletal Care. 2010;8(2):99–106.
11. Treharne GJ, Lyons AC, Kitas GD. Suicidal ideation in patients with rheumatoid arthritis. Research may help identify patients at high risk. BMJ. 2000;321(7271):1290.
12. Mattey DL, Dawes PT, Hassell AB, Brownfield A, Packham JC. Effect of psychological distress on continuation of anti-tumor necrosis factor therapy in patients with rheumatoid arthritis. J Rheumatol. 2010;37(10):2021–4.
13. Margaretten M, Julian L, Katz P, Yelin E. Depression in patients with rheumatoid arthritis: description, causes and mechanisms. Int J Clin Rheumtol. 2011;6(6):617–23.
14. Li X, Gignac MA, Anis AH. The indirect costs of arthritis resulting from unemployment, reduced performance, and occupational changes while at work. Med Care. 2006;44(4):304–10.
15. Nagyova I, Stewart RE, Macejova Z, van Dijk JP, van den Heuvel WJ. The impact of pain on psychological well-being in rheumatoid arthritis: the mediating effects of self-esteem and adjustment to disease. Patient Educ Couns. 2005;58(1):55–62.
16. Sleath B, Chewning B, de Vellis BM, Weinberger M, de Vellis RF, Tudor G, Beard A. Communication about depression during rheumatoid arthritis patient visits. Arthritis Rheum. 2008;59(2):186–91.
17. Takeda T, Morimoto N, Kinukawa N, Nagamine R, Shutou T, Tashiro N. Factors affecting depression and anxiety in female Japanese patients with rheumatoid arthritis. Clin Exp Rheumatol. 2000;18(6):735–8.
18. Matsuda Y, Singh G, Yamanaka H, Tanaka E, Urano W, Taniguchi A, Saito T, Hara M, Tomatsu T, Kamatani N. Validation of a Japanese version of the Stanford health assessment questionnaire in 3,763 patients with rheumatoid arthritis. Arthritis Rheum. 2003;49(6):784–8.
19. Suzuki K, Kumei S, Ohhira M, Nozu T, Okumura T. Screening for major depressive disorder with the patient health questionnaire (PHQ-9 and PHQ-2) in an outpatient clinic staffed by primary care physicians in Japan: a case control study. PLoS One. 2015;10(3):e0119147.
20. Bot AGJ, Menendez ME, Neuhaus V, Mudgal CS, Ring D. The comparison of paper- and web-based questionnaires in patients with hand and upper extremity illness. Hand (N Y). 2013;8(2):210–4.
21. Saijo Y, Chiba S, Yoshioka E, Kawanishi Y, Nakagi Y, Itoh T, Sugioka Y, Kitaoka-Higashiguchi K, Yoshida T. Effects of work burden, job strain and support on depressive symptoms and burnout among Japanese physicians. Int J Occup Med Environ Health. 2014;27(6):980–92.
22. Marion CE, Balfe LM. Potential advantages of Interprofessional Care in Rheumatoid Arthritis. J Manag Care Pharm. 2011;17(9 Suppl B):S25–9.
23. Margaretten M, Yelin E, Imboden J, Graf J, Barton J, Katz P, Julian L.

Predictors of depression in a multiethnic cohort of patients with rheumatoid arthritis. Arthritis Rheum. 2009;61(11):1586–91.

22. Marion CE, Balfe LM. Potential advantages of Interprofessional Care in Rheumatoid Arthritis. J Manag Care Pharm. 2011;17(9 Suppl B):S25–9.

23. Margaretten M, Yelin E, Imboden J, Graf J, Barton J, Katz P, Julian L. Predictors of depression in a multiethnic cohort of patients with rheumatoid arthritis. Arthritis Rheum. 2009;61(11):1586–91.

24. Sato E, Nishimura K, Nakajima A, Okamoto H, Shinozaki M, Inoue E, Taniguchi A, Momohara S, Yamanaka H. Major depressive disorder in patients with rheumatoid arthritis. Mod Rheumatol. 2013;23(2):237–44.

25. Statistics and Information Department Minister's Secretariat Ministry of Health Labour and Welfare. Patient survey 2014. Tokyo: Health and Welfare Statistics Association; 2016.

26. Fushimi M. Prevalence of depressive symptoms and related factors in Japanese employees: a comparative study between surveys from 2007 and 2010. Psychiatry J. 2015;2015(Article ID 537073):7.

27. Hare DL, Toukhsati SR, Johansson P, Jaarsma T. Depression and cardiovascular disease: a clinical review. Eur Heart J. 2014;35(21):1365–72.

28. Watson K, Summers KM. Depression in patients with heart failure: clinical implications and management. Pharmacotherapy. 2009;29(1):49–63.

29. Liu YL, Szklo M, Davidson KW, Bathon JM, Giles JT. Differential Association of Psychosocial Comorbidities with Subclinical Atherosclerosis in rheumatoid arthritis. Arthritis Care Res (Hoboken). 2015;67(10):1335–44.

30. Kaplan MJ. Cardiovascular complications of rheumatoid arthritis - assessment, prevention and treatment. Rheum Dis Clin N Am. 2010;36(2):405–26.

31. Kekow J, Moots R, Khandker R, Melin J, Freundlich B, Singh A. Improvements in patient reported outcomes, symptoms of depression and anxiety, and their association with clinical remission among patients with moderate-to-severe active early rheumatoid arthritis. Rheumatology (Oxford). 2011;50(2):401–9.

32. Lee YC, Frits ML, Iannaccone CK, Weinblatt ME, Shadick NA, Williams DA, Cui J: Subgrouping of rheumatoid arthritis patients based on pain, fatigue, inflammation and psychosocial factors. Arthritis & rheumatology. Arthritis Rheumatol. 2014, 66(8):2006-2014.

33. Salaffi F, Cimmino MA, Leardini G, Gasparini S, Grassi W. Disease activity assessment of rheumatoid arthritis in daily practice: validity, internal consistency, reliability and congruency of the disease activity score including 28 joints (DAS28) compared with the Clinical Disease Activity Index (CDAI). Clin Exp Rheumatol. 2009;27(4):552–9.

34. Covic T, Adamson B, Spencer D, Howe G. A biopsychosocial model of pain and depression in rheumatoid arthritis: a 12-month longitudinal study. Rheumatology (Oxford). 2003;42(11):1287–94.

35. Miller AH, Maletic V, Raison CL. Inflammation and its discontents: the role of cytokines in the pathophysiology of major depression. Biol Psychiatry. 2009;65(9):732–41.

36. Alesci S, Martinez PE, Kelkar S, Ilias I, Ronsaville DS, Listwak SJ, Ayala AR, Licinio J, Gold HK, Kling MA, et al. Major depression is associated with significant diurnal elevations in plasma interleukin-6 levels, a shift of its circadian rhythm, and loss of physiological complexity in its secretion: clinical implications. J Clin Endocrinol Metab. 2005;90(5):2522–30.

37. Kahl KG, Greggersen W, Rudolf S, Stoeckelhuber BM, Bergmann-Koester CU, Dibbelt L, Schweiger U. Bone mineral density, bone turnover, and osteoprotegerin in depressed women with and without borderline personality disorder. Psychosom Med. 2006;68:669–74.

38. Valkanova V, Ebmeier KP, Allan CL. CRP, IL-6 and depression: a systematic review and meta-analysis of longitudinal studies. J Affect Disord. 2013; 150(3):736–44.

39. Wang D, Sun Y, Salvadore G, Singh J, Hsu B, Curran M, Caers I, Kent J, Drevets WC, Wittenberg GM, et al. P.2.h.016 Interleukin-6 antibody Sirukumab improves depressive symptoms in a randomized, placebo-controlled, phase 2 study in patients with rheumatoid arthritis. Eur Neuropsychopharmacol. 2015;25(Supplement 2):S462.

40. Yarlagadda A, Alfson E, Clayton AH. The blood brain barrier and the role of cytokines in neuropsychiatry. Psychiatry (Edgmont). 2009;6(11):18–22.

41. Mahlich J, Sruamsiri R. Treatment patterns of rheumatoid arthritis in Japanese hospitals and predictors of the initiation of biologic agents. Curr Med Res Opin. 2017;3(1):101–7.

7

An evaluation of gout visits in the United States for the years 2007 to 2011

Kristen E. Castro, Kaitlyn D. Corey, Diana L. Raymond, Michael R. Jiroutek* and Melissa A. Holland

Abstract

Background: This study analyzed visits for and factors associated with gout and gout medication treatment trends for the years 2007–2011 in the United States given the introduction of febuxostat, the first new treatment option for gout in over 40 years, which was introduced to the market in 2009.

Methods: This study was a retrospective, cross-sectional, observational study of patients age 20 and older seen by providers who participated in the National Ambulatory Medical Care Survey (NAMCS), the National Hospital Ambulatory Medical Care Survey Outpatient Department (NHAMCS-OPD) or Emergency Department (NHAMCS-ED) in the United States. The outcome of interest was visits for gout diagnosis and visits where a gout medication was prescribed.

Results: Approximately 1.2% of visits had a diagnosis of gout. There was a significant increase in the percentage of visits with a diagnosis of gout in years 2009–2011 compared to 2007–2008, which remained after adjusting for covariates of interest. Groups more likely to have a visit with gout included those ≥65 and 45–64 (both as compared to those 20–44), the African-American and 'Other' race groups (as compared to Caucasians) and those on a diuretic. Groups less likely to have a visit with gout included females, Hispanic/Latinos, those with insurance type of 'Other' and Medicaid (both as compared to private insurance) and visits to a hospital emergency setting (as compared to physician's office visits).

Conclusion: Although there was a significant increase in visits where gout is diagnosed across study years, the overall percentage of visits with a gout diagnosis is low in the US population. Treatment trends over the study years has remained consistent, with the introduction of febuxostat appearing to have little impact for the study years through 2011.

Keywords: Gout, Febuxostat, NAMCS, NHAMCS-OPD, NHAMCS-ED

Background

Gout is a type of inflammatory arthritis associated with the formation of urate crystals in the joints. It is estimated that approximately 4% of Americans are affected, but previous research has shown the prevalence of gout is increasing [1]. Contributing factors to gout include increase in obesity, hypertension, and purine-rich diets [2]. The severity and progression of gout has been directly correlated to an increase in age. [3] Gout is known to be more predominant in males, but is seen in postmenopausal women. The prevalence of gout is higher in African Americans as compared to Caucasians, with increasing prevalence overall across all demographics [3]. Prior to 2009, pharmacological treatment options for gout had not changed in many years. A new treatment option, febuxostat, was approved by the Food and Drug Administration in February 2009 [4].

No studies have evaluated the proportion of visits with a gout diagnosis since 2009 when febuxostat was introduced to the market. Previous studies have shown that an above normal BMI, hypertension, dyslipidemia, use of a diuretic and older age are associated with an increased risk of gout [5–10].

With the first new gout therapy in over 40 years introduced to the market in 2009, this study sought to evaluate changes in gout-related ambulatory and emergency department visits for the years 2007 through 2011 (the

* Correspondence: jiroutekm@campbell.edu
Campbell University College of Pharmacy & Health Sciences, 180 Main Street PO Box 1090, Buies Creek, NC 27506, USA

most recent data available) as well as assess factors associated with gout [11]. Additionally, gout treatment trends were plotted to determine the impact of febuxostat on gout therapy since its introduction to the market.

Methods

This retrospective, cross-sectional, observational study analyzed data collected in the National Ambulatory Medical Care Survey (NAMCS) and the National Hospital Ambulatory Medical Care Survey Outpatient Department & Emergency Department (NHAMCS-OPD/NHAMCS-ED) during the years 2007–2011. Hundreds of reports, manuscripts and books based on data from these widely utilized and respected surveys have been published since the 1970s (https://www.cdc.gov/nchs/data/ahcd/namcs_nhamcs_publication_list.pdf).

The NHAMCS is an annual, national probability sample of ambulatory visits made to non-federal, general, and short-stay hospitals in the US conducted by the Centers for Disease Control and Prevention, National Center for Health Statistics (NCHS). The multi-staged sampling design is composed of four stages and includes visits to both selected emergency care departments as well as hospital outpatient departments [12–14]. The NAMCS is an annual, national probability sample of visits made to the offices of non-federally employed physicians classified by the American Medical Association or the American Osteopathic Association as "office-based, patient care" (excluding anesthesiologists, pathologists and radiologists) [12–14]. For more information regarding the survey instruments, scope and sample design, data collection and processing, estimation procedures and reliability of survey estimates, go to http://www.cdc.gov/nchs/ahcd/ahcd_questionnaires.htm.

NAMCS, NHAMCS-OPD and NHAMCS-ED datasets covering five years (2007–2011) were included in this study. Patients 20 or older from any of the three databases were coded as included in the final analysis dataset. There were no exclusions for the study. Across all five years a total of 128,734 raw records in the NHAMCS-OPD, 126,836 raw records in the NHAMCS-ED and 126,651 in the NAMCS databases met the inclusion criteria (382,221 combined). The study was submitted to the Campbell University Institutional Review Board and received an exemption due to the data sources used being publicly available and de-identified. As such, since this research was based solely on the analysis of previously collected, de-identified data, it complies with the Helsinki Declaration.

The survey data were analyzed using the sampled visit weight that is the product of the corresponding sampling fractions at each stage in the sample design. The sampling weights have been adjusted by NCHS for survey nonresponse as appropriate within each database,

yielding unbiased national annual estimates of visit occurrences, percentages, and characteristics [12].

Because of the complex sample design, sampling errors were determined using the SAS SURVEYFREQ and SURVEYLOGISTIC procedures which take into account the clustered nature of the sample [15]. The appropriate NOMCAR and DOMAIN statements/options were implemented in these procedures as recommended by the NCHS [12].

The dependent variable of interest was a diagnosis of gout, where the denominator is the number of visits meeting the inclusion/exclusion criteria. A diagnosis of gout was defined by the appropriate diagnosis codes found in any of the DIAG1-DIAG3 diagnosis fields or appropriate gout medication codes for allopurinol, febuxostat, colchicine, probenecid, and colchicine-probenecid found in any of the DRUGID1-DRUGID8 medication fields.

Rao-Scott chi-square tests were used to analyze whether the proportion of visits with a diagnosis of gout differs by year group (2007–2008 vs. 2009–2011) and whether any association exists between visits with a diagnosis of gout and each of the following variables: age, sex, race, ethnicity, region (US geographic regions included Northeast, Midwest, South, and West), metropolitan statistical area (MSA), insurance status (private, Medicaid or Children's Health Insurance Program [CHIP]/State Children's Health Insurance Program [SCHIP], Medicare, and other [worker's compensation, self-pay, no charge/charity, other], setting type (physician office, hospital outpatient department, hospital emergency department) and diuretic use. These variables were grouped for analysis as shown in Table 1. Odds ratios (ORs), corresponding 95% confidence intervals (CIs) and p-values were reported.

A multivariable logistic regression model was also constructed in order to evaluate the predictive value of all the independent variables of interest simultaneously on visits with a diagnosis of gout, adjusting for covariates of interest. As a primary model filter, only variables with an overall chi-square test of association p-value < 0.2 were included in the multivariable model (year group was included regardless). ORs with corresponding 95% CIs and p-values for each level of each variable included in the model (in comparison to each variable's reference group) were reported. No collinearity issues between the independent variables included in the model were found. All analyses were generated using SAS software, version 9.3. Plots of the percentage of visits per year with gout medication by drug class and individual drug were constructed to descriptively assess gout treatment trends.

Per NCHS recommendations, any variable with a survey estimate based on either less than 30 records, a

Table 1 Demographics and Patient Characteristics (N = 382,221)[a]

Characteristic	No. (%) of Patient Visits[b]
Observation Period	
2009–2011	588,791,594 (61)
2007–2008	375,839,802 (39)
Age (years)	
Mean (SE)	53.9 (0.23)
Age Group	
≥65	299,032,423 (31)
45–64	351,209,142 (36)
20–44	314,389,831 (33)
Sex	
Female	587,394,025 (61)
Male	377,237,371 (39)
Race	
Other	33,516,436 (5)
African-American	99,604,070 (14)
Caucasian	602,374,076 (82)
Ethnicity	
Hispanic/Latino	79,262,491 (11)
Non-Hispanic/Latino	630,345,157 (89)
Region	
Northeast	189,690,837 (20)
Midwest	206,775,296 (21)
West	201,670,759 (21)
South	366,494,504 (38)
MSA	
Non-MSA	120,846,147 (13)
MSA	843,785,249 (87)
Insurance Status	
Other	98,736,670 (11)
Medicaid	88,374,398 (10)
Medicare	280,902,288 (30)
Private Insurance	461,730,141 (49)
Setting Type	
Hospital Emergency	94,712,528 (10)
Hospital Outpatient	78,137,131 (8)
Physician's Office	791,781,738 (82)
Diuretic Use	
Yes	71,243,249 (7)
No	893,388,147 (93)
Gout	
Yes	11,769,697 (1)
No	952,861,700 (99)

MSA Metropolitan Statistical Area
[a]Unweighted, raw study sample size
[b]Survey weighting and clusters accounted for reflecting unbiased, national annual estimates of visit occurrences for the portion of the population meeting the study inclusion/exclusion criteria

relative standard error of more than 30%, or more than 30% missing data was excluded from the analyses due to potential unreliability [12]. As a result, the variables of interest weight status, tobacco use, depression, hypertension, and diabetes were excluded from all analyses due to not meeting one or more of the above listed criteria. Missing values were treated as missing in the statistical evaluation. No adjustments for multiple comparisons were made and p-values < 0.05 were considered statistically significant.

Results

During the study period (2007–2011), the NAMCS, NHAMCS-OPD, and NHAMCS-ED datasets include a total of 495,370 patient visits (unweighted, raw data). A total of 382,221 patient visits within this five-year period met the inclusion criteria and were included in this study (Table 1). Most variables had no missing data, however, ethnicity, race and insurance status were missing 21, 16 and 5%, respectively. Gout was diagnosed in just over 1.2% of all patient visits. More patient visits occurred during the more recent half of the study period (61% in the years 2009–2010). The mean age (SE) was 53.9 (0.23) years, with a similar percentage of patients in each of the three age groups. Of the patient visits included in the analyses, 61% were female, 82% were Caucasian, 14% were African-American, and 11% were Hispanic/Latino. Nearly twice as many visits occurred in the South (38%) as compared to the other regions (21% in the Midwest, 21% in the West and 20% in the Northeast). However, visits in metropolitan areas represented 87% of the study total. Private insurance was presented at the majority of all patient visits (50%), with Medicare presented at 30% of visits and Medicaid at 10%. The vast majority of visits occurred in a physician's office (82%), reflecting the NAMCS survey data (collected in physician offices). Only 7% of patient visits reported diuretic use.

The primary analysis showed a 30% relative increase in the percentage of patients who had a visit with a diagnosis of gout in the years 2009–2011 compared to 2007–2008 (1.3% vs. 1.0%, respectively; OR 1.28, 95% CI 1.10–1.49) (Table 2). The individual chi-square tests of the other covariates of interest that comprised the first part of the secondary analysis, showed a significant association between visits with a diagnosis of gout and the following variables: age, sex, ethnicity, race group, insurance status, setting type, region and diuretic use. See the univariable columns in Table 2 for the details of these individual associations with visits for a diagnosis of gout.

The weighted multivariable logistic regression model, allowing adjustment for the effect of potentially

Table 2 Gout Predictor Variables, Univariable and Multivariable Analyses* Data are given as number (%) of patients

Parameter	Gout (%)	No Gout (%)	Univariable		Multivariable	
			OR (95% CI)	P	OR (95% CI)	P
Observation Period						
2009–2011	7,849,421 (1.3)	580,942,174 (98.7)	1.28 (1.10–1.49)	0.0010	1.24 (1.02–1.52)	0.0346
2007–2008	3,920,276 (1.0)	371,919,526 (99.0)	Referent	–	Referent	–
Age Group (years)						
≥ 65	7,113,034 (2.4)	291,919,369 (97.6)	8.64 (7.04–10.60)	< 0.0001	4.94 (3.69–6.62)	< 0.0001
45–64	3,772,290 (1.1)	347,436,851 (98.9)	3.85 (3.11–4.77)	< 0.0001	2.52 (1.97–3.21)	< 0.0001
20–44	884,372 (0.3)	313,505,459 (99.7)	Referent	–	Referent	–
Sex						
Female	3,055,558 (0.5)	584,338,467 (99.5)	0.22 (0.20–0.25)	< 0.0001	0.20 (0.18–0.24)	< 0.0001
Male	8,714,139 (2.3)	368,523,233 (97.7)	Referent	–	Referent	–
Race						
Other	574,306 (1.7)	32,942,130 (98.3)	1.43 (1.03–1.99)	0.0332	2.02 (1.47–2.77)	< 0.0001
African-American	1,226,437 (1.2)	98,377,632 (98.8)	1.02 (0.82–1.27)	0.8513	1.33 (1.03–1.72)	0.0271
Caucasian	7,264,368 (1.2)	595,109,707 (98.8)	Referent	–	Referent	–
Ethnicity						
Hispanic/Latino	511,614 (0.6)	78,750,878 (99.4)	0.49 (0.36–0.67)	< 0.0001	0.64 (0.48–0.86)	0.0032
Non-Hispanic/Latino	8,252,946 (1.3)	622,092,211 (98.7)	Referent	–	Referent	–
Region						
Northeast	2,019,734 (1.1)	187,761,102 (98.9)	0.90 (0.72–1.13)	0.3629	0.80 (0.62–1.03)	0.0823
Midwest	3,053,963 (1.5)	203,721,333 (98.5)	1.25 (1.04–1.52)	0.0169	1.16 (0.95–1.43)	0.1501
West	2,367,739 (1.2)	199,303,020 (98.8)	0.99 (0.80–1.24)	0.9580	0.86 (0.67–1.10)	0.2296
South	4,328,261 (1.2)	362,166,243 (98.8)	Referent	–	Referent	–
MSA						
Non-MSA	1,709,090 (1.4)	119,137,057 (98.6)	1.18 (0.93–1.52)	0.1636	1.01 (0.77–1.32)	0.9462
MSA	10,060,607 (1.2)	833,724,642 (98.8)	Referent	–	Referent	–
Insurance Status						
Other	407,967 (0.4)	98,328,703 (99.6)	0.43 (0.32–0.58)	< 0.0001	0.51 (0.36–0.72)	0.0001
Medicaid	407,549 (0.5)	87,966,848 (99.5)	0.48 (0.35–0.66)	< 0.0001	0.56 (0.39–0.80)	0.0014
Medicare	6,193,910 (2.2)	274,708,378 (97.8)	2.35 (2.07–2.68)	< 0.0001	0.93 (0.74–1.15)	0.4846
Private Insurance	4,382,477 (0.9)	457,347,665 (99.1)	Referent	–	Referent	–
Setting Type						
Hospital Emergency	353,199 (0.4)	94,359,329 (99.6)	0.28 (0.23–0.33)	< 0.0001	0.42 (0.34–0.51)	< 0.0001
Hospital Outpatient	892,347 (1.1)	77,244,784 (98.9)	0.86 (0.71–1.03)	0.0994	1.05 (0.88–1.26)	0.5718
Physician Office	10,524,151 (1.3)	781,257,587 (98.7)	Referent	–	Referent	–
Diuretic Use						
Yes	3,575,442 (5.0)	67,667,807 (95.0)	5.71 (5.04–6.47)	< 0.0001	4.00 (3.37–4.75)	< 0.0001
No	8,194,254 (0.9)	885,193,893 (99.1)	Referent	–	Referent	–

MSA Metropolitan Statistical Area

* Survey weighting and clusters accounted for reflecting unbiased, national annual estimates of visit occurrences for the portion of the population meeting the study inclusion/exclusion criteria

Note that per the model fitting criterion described in the methods section, no variables were excluded from the multivariable model

important variables, demonstrated that significant associations remained between visits with a gout diagnosis and age group (≥65 and 45–64 vs. 20–44), sex, ethnicity, race group ('Other' vs. Caucasian as well as now African-American vs. Caucasian), insurance status (Other and Medicaid vs. private insurance, but no longer

Medicare vs. private insurance), hospital emergency departments (vs. physician office visits) and diuretic use. However, the associations between visits with a gout diagnosis and region[1] of the country and as well as gout visits and Medicare (vs. private insurance) did not remain significant following adjustment for the effect of the other covariates of interest in the model. A diagnosis of gout remained more likely for patient visits in 2009–2011 as compared to visits in 2007–2008 (OR 1.24, 95% CI 1.02–1.52). Additionally, a diagnosis of gout remained more likely for visits with patients 65 and older and patients 45–64 as compare to visits for those 20–44 (OR 4. 94, 95% CI 3.69–6.62 and OR 2.52, 95% CI 1.97–3.21, respectively). Gout was less likely to be diagnosed at visits for females as compared to males (OR 0.20, 95% CI 0.18–0.24) and Hispanic/Latino patients as compared to Non-Hispanic/Latino patients (OR 0.64, 95% CI 0.48–0.86), while gout was more likely to be diagnosed at visits for those on a diuretic as compared to those not on a diuretic (OR 4.00, 95% CI 3.37–4.75). Gout was less likely to be diagnosed at patient visits with an insurance status of "Other" and Medicaid as compared to those with private insurance (OR 0.51, 95% CI 0.36–0.72 and OR 0.56, 95% CI 0.39–0.80, respectively). Patients whose visit was recorded in an emergency department were less likely (OR 0.42, 95% CI 0.34–0.51) to be diagnosed with gout as compared to those with a physician's office visit (Table 2). Second order interaction terms were investigated, found to contribute nothing significant to the understanding of the overall results and were excluded from the final reported model.

Finally, plots of the percentage of patient visits with gout by year for medication class and individual drug showing the most common gout treatments can be seen in Figs. 1 and 2. The percent of gout visits in each drug class appears similar across the years studied. Antigout (80–86%) and antihyperuricemic (67–75%) medications were consistently the most common treatment while NSAIDs (14–20%) and steroids (6–12%) were a distant third and fourth, respectively.

Among individual medications, allopurinol (67–74%) is clearly the most common, three to four times as likely as the next closest (colchicine). Febuxostat, probenecid and colchicine-probenecid were infrequently prescribed (all less than 5%). Allopurinol and colchicine dominate the market, their use appears consistent across the years studied, while probenecid's use has decreased over time. Uptake does appear to be slow for febuxostat, the newest gout medication, as two years after entering the market, the percentage of patients with gout taking the drug remains around 3%.

Discussion

The proportion of patient visits with a diagnosis of gout increased between 2007 and 2011, and this increase was significant. It is hypothesized that gout visits are on the rise due to increases in obesity, hypertension, and purine-rich diets [1, 2]. Obesity increases the production of serum urate (sUA) levels and also decreases urate excretion while weight reduction has been associated with uric acid level declination [16]. Along with risk factors, there are many disease associations with gout including metabolic syndrome, hypertension, and cardiovascular disease [16]. Metabolic syndrome has been strongly associated with gout; 60% of US population with gout also has metabolic syndrome, a prevalence three times higher in those with gout [17]. Metabolic syndrome has likely

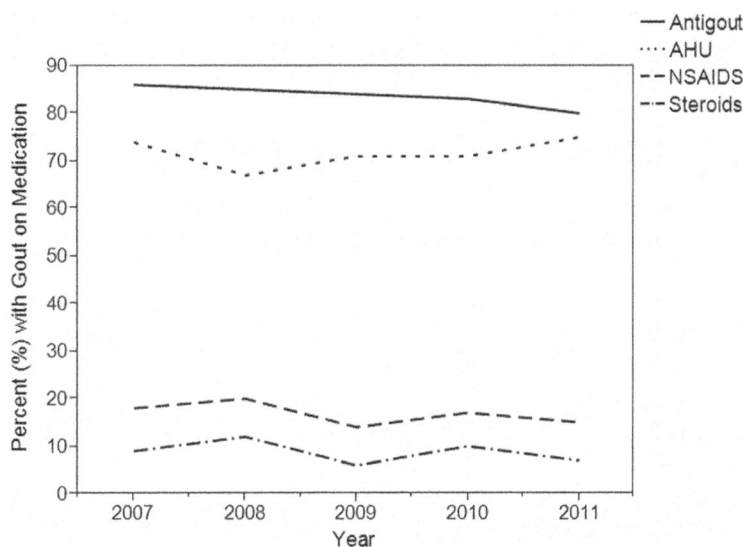

Fig. 1 Gout Prescription Trends by Drug Class, 2007–2011

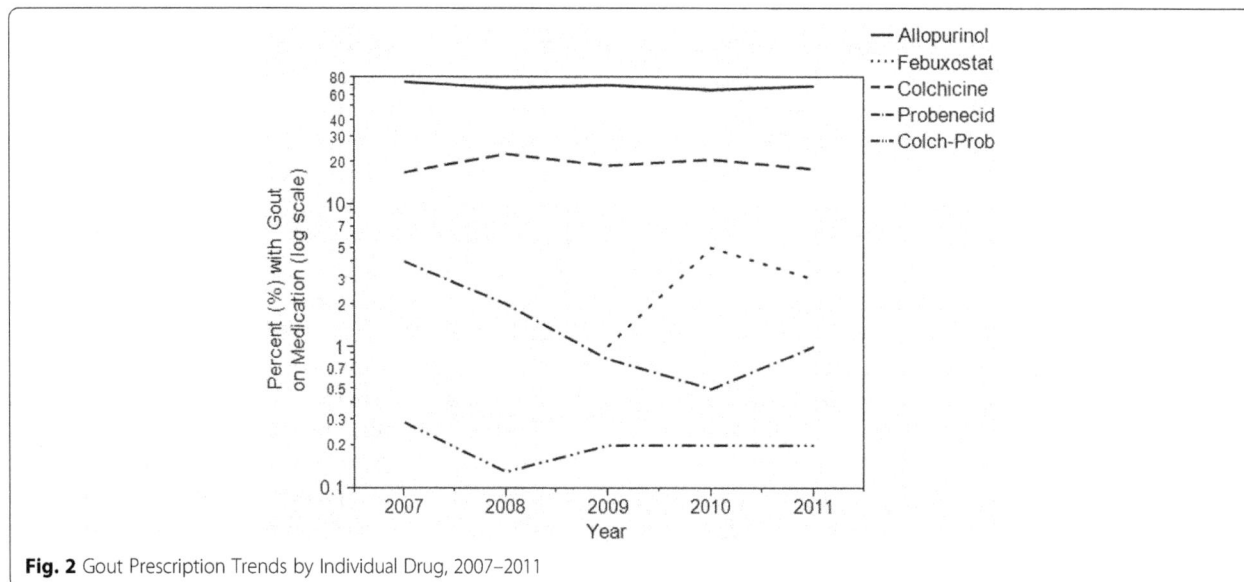

Fig. 2 Gout Prescription Trends by Individual Drug, 2007–2011

increased over the study years, helping explain the rise in gout diagnoses [18].

The number of gout visits in this study was not as high as noted in a similar prior study, [8] which could be attributed to several different factors. Although not specified in their methods, the Krishnan and Chen study appears to have used aggregated estimates for the years and databases studied, rather than the average annual estimates used in this study. Additionally, Krishnan and Chen only utilized NAMCS and NHAMCS-OPD, whereas this study also utilized NHAMCS-ED. Despite approximately 95 million visits attributed to the NHAMCS-ED, visits for gout in the ED were less likely. This likely increased the total number of overall visits without adding a commensurate number of gout-specific visits to the numerator. Further, while only 31% of the study population was aged 65 or older, 61% was female and the prevalence of gout is known to both increase with age and be more prevalent in males [3].

Another prior study with higher gout estimates by Zhu, et al. was based on participant reported data from the National Health and Nutrition Examination Survey (NHANES), which lends itself to estimating true prevalence [1]. This study is based on provider reported ambulatory, outpatient and emergency visits, therefore limiting the ability to estimate the true prevalence of gout. This database distinction helps explain this difference in gout estimates. It is worth noting that NHANES as well as the data sources used for this study are all population-based surveys.

The study results are consistent with several international epidemiology studies which examined the prevalence of gout [19–23]. The prevalence of gout has increased significantly in the United Kingdom (UK) over

the years of 1997 through 2012 according to a study which utilized the Clinical Practice Datalink [19]. Another study which looked at gout prevalence in the UK and Germany from 2000 to 2005 with the IMS Disease Analyzer found a prevalence of 1.4% [20]. A study of the Canadian province of British Columbia from 2000 to 2012 using PopulationDataBC found a prevalence of 3.8% in 2012, and there was a noted increase over the study period [21]. A Swedish study examined gout trends from 2002 to 2012 and found a prevalence of 1.8% in 2012 as well as an increase over the study period. [22] A study in Taiwan utilizing the National Health Insurance Research Database found a higher prevalence rate of 6.24% over the study period of 2005 to 2010 [23]. With the exception of the Taiwan study [23], all studies were consistent with this study's findings with regards to gout prevalence and increasing prevalence over the years.

This study demonstrated an association between age, sex, race group and gout visits, with an increased proportion among older age groups (≥45 years of age), males, African American and 'Other' race groups. These finding are consistent with previous studies [1, 3, 8, 10] showing that the risk of developing gout is age-related, [1, 8] and that estrogen is protective in premenopausal women due to its uricosuric effect [10]. 'Other' race within the databases consists of Asian, Native Hawaiian or other Pacific Islander, American Indian or Alaska Native, or more than one race reported. A higher prevalence of gout is well known in Asians and Pacific Islanders, as well as African Americans with genetics playing a role due to hyperuricemia-associated DNA sequence variations [24, 25]. However, diet and the presence of co-morbidities cannot be ruled out.

Hispanic/Latino individuals were found to be less likely to have a visit with gout than Non-Hispanic/Latinos. One possible explanation is related to diet. A previous study showed that Non-Hispanic/Latinos consume more red meat and seafood when compared to Hispanic/Latinos. [26] Diets rich in red meat and seafood are widely known to be associated with the production of uric acid [2]. Given that Hispanic/Latino diets are typically more heavily based on grains and beans along with fresh fruits and vegetables, Hispanic/ Latinos may produce less uric acid resulting in a lower incidence of gout [27].

Patient visits with Medicaid and 'Other' insurance were less likely to have a diagnosis of gout. Despite the lack of statistically significant interaction effects in the multivariable model, this could be attributed to the role of age with the risk of developing gout [1, 8]. 'Other' insurance consisted of worker's compensation, self-pay, no charge/charity, and other, while Medicaid also included the Children's Health Insurance Program. Patients with 'Other' insurance or Medicaid are less likely to be older, the age group at the highest risk for gout.

Individuals were significantly less likely to have a visit with a diagnosis of gout in a hospital emergency setting than they were in a physician's office. Patients are more likely to visit a provider's office for routine check-ups and for chronic conditions like gout. While individuals may visit a hospital for an initial or particularly severe attack of gout, they are presumably more likely to visit their provider when simply attempting to help keep their gout under control. Furthermore, patients with gout are much more likely to visit their provider if they are being prescribed gout prophylaxis medication.

A study by Garg, et al. looked at gout-related health care utilization in US emergency departments utilizing the National Emergency Department Sample (NEDS) from 2006 to 2008 [28]. The Garg study found approximately 0.7% of ED visits to be gout-related, slightly higher than 0.4% found in this study [28]. A similar study by Jinno, et al. also utilized NEDS and examined gout ED visits from 2006 to 2012 [29]. This study found 0.19% of visits with a primary diagnosis of gout [29]. Although not exactly comparable to this study, which includes non-ED databases in addition to the NHAMCS-ED, similar findings with both of these studies include gout-related ED visits being more likely with men, and increasing age; and less likely with different insurance types [28, 29].

Diuretic use was four times more likely to be associated with a gout visit. Previous research has shown that individuals who have high blood pressure and are also taking a diuretic have an increased risk for acquiring gout [6]. The diuretics' mechanism of action is thought to contribute to gout, increasing uric acid reabsorption [30].

The graph of gout medication class by year showed consistency in use among the drug classes over the years. Antigout and antihyperuricemic medication classes remained the two most commonly prescribed treatments, while NSAIDs and steroids were used less. It is worth noting that due to drug class coding within the databases some medications could have been coded in both the antigout and antihyperuricemic class (i.e., allopurinol and febuxostat) since drugs may be coded in as many as four different medication classes. This might explain why the antigout percentage is greater than the antihyperuricemics. However, the findings in this study are consistent with the prior NAMCS and NHAMCS-OPD study which looked at gout treatment trends up through 2009 [8]. These treatment trends can also be explained by typical prescribing patterns for a gouty attack versus prophylaxis treatment to prevent gout flare. NSAIDs and steroids are typically only used for gouty attacks and patients are treated prophylactically after an initial gout attack to prevent future attacks [2, 31]. In addition, the risk of side effects with NSAIDs such as gastrointestinal bleeds, renal failure, and hypertension likely impacted their use in treatment, especially in the case when chronic treatment is warranted [32, 33].

As evident from the figure showing the percentage of visits by year for individual gout drugs, allopurinol continues to be the most prescribed treatment with colchicine second, a finding also consistent with Krishnan and Chen [8]. Allopurinol dominated the market as the only medication to reduce uric acid synthesis until the introduction of febuxostat in 2009 [2, 4, 11]. As expected, the percentage of visits with febuxostat increased following its approval. Despite this, allopurinol and colchicine use changed little from 2009 through 2011, evidence that febuxostat introduction had minimal impact on the treatment trends for the study years. Probenecid use has declined over the years which can be explained by its potential for drug-drug interactions as well as less favorable side effect profile, including risk of urolithiasis [2, 11, 34].

The previously mentioned international studies showed similar treatment trends. Allopurinol was prescribed for most patients in UK and Germany at 89 and 93% respectively; while colchicine use was only around 15–16% for both [20]. Probenecid use was minimal (< 1%), but NSAIDs were utilized 80–90% for prophylaxis. [20]. Allopurinol was also most commonly prescribed in British Columbia, Canada, with less than 1% use of febuxostat and probenecid [21]. Colchicine and steroid use increased in British Columbia over the study period, while NSAID use declined by 31% [21]. A study in Australia in 2005 found allopurinol to comprise 98.4% of all urate lowering therapy with probenecid at < 1% [35]. There was a common theme from these studies of the overall underutilization of urate-lowering treatment for gout [19–23, 35].

The study is not without limitations. The observational, cross-sectional nature of the study design limited the authors to statements of association between visits with gout diagnosis and the factors of interest. No claims of causality can be made. Furthermore, the cross-sectional nature of the data sources used did not allow for repeated measurements on patients over time. Several variables of interest, including alcoholism, Parkinson's disease, depression, hypertension, weight status, tobacco use, and losartan use had to be excluded from all analyses due to missing data and/or reliability issues. This is particularly unfortunate for variables such as hypertension and weight status, both known to be significantly associated with gout. All of the databases utilized are limited to three diagnoses. The NAMCS and NHAMCS-OPD include a data field to collect other specific disease states (includes hypertension, diabetes, and depression), but NHAMCS-ED does not and only collects the diabetes variable of interest in their other specific disease field. This likely contributed to the missing data for such highly prevalent conditions like hypertension and diabetes. The NAMCS and NHAMCS databases do not include federal offices or hospitals, including Veterans Affairs facilities where gout can be prevalent. In addition, the databases do not provide a true prevalence of gout, but rather a surrogate via visits for gout based on diagnostic codes from the three recorded diagnoses and gout medications prescribed at the visits. It is not uncommon for epidemiological studies to rely on diagnostic codes for estimating prevalence. Those studies which have relied on such codes have shown good accuracy. In addition, although gout medications were also used to identify gout visits, there is a chance that medications like colchicine and probenecid were used for conditions other than gout. However, such alternative uses are rare. Study strengths include the use of nationally representative, population-based surveys which allow for generalizing findings to the portion of the US population that is commensurate with the study population. Further, the databases are provider reported data which allows for more reliability of results as compared to patient reported data. This is the first study known to the authors to investigate febuxostat in the treatment of gout since its approval in 2009 [4].

Conclusion

This study found that the proportion of visits with a diagnosis of gout continues to increase, although the overall percentage of gout remains low in the US population. Individuals who are male, aged 45–64 or 65 and older, non-Hispanic/Latino, African American or of 'Other' race, use private insurance, present to a physician's office, or use a diuretic are more likely to have a visit with a diagnosis of gout. Treatment trends over the study years by medication class and individual gout medications have remained consistent, with the introduction of febuxostat having little impact for the study years through 2011.

Poster presentations 2016 Wiggins Academic Symposium, Campbell University, Buies Creek, NC.

2017 Interprofessional Health Sciences Research Symposium, Campbell University, Buies Creek, NC.

Endnotes

[1]The NAMCS and NHAMCS surveys define the four regions that comprise this variable as follows:Northeast: Connecticut, Maine, Massachusetts, New Hampshire, New Jersey, New York, Pennsylvania, Rhode Island, Vermont; Midwest: Illinois, Indiana, Iowa, Kansas, Michigan, Minnesota, Missouri,Nebraska, North Dakota, Ohio, South Dakota, Wisconsin; South: Alabama, Arkansas, Delaware, District of Columbia, Florida, Georgia, Kentucky, Louisiana, Maryland, Mississippi, North Carolina,Oklahoma, South Carolina, Tennessee, Texas, Virginia, West Virginia; West: Arizona, California, Colorado, Idaho, Montana, Nevada, New Mexico, Oregon, Utah, Washington, Wyoming, Alaska, Hawaii

Abbreviations

CIs: Confidence intervals; MSA: Metropolitan statistical area; NAMCS: National Ambulatory Medical Care Survey; NCHS: National Center for Health Statistics; NEDS: National Emergency Department Sample; NHAMCS-OPD/NHAMCS-ED: National Hospital Ambulatory Medical Care Survey Outpatient Department & Emergency Department; NHANES: National Health and Nutrition Examination Survey; ORs: Odds ratios; sUA: Serum urate

Authors' contributions

KEC, KDC, DR, and MH wrote the Background, Discussion, Results, and Conclusions sections of the manuscript. MJ conducted all analyses and wrote the Methods section of the manuscript. All authors read and approved the final manuscript.

Ethics approval and consent to participate

The study was submitted to the Campbell University Institutional Review Board and received an exemption due to the data sources used being publicly available and de-identified. As such, since this research was based solely on the analysis of previously collected, de-identified data, it complies with the Helsinki Declaration.

Competing interests

The authors declare that they have no competing interests.

References

1. Zhu Y, Pandya BJ, Choi HK. Prevalence of gout and hyperuricemia in the US general population. Arthritis Rheum. 2011;63:3136–41.
2. Rymal E, Rizzolo D. Gout a comprehensive review. JAAPA. 2014;27:26–31.
3. Sunkureddi PS, Nguyen-Oghalai TU, Karnath BM. Clinical signs of gout. Hospital Physician. 2006;42:39–42,47.
4. U.S. Food and Drug Administration. FDA Approved Drug Products. http://www.accessdata.fda.gov/scripts/cder/drugsatfda/index.cfm?fuseaction=Search.DrugDetails. Accessed 10 Aug 2016.
5. Choi HK, Atkinson K, Karlson EW, Curhan G. Obesity, weight change, hypertension, diuretic use, and risk of gout in men: the health professionals follow-up study. Arch Intern Med. 2005;165:742–8.

6. Primatesta P, Plana E, Rothenbacher D. Gout treatment and comorbidities: a retrospective cohort study in a large US managed care population. BMC Musculoskelet Disord. 2011;12:103.

7. Juraschek SP, Miller ER, Gelber AC. Body mass index, obesity, and prevalent gout in the United States in 1988-1994 and 2007-2010. Arthritis Care Res. 2013;65:127–32.

8. Krishnan E, Chen L. Trends in physician diagnosed gout and gout therapies in the US: results from the national ambulatory health care surveys 1993 to 2009. Arthritis Res Ther. 2013;15:R181.

9. Lee SJ, Hirsch JD, Terkeltaub R, Khanna D, Singh JA, Sarkin A, et al. Perceptions of disease and health-related quality of life among patients with gout. Rheumatology (Oxford). 2009;48:582–6.

10. Bhole V, de Vera M, Rahman M, Krishnan E, Choi H. Epidemiology of gout in women: fifty-two-year followup of a prospective cohort. Arthritis Rheum. 2010;62:1069–76.

11. Baker JF, Schumacher HR. Update on gout and hyperuricemia. Int J Clin Pract. 2010;64:371–7.

12. McCaig LF, Burt CW. Understanding and interpreting the National Hospital Ambulatory Medical Care survey: key questions and answers. Ann Emerg Med. 2012;60:716–21.

13. Sample text for describing NHAMCS in a research article. https://www.cdc.gov/nchs/data/ahcd/Sample_Text_for_Describing_NHAMCS_in_Research_Article.pdf. Accessed 1 Mar 2018.

14. National Center for Health Statistics. Scope and sample design. http://www.cdc.gov/nchs/ahcd/ahcd_scope.htm#namcs_scope. Accessed 1 Mar 2018.

15. SAS Institute Inc. SAS/STAT 9.3 User's Guide. Cary: SAS Institute Inc; 2011.

16. Saag KG, Choi H. Epidemiology, risk factors, and lifestyle modifications for gout. Arthritis Res Ther. 2006;8(1):S2.

17. Choi HK, Ford ES, Li C, Curhan G. Prevalence of the metabolic syndrome in patients with gout: the third National Health and nutrition examination survey. Arthritis Rheum. 2007;57:109–15.

18. Aguilar M, Bhuket T, Torres S, Liu B, Wong RJ. Prevalence of the metabolic syndrome in the United States, 2003-2012. JAMA. 2015;313:1973–4.

19. Kuo CF, Grainge MJ, Mallen C, Zhang W, Doherty M. Rising burden of gout in the UK but continuing suboptimal management: a nationwide population study. Ann Rheum Dis. 2015;74:661–7.

20. Annemans L, Spaepen E, Gaskin M, Bonnemaire M, Malier V, Gilbert T, et al. Gout in the UK and Germany: prevalence, comorbidities and management in general practice 2000-2005. Ann Rheum Dis. 2008;67:960–6.

21. Rai SK, Avina-Zubieta JA, McCormick N, De Vera MA, Shojania K, Sayre EC, et al. The rising prevalence and incidence of gout in British Columbia, Canada: population-based trends from 2000 to 2012. Semin Arthritis Rheum. 2017;46:451–6.

22. Dehlin M, Drivelegka P, Sigurdardottir V, Svard A, Jacobsson LTH. Incidence and prevalence of gout in western Sweden. Arthritis Res Ther. 2016;18:164.

23. Kuo CF, Grainge MJ, See LC, Yu KH, Luo SF, Zhang W, et al. Epidemiology and management of gout in Taiwan: a nationwide population study. Arthritis Res Ther. 2015;17:13.

24. Reginato AM, Mount DB, Yang I, Choi HK. The genetics of hyperuricaemia and gout. Nat Rev Rheumatol. 2012;8:610–21.

25. Yang Q, Köttgen A, Dehghan A, Smith AV, Glazer NL, Chen MH, et al. Multiple genetic loci influence serum urate levels and their relationship with gout and cardiovascular disease risk factors. Circ Cardiovasc Genet. 2010;3:523–30.

26. Winkleby MA, Albright CL, Howard-Pitney AB, Lin J, Fortmann SP. Hispanic/white differences in dietary fat intake among low educated adults and children. Prev Med. 1994;23:465–73.

27. Diet.com. Hispanic and latino diet. http://www.diet.com/g/hispanic-and-latino-diet. Accessed 1 Mar 2018.

28. Garg R, Sayles HR, Yu F, Michaud K, Singh J, Saag KG, et al. Gout-related health care utilization in US emergency departments, 2006 through 2008. Arthritis Care Res. 2013;65:571–7.

29. Jinno S, Hasegawa K, Neogi T, Goho T, Dubreuil M. Trends in emergency department visits and charges in the United States between 2006 and 2012. J Rheumatol. 2016;43:1589–92.

30. Pascual E, Perdiguero M. Gout, diuretics and the kidney. Ann Rheum Dis. 2006;65:981–2.

31. Rees F, Hui M, Doherty M. Optimizing current treatment of gout. Nat Rev Rheumatol. 2014;10:271–83.

32. Moon KW, Kim J, Kim JH, Song R, Lee EY, Song YW, et al. Risk factors for acute kidney injury by non-steroidal anti-inflammatory drugs in patients with hyperuricemia. Rheumatology. 2011;50:2278–82.

33. Madhok R, Wu O, McKellar G, Singh G. Non-steroidal anti-inflammatory drugs-changes in prescribing may be warranted. Rheumatology. 2006;45:1458–60.

34. Reinders MK, van Roon EN, Jansen TL, Deising J, Griep EN, Hoekstra M, et al. Efficacy and tolerability of urate-lowering drugs in gout: a randomized controlled trial of benzbromarone versus probenecid after failure of allopurinol. Ann Rheum Dis. 2009;68:51–6.

35. Chung Y, Lu CY, Graham GG, Mant A, Day RO. Utilization of allopurinol in the Australian community. Int Med J. 2008;38:388–95.

8

High prevalence of protein tyrosine phosphatase non-receptor N22 gene functional variant R620W in systemic lupus erythematosus patients from Kuwait: implications for disease susceptibility

Adel M. Al-Awadhi[1,2], Mohammad Z. Haider[3]* (iD), Jalaja Sukumaran[3] and Sowmya Balakrishnan[3]

Abstract

Background: Systemic lupus erythematosus (SLE) is an autoimmune inflammatory disease which involves the loss of self-tolerance with hyperactivation of autoreactive T- and B-cells. Protein tyrosine phosphatase non-receptor type 22 (PTPN22) encodes for lymphoid specific phosphatase (LYP) which is a key negative regulator of T lymphocyte activation. The aim of this study was to investigate the association between *PTPN22* gene functional variant R620W and systemic lupus erythematosus (SLE) by comparing its prevalence in Kuwaiti SLE patients and controls.

Methods: The study included 134 SLE patients and 214 controls from Kuwait. The genotypes of *PTPN22* gene functional variant R620W were determined by PCR-RFLP and confirmed by DNA sequence analysis in both SLE patients and the controls.

Results: A relatively high prevalence of the variant 620 W (T-allele) of the *PTPN22* gene was detected in the SLE patients from Kuwait. 35.7% of the SLE patients had at least one variant allele (T-allele) compared to 15.9% in the controls. A statistically significant difference was detected in the frequency of variant genotypes, TT and CT between SLE patients and the controls ($p < 0.0001$). No association was detected between the *PTPN22* gene variant and the Raynaud's phenomenon, renal involvement and severity of the SLE.

Conclusions: The frequency of *PTPN22* gene functional variant R620W reported in this study is amongst the highest compared to other world populations. A high prevalence of this variant in SLE patients in comparison to the healthy controls suggests its significant contribution in conferring susceptibility to SLE together with other factors.

Keywords: Protein tyrosine phosphatase non receptor-22, Systemic lupus erythematosus, Kuwait, Gene, Functional variant

Background

Systemic lupus erythematosus (SLE; MIM 152700) is a common, complex autoimmune disease with multiple-organ involvement, characterized by the production of pathogenic autoantibodies directed against cytoplasmic and nuclear cellular components [1]. It occurs predominantly in women (> 90%) and is distinguished by a loss of tolerance to self-antigens, the deposition of immune complexes and tissue inflammation and destruction. There are variable clinical manifestations associated with SLE which include arthralgia, rashes, alopecia, serositis, leukopenia and renal involvement [2, 3]. Unrestricted hyper-activation of the immune system may lead to the overproduction of autoantibodies, immune complex deposition, inflammatory cytokine release and eventually organ damage in SLE pathogenesis [4, 5]. The causes of SLE are not completely understood at present. It is thought that the onset of SLE results from multifactorial etiology, involving hormonal factors, environmental triggers and genetic susceptibility [6]. Systemic autoimmune

* Correspondence: haider@hsc.edu.kw
[3]Department of Pediatrics, Faculty of Medicine, Kuwait University, P. O. Box 24923, 13110 Safat, Kuwait
Full list of author information is available at the end of the article

diseases e.g. SLE and many others are thought to share common genetic causative factors in populations of different ethnic or racial origin [7]. The involvement of major histocompatibility complex (MHC) also supported this hypothesis. However, non-MHC alleles such as a functional polymorphism (rs2476601, Arginine 620 Tryptophan, R620W) in protein tyrosine phosphatase non-receptor type 22 (PTPN22), which encodes the lymphoid PTP (LYP), was reported to be significantly associated with multiple autoimmune disorders including type 1 diabetes mellitus (T1DM; [8]), rheumatoid arthritis [9], SLE [10], Hashimoto thyroiditis [11], autoimmune thyroid disease [12] and Grave's disease [13].

The *PTPN22* gene encodes a lymphoid-specific phosphatase (LYP) which has been shown to be a negative regulator of T cell activation [14]. The LYP contribute to T cell activation by binding to the regulatory Src tyrosine kinase (Csk) [14]. It has been reported that a functional variant R620W (C1858T polymorphism) of the *PTPN22* gene is located in a motif which facilitate binding of the LYP with Csk [15]. The variant form, 620 W carries a tryptophan residue in place of arginine (R) and affects the binding of LYP and Csk thereby disrupting the regulation of T cell receptor-signaling kinases e.g. Lck, Fyn and ZAP70 [14–16]. It has been postulated that the individuals carrying the variant allele (620 W) have an altered threshold for thymic selection, with increased numbers of autoreactive T cells escaping the negative selection, thus persisting in the circulation, and are prone to autoimmunity [17]. The C1858T variant has also been shown to be associated with changes in cytokine profile in SLE patients in vivo [18].

In spite of a large number of reports linking the *PTPN22* gene R620W functional variant with a number of autoimmune diseases, conflicting results have appeared in the literature about its prevalence in different world populations [3, 5, 7, 19–22]. In view of these diverse findings on prevalence and relationship of the *PTPN22* gene R620W functional variant with SLE, we carried out this study in SLE patients from Kuwait to investigate its possible association with susceptibility to SLE in a completely different population/ethnic group.

Methods

The SLE patients were recruited from two major teaching hospitals (Amiri and Mubarak Al-Kabeer) from Kuwait. The inclusion criteria described by the American College of Rheumatology (ACR) for the diagnosis of SLE was used [23]. For the patients included in the study, a diagnosis of SLE had been made at least 2–3 months prior to their recruitment. The information collected from the patients included age, age-at-onset, gender, clinical manifestations associated with SLE and disease severity. The evaluation of SLE severity was

made as follows: the patients were considered to have a 'mild disease' if they presented muco-cutaneous serositis, and/or arthritis and 'mild-severe' disease if the patients had hematological, renal and neurological manifestations. The renal disease associated with SLE was ascertained if the 24 h urine protein excretion exceeded 500 mg or hematouria was detected (> 5 red blood cells/field). The hematological abnormalities associated with SLE included the presence of hemolytic anemia with reticulocytosis, or leucopenia ($< 4000/mm^3$ on > two occasions), or lymphopenia ($< 1500 \ mm^3$ on > two occasions) or thrombocytopenia ($< 100,000/mm^3$ in the absence of drugs). The presence of seizures or psychosis without the use of drugs or metabolic derangement were considered as the neurological presentations associated with SLE. The frequency of *PTPN22* gene polymorphism in SLE patients was compared to that in a group of 214 healthy controls, matched for age and sex with the patients. The controls subjects were unrelated to the patients; were otherwise healthy and were seen at hospital outpatient clinics for minor illnesses. The controls were thoroughly examined by a specialist to ascertain their health status before recruitment in the study.

Identification of genotypes for *PTPN22* gene functional variant (R620W)

The *PTPN22* gene polymorphism genotypes were determined in 126 patients with SLE and 214 healthy controls. Approximately 5 ml blood was collected from all the study subjects in appropriate tubes. For molecular studies, blood was anti-coagulated in the presence of EDTA. Total genomic DNA was isolated by using a standard method [24]. The genotypes for a non-synonymous single nucleotide polymorphism (SNP) +1858C→T (rs2476601) in the *PTPN22* gene were identified by polymerase chain reaction-restriction enzyme fragment length polymorphism (PCR-RFLP) method as described earlier [25]. A 218 bp DNA fragment was amplified by using the primers: Forward primer: 5'-ACTGATAATGTTGCTTCAACGG-3' and reverse primer: 5-TCACCAGCTTCCTCAACCAC-3'. The PCR mixture contained 10× PCR buffer (Applied BioSystems, Foster City, USA); 1.5 mM $MgCl_2$; 0.2 mM of each of the dNTPs (deoxyribonucleotide triphosphates); 20 pmol of each primer, 250 ng template DNA and 1 U AmpliTaq DNA polymerase (Applied BioSystems). The amplification conditions used were denaturation at 94 °C for 5 min followed by 35 cycles of 94 °C for 30 s, 60 °C for 30 s and 72 °C for 30 s and an extension step at 72 °C for 5 min. The PCR product was digested with restriction enzyme *Rsa*I at 37 °C for 90 min. The cleavage products were analyzed by 2% agarose gel electrophoresis and visualized under UV light after staining with ethidium bromide. The 218 bp PCR product did not have an *Rsa*I cleavage site when 1858 T allele (620 W variant) was present and the presence of C1858 allele (R620) was associated with the presence of 176 bp and 42 bp cleavage products. In case of a heterozygous individual both the 218 and 176 bp bands were detected. The PCR amplicons were sequenced in a blinded manner on ABI 3130 genetic analyzer to confirm the genotypes. Genotypes could not be done in 8 SLE patients due to low volume of the blood samples obtained. The study was carried out according to the Helsinki declaration and was approved by the Institutional Ethics Committee for the protection of human subjects in research. Written informed consent was obtained from all the study subjects.

Statistical analysis

The information and the data collected from and on the study subjects was analyzed using the Statistical Package for the Social Sciences version 24 (SPSS, Chicago IL, USA). The frequencies of various genotypes and alleles detected among the SLE patients and controls were calculated by direct counting. The significance of their association was evaluated by using the Chi-square test, Fisher's Exact test and p-values were regarded significant when < 0.05. The strength of association was estimated by the odds ratios which were calculated at 95% confidence interval. The genotype distribution was also tested for Hardy Weinberg equilibrium by goodness of fit method using MSTAT software.

Results

This study included 134 SLE patients and 214 controls. In the patients group (n = 134), there were 123 (91.8%) females and 11 (8.2%) males. In the control group, there were 199 females. In the SLE patients group, the age of onset information was available in 118 cases. When stratified on the basis of age of onset, 16/118 (14%) patients were aged between 1 and 14 years, 25/118 (21%) between 15 and 24 years, 26/118 (22%) between 25 and 34 years, 34/118 (29%) between 35 and 44 years and 17/118 (14%) > 45 years respectively. The data on SLE patient characteristics and clinical manifestations has been presented in Table 1. The genotype and allele frequencies of PTPN22 gene R620W functional variant amongst the SLE patients and controls have been presented in Table 2. A comparison of genotype frequency between SLE patients and the controls showed statistically significant differences in the case of CC and TT genotypes (Table 2). Similarly, the frequencies of C- and T-alleles were also significantly different between the SLE patients and controls (Table 2). Statistically significant differences were detected in all the three genotypes (CC, CT, TT) between females and male SLE patients (P < 0.0001 in case of all three genotypes). However, as it is generally the case, the incidence of SLE was much higher in females than in the males in our study group. A comparison was also made for the genotype distribution on the basis of gender between the

Table 1 The characteristics of systemic lupus erythematosus (SLE) patients included in the study (n = 134). S.D., standard deviation; ANA, anti-nuclear antibody

Gender ratio (Female: Male)	11: 1 (123/11)
Mean age (± S.D.), years	36.7 (± 9.3)
Mean age at diagnosis (± S.D.), years	30.6 (± 8.3)
Mean disease duration (range), months	48 (6–280)
Clinical manifestations: n (%)	
Malar rash	73 (54.4)
Mouth ulcers	26 (19.4)
Photosensitivity	25 (18.7)
Discoid rash	9 (6.7)
Raynaud's phenomenon	22 (16.4)
Arthritis	128 (95.5)
Serositis	29 (21.6)
Renal involvement	22 (16.4)
Hematological abnormalities	51 (38)
Neurological disorders	5 (3.7)
Immunological abnormalities[a]	95 (70.9)
ANA[b]	134 (100)
Hypertension[c]	7 (5.2)

[a]As per criteria of the American College of Rheumatology (ACR) [23]
[b]A standard indirect immunofluorescence method was used for detection and ascertainment as per ACR criteria and cutoff limits [23]
[c]Blood Pressure > 140/90 mmHg (or > 130/80 mmHg in the case of renal insufficiency)

SLE patients and the controls (Table 3). For the CC and CT genotypes, the difference was statistically significant both for the females and males between the SLE patients and that in the controls. However, in the case of TT genotype, there was no significant difference between the genotype distribution between SLE patients and the controls in relation to their gender (Table 3). It may be mentioned here that in the case of controls, only 2/214 subjects had a TT genotype and of these, one was male and the second a female. We did not find an association between T-allele of the PTPN22 gene functional variant and the Raynaud's

Table 2 Genotype and allele frequency of PTPN22 gene R620W functional variant in SLE patients and controls

Genotype/ Allele	SLE patients N = 126 (%)	Controls N = 214 (%)	OR (95% CI)[a]	P-value*
CC	81 (64.3)	180 (84.1)	0.34 (0.20–0.57)	< 0.0001
CT	23 (18.3)	32 (15)	1.27 (0.70–2.28)	0.51
TT	22 (17.4)	2 (0.9)	22.42 (5.17–97.21)	< 0.0001
Distribution of Alleles				
C – allele	185/252 (73.4)	392/428 (91.6)	0.25 (0.16–0.39)	< 0.0001
T – allele	67/252 (26.6)	36/428 (8.4)	3.94 (2.53–6.13)	< 0.0001

[a]OR, odds ratio at 95% confidence interval
*P-values were considered significant when < 0.05

Table 3 Comparison of genotypes of *PTPN22* gene R620W functional variant between SLE patients group and controls stratified according to gender

Genotype/Gender	SLE patients N (%)	Control N (%)	P-value[a]
CC	(N = 76)	(N = 177)	< 0.001*
Female	70 (92.1)	115 (65)	
Male	6 (7.9)	62 (35)	
CT	(N = 21)	(N = 32)	< 0.001*
Female	21 (100)	19 (59.4)	
Male	0 (0)	13 (40.6)	
TT	(N = 21)	(N = 2)	0.25
Female	19 (90.5)	1 (50)	
Male	2 (9.5)	1 (50)	

[a]Chi-square test of the full cohort
*P-value were considered significant when < 0.05

phenomenon, nephritis or the disease severity in SLE or any of its other manifestations in patients from Kuwait (data not shown).

Discussion

The most significant finding in this study is that a relatively high frequency of *PTPN22* gene functional variant 620 W was detected in the SLE patients (17.4%) compared to 0.9% in the controls. When taken together, the homozygous and heterozygous combinations of this variant allele were detected in 35.7% of the SLE patients from Kuwait. This is significantly higher than previous reports from other populations/ethnic groups. Machado-Contreras et al. [5], did not find homozygous TT genotype in any of their Mexican SLE patients, however heterozygous CT genotype was detected in 6% Mexican SLE patients. Similarly, in a Greek study on the SLE patients from the Island of Crete, TT genotype was not detected at all while CT genotype was detected in 5.39% cases. In a report on SLE patients from Egypt [26], the authors could not detect a homozygous TT genotype but did find heterozygous CT genotype in 52.5% SLE cases. A comprehensive *PTPN22* gene association study [3], reported minor allele frequency (MAF) of 11.9% in European Americans, 2.1% in African Americans and 7.6% in Hispanics. This study also reported that the association of the 1858 T allele with SLE was greater in European American patients with familial SLE (11.9%) compared to the sporadic SLE (8.2%). A study from Poland [21] found a positive association between the variant allele of the *PTPN22* gene and SLE. Aksoy et al. [22] did not find the TT genotype in Turkish SLE patients while the CT genotype was detected in 7% cases. Another study, on white Americans [27], reported that the TT genotype was detected in 2.5% SLE patients while the CT genotype was found in 20.4% SLE patients. In this study, the overall risk-allele frequency was found to be 12.67% compared to

8.64% in the white American controls. Positive association between *PTPN22* gene polymorphism and SLE susceptibility has been reported from Sweden [28] and Spain [29]. Namjou et al. [29] reported findings from genotyping of ten SNPs in four large multi-ethnic populations and using their results in conjunction with data from the Hap-Map project, concluded that SLE association with *PTPN22* was largely accounted for by the R620W variant (rs2476601) in individuals of European ancestry [21–26, 30, 31]. A strong North-South gradient in the risk-allele frequency has also been reported in Europe [32].

Recent reports provide information on the mechanism of R620W functional variant of the *PTPN22* gene [33–38]. In the light of postulated scheme for involvement of R620W variant in the molecular mechanism of auto-immunity [33, 34], our data from SLE patients from Kuwait supports and highlights its role as a significant determinant of the SLE susceptibility. However, it may also be appropriate to mention that the genetic factors which contribute to susceptibility/protection to develop SLE most likely involve multiple genes. Kuwait is a small country located in the North of Arabian Gulf. The population of Kuwait is quite diverse; Kuwaiti Arabs constitute nearly 45% of the population. There is a high incidence of consanguinity (54%; [39]), which often results in familial clustering of common chronic disorders. The incidence of diseases with autoimmune etiology such as type 1 diabetes mellitus is amongst the highest in the region and bordering with the high-incidence countries of the world [40, 41]. The original settlers of Kuwait were immigrants from Najd, an area that now constitute eastern and central Saudi Arabia. The ethnic origin of Kuwaiti Arabs is quite varied; 50% are of Arab origin, some are Bedouins and nearly 50% are immigrants [42]. The Arabs residing in most of the Gulf countries are a result of an admixture with other populations such as Persians, Turks, South Asians, Europeans and Africans [42]. The genotype frequency of variant 620 W reported in our SLE patient group from Kuwait is amongst the highest (TT, 17.4% and combined TT and CT in 35.7% patients) compared to any of the other populations/ethnic groups. This can possibly be due to a cumulative effect of unique genetic/ethnic background along with a very high rate of consanguinity (54%) in the Kuwaiti population and can at least in part, explain the high incidence of autoimmune diseases including SLE in the country.

Conclusions

The frequency of *PTPN22* gene functional variant R620W reported in this study is amongst the highest compared to other world populations. A high prevalence of this variant in SLE patients in comparison to controls suggests its significant contribution in conferring susceptibility to SLE along with other factors.

Abbreviations

Csk: Src tyrosine kinase; DNA: Deoxyribonucleic acid; dNTP: Deoxyribonucleotide triphosphate; LYP: Lymphoid specific phosphatase; MHC: Major histocompatibility complex; PCR: Polymerase chain reaction; PTPN22: Protein tyrosine phosphatase non-receptor type 22; R: Arginine; RA: Rheumatoid arthritis; RFLP: Restriction fragment length polymorphism; SLE: Systemic lupus erythematosus; SNP: Single nucleotide polymorphism; T1DM: Type 1 diabetes mellitus; W: Tryptophan

Acknowledgements

The assistance of hospital staff who helped in sample and data collection is thankfully acknowledged. We thank Mrs. Asiya Ibrahim for help in statistical analysis.

Funding

The project was funded by Kuwait University and the funding body had no role in study design, collection and analysis of data and writing the manuscript.

Authors' contributions

All authors have read the manuscript and approve its submission for publication. AMA contributed in study design, recruitment and clinical evaluation of the study subjects and in writing the manuscript. MZH along with AMA conceived and designed the study, supervised the laboratory/analytical procedures, analyzed clinical and laboratory data and wrote the manuscript. JS and SB Carried out laboratory and experimental studies and compiled the data.

Competing interests

The authors declared that they have no competing interests.

Author details

[1]Department of Medicine, Faculty of Medicine, Kuwait University, Jabriya, Kuwait. [2]Rheumatic Disease Unit, Al-Amiri Hospital, Dasman, Kuwait. [3]Department of Pediatrics, Faculty of Medicine, Kuwait University, P. O. Box 24923, 13110 Safat, Kuwait.

References

1. Choi J, Kim ST, Craft J. The pathogenesis of systemic lupus erythematosus – an update. Curr Opin Immunol. 2012;24:651–7.
2. Lahita RG. Systemic lupus erythematosus. 4th ed. New York, USA: Academic Press; 2004.
3. Kaufman KM, Kelly JA, Herring BJ, Adler AJ, Glenn SB, et al. Evaluation of the gene association of the PTPN22 R620W polymorphism in familial and sporadic Systemic lupus erythematosus. Arthritis Rhem. 2006;54:2533–40.
4. Anaya J-M, Shoenfeld Y, Cervera R. Systemic lupus erythematosus-2014. Autoimmune Dis. 2014, 274323. DOI: https://doi.org/10.1155/2014/274323.
5. Machado-Contreras JR, Munoz-Valle JF, Cruz A, Salazar-Camarena DC, Marin-Rosales M, et al. Distribution of PTPN22 polymorphisms in SLE from western Mexico: correlation with mRNA expression and disease activity. Clin Exp Med. 2016;16:399–406.
6. O'Neill S, Cerevera R. Systemic lupus erythematosus. Best Pract Res Clin Rheumatol. 2010;24:841–55.
7. Tang L, Wang Y, Zheng S, Bao M, Zhang Q, Jianming L. PTPN22 polymorphisms, but not R620W, were associated with the genetic susceptibility of systemic lupus erythematosus and rheumatoid arthritis in a Chinese Han population. Hum Immunol. 2016;77:692–8.
8. Aarnisalo J, Treszl A, Svec P. Reduced CD4(+) T cell activation in children with type 1 diabetes carrying the PTPN22/Lyp 620Trp variant. J Autoimmun. 2008;31:13–21.
9. Rodriguez-Rodriguez WR, Tai R, Topless S, Steer MF, Gonzales-Escribano A, et al. The PTPN22 R263Q polymorphism is a risk factor for rheumatic arthritis in Caucasian case-control samples. J Arthritis Rheum. 2011;63:365–72.
10. Baca V, Velazquez-Cruz R, Salas-Martinez G, Espinosa-Rosales Y, Saldana-Alvarez L, et al. Association analysis of the PTPN22 gene in childhood-onset systemic lupus erythematosus in Mexican population. Genes Immun. 2006;7:693–5.
11. Criswell LA, Pfeiffer KA, Lum RF, Gonzales B, Novitzke J, et al. Analysis of families in the multiple autoimmune disease genetics consortium (MADGC) collection: the PTPN22 620W allele associates with multiple autoimmune phenotypes. Am J Hum Genet. 2005;76:561 71.
12. Wu H, Cantor RM, Cunninghame DS, Graham DS, Lingren CM, et al. Association analysis of the R620W polymorphism of the protein tyrosine phosphatase PTPN22 in systemic lupus erythematosus patients with autoimmune thyroid disease. Arthritis Rheum. 2005;52:2396–2402.
13. Heward M, Brand OJ, Barrett JC, Carr-Smith JA, Franklyn SC, et al. Association of PTPN22 haplotypes with Grave's disease. J Clin Endocrinol Metab. 2007;92:685–90.
14. Bottini N, Musumeci L, Alonso A, Rahmouni K, Nika M, et al. A functional variant of lymphoid tyrosine phosphatase is associated with type 1 diabetes. Nat Genet. 2004;36:337–8.
15. Cloutier JF, Veillette A. Cooperative inhibition of T-cell antigen receptor signaling by a complex between a kinase and a phosphatase. J Exp Med. 1999;198:111–21.
16. Bogovich AB, Carlton VE, Honigberg LA, Schrodi SJ, Chokkalingam AP, et al. A missense single nucleotide polymorphism in a gene encoding a protein tyrosine phosphatase (PTPN22) is associated with rheumatoid arthritis. Am J Hum Genet. 2004;75:330–7.
17. Bottini N, Vang T, Cucca F, Mustelin T. Role of PTPN22 in type 1 diabetes and other autoimmune diseases. Semin Immunol. 2006;18:207–13.
18. Kariuki SN, Crow MK, Niewold TB. The PTPN22 C1858T polymorphism is associated with skewing of cytokine profiles towards high interferon-alpha activity and low tumor necrosis factor alpha levels in patients with lupus. Arthritis Rheum. 2008;58:2818–23.
19. Eliopoulos E, Zervou MI, Andreou A, Dimopoulou N, Cosmidis N, et al. Association of the PTPN22 R620W polymorphism with increased risk for SLE in the genetically homogeneous population of Crete. Lupus. 2011;20(5):501–6.
20. Maalej A, Chabchoub G, Glikmans E. Association study of PTPN22 gene with Rheumatoid Arthritis in the Tunisian population. Eur J Hum Genet. 2006;14(Suppl.1):326.
21. Piotrowski P, Lianeri M, Wudarski M, Lacki JK, Jagodzinski PP. Contribution of the R620W polymorphism of protein tyrosine phosphatase non-receptor 22 to systemic lupus erythematosus in Poland. Clin Exp Rheumatol. 2008;26(6):1099–102.
22. Aksoy R, Duman T, Keskin O, Duzgun N. No association of PTPN22 R620W gene polymorphism with rheumatic heart disease and systemic lupus erythematosus. Mol Biol Rep. 2011;38:5393–6.
23. Tan EM, Cohen AS, Fries JF, Masi AT, McShane DJ, et al. The 1982 revised criteria for the classification of systemic lupus erythematosus. Arthritis Rheum. 1982;25:1271–7.
24. Sambrook J, Freitsch EF, Maniatis T. Molecular Cloning: A Laboratory Manual. 2nd ed. New York, USA: Cold Spring Harbor Laboratory; 1989.
25. Saccucci P, Del Duca E, Rapini N, Verrotti A, Piccinini S, et al. Association between PTPN22 C1851T and type 1 diabetes: a replication in continental Italy. Tissue Antigens. 2008;71:234–7.
26. Moez P, Soliman E. Association of PTPN22 gene polymorphism and systemic lupus erythematosus in a cohort of Egyptian patients: impact on clinical and laboratory results. Rheumatol Int. 2012;32:2753–8.
27. Kyogoku C, Langefeld CD, Ortman WA, Lee A, Selby S, et al. Genetic association of the R620W polymorphism of protein tyrosine phosphatase PTPN22 with human SLE. Am J Hum Genet. 2004;75:504–7.
28. Reddy MV, Johansson M, Sturfelt G, Jinsen A, Gunnarsson I, et al. The R620W C/T polymorphism of the gene PTPN22 is associated with SLE independently of the association of PDCD1. Genes Immun. 2005;6:658–62.
29. Namjou B, Kin-Howard X, Sun C, Adler A, Chung SA, et al. PTPN22 association in systemic lupus erythematosus (SLE) with respect to individual ancestry and clinical sub-phenotypes. PLoS One. 2013;8:e69404.
30. Lea W, Lee Y. The association between the PTPN22 C1858T polymorphism and systemic lupus erythematosus: a meta-analysis update. Lupus. 2011;20:51–7.
31. Orozco G, Sanchez E, Gonzalez-Gay MA, Lopez-Nevot MA, Torres B, et al. Association of a functional single-nucleotide polymorphism of PTPN22 encoding lymphoid protein phosphatase, with rheumatoid arthritis and systemic lupus erythematosus. Arthritis Rheum. 2005;52:219–24.
32. Manjarrez-Orduno N, Marasco E, Chung SA, Katz MS, Kiridly JF, et al. CSK regulatory polymorphism is associated with systemic lupus erythematosus and influence B-cell signaling and activation. Nat Genet. 2012;44:1227–30.
33. Behrens TW. Lyp breakdown and autoimmunity. Nat Genet. 2011;43:821–2.
34. Zhang J, Zahir N, Jiang Q, Miliotis H, Heyrand S, et al. The autoimmune disease-associated PTPN22 variant promotes calpain-mediated Lyp/Pep degradation associated with lymphocyte and dendritic cell hyperresponsiveness. Nat Genet. 2011;43:902–7.

35. Vang T, Congia M, Macis MD, Masumeci L, Orru V, et al. Autoimmune-associated lymphoid tyrosine phosphatase is a gain-of-function variant. Nat Genet. 2005;37:1317–9.

36. Arechiga AF, Habib T, He Y, Zhang X, Zhang ZY, et al. Cutting edge: the *PTPN22* allele variant associated with autoimmunity impairs B cell signaling. J Immunol. 2009;182:3343–7.

37. Dai X, James RG, Habib T, Singh S, Jackson S, et al. A disease-associated *PTPN22* variant promotes systemic autoimmunity in murine models. J Clin Invest. 2013;123:2024–36.

38. Cambier JC. Autoimmunity risk alleles: hot spots in B cell regulatory signaling pathways. J Clin Invest. 2013;123:1928–31.

39. Al-Awadi SA, Moussa MA, Naguib KK, Farag TI, Teebi AS, et al. Consanguinity among the Kuwaiti population. Clin Genet. 1985;27:483–6.

40. Shaltout AA, Moussa MAA, Qabazard M, Abdella N, Karvonen M, et al. Further evidence for the rising incidence of childhood type-1 diabetes in Kuwait. Diabet Med. 2002;19(6):522–5.

41. Rasoul MA, Al-Mahdi M, Al-Kandari H, Dhaunsi GS, Haider MZ. Low serum vitamin D status is associated with high prevalence and early onset of type-1 diabetes mellitus in Kuwaiti children. BMC Pediatr. 2016;16:95. https://doi.org/10.1186/s12887-016-0629-3.

42. Teebi AS, Farag TI. Population dimensions in Arab World. In: Teebi AS, Farag TI, editors. Genetic disorders among Arab populations. Oxford, UK: Oxford University Press; 1997. p. 29–51.

9

A prospective, open-label, non-comparative study of ambrisentan with anti-fibrotic agent combination therapy in the treatment of diffuse systemic sclerosis

Annemarie Schorpion[1], Max Shenin[2], Robin Neubauer[1] and Chris T. Derk[1,3*] (iD)

Abstract

Background: Systemic Sclerosis is a multifactorial autoimmune rheumatic disease characterized by inflammation, fibrosis, immune dysregulation and vascular dysfunction.

Methods: An open label, prospective, non-comparative study evaluating ambrisentan with an antifibrotic agent in diffuse cutaneous systemic sclerosis (dcSSc). Recruited 15 consecutive patients with dcSSc who were already on a stable dose of an antifibrotic agent and if they met inclusion criteria they were initiated on ambrisentan 5 mg/day for 12 months. Primary outcome measure was the modified Rodnan skin score (mRSS) while secondary measures were the short form 36 (SF-36) questionnaire, the Medsger severity score and pulmonary function studies.

Results: Fifteen patients were recruited and ten patients completed all 12 months of the study. An intention to treat was used to analyze the data. There was statistical improvement of the mean mRSS and the perceived change in health component of the SF-36. The Medsger severity score and pulmonary function studies remained unchanged over the course of the study.

Conclusion: Patients who tolerated the combination of an antifibrotic with ambrisentan had an improvement of their mRSS over the course of the study as well as an improvement of their perceived health.

Keywords: Systemic sclerosis, Scleroderma, Ambrisentan, Combination therapy, Therapy, Mycophenolic mofetil, Treatment, Open label, Endothelin receptor blocker, Endothelin

Background

Systemic Sclerosis (SSc) is an autoimmune rheumatic disorder of unknown etiology characterized by immune activation with autoantibody production, endothelial injury which leads to vascular dysfunction, and tissue fibrosis of both the cutaneous and visceral organs [1, 2]. It is believed that endothelial injury is the initial event which leads to vessel wall abnormality and an up-regulation of adhesion molecules that in turn attract inflammatory cells which transmigrate through the damaged vessel wall. Once these inflammatory cells migrate into the vessel wall they lead to local production of cytokines and growth factors. Tissue growth factor β (TGFβ) connective tissue growth factor (CTGF), inter-leukin (IL)-13 and IL-6 are just some of the cytokines and growth factors that are locally released in the vessel wall. On the other hand the injured endothelial cells release endothelin (ET)-1 and other vasoconstrictive chemokines. Platelets also play a significant role in the early steps of the pathogenesis of this disorder and they too are attracted to the injured endothelium and they in turn release platelet derived growth factor (PDGF), thrombin and thromboxane which in combination with the above mentioned growth factors and cytokines lead to fibroblast activation, with increased collagen synthesis and

* Correspondence: Chris.Derk@uphs.upenn.edu
[1]Hospital of the University of Pennsylvania, Philadelphia, USA
[3]Division of Rheumatology, University of Pennsylvania, 5th Floor White Building, 3400 Spruce Street, Philadelphia, PA 19107, USA
Full list of author information is available at the end of the article

other extracellular matrix proteins that deposit in the vessel wall, and a subsequent transformation of fibroblasts into myofibroblasts. This results in functional and structural abnormalities of the vessel which in turn is theorized to cause similar changes to the organs that these vessels supply, such as the cutaneous tissue and the visceral organs [2–4]. Endothelin is one of the key pathogenic mediators in SSc having both a vascular and a fibrotic effect. There are three vasoactive peptides ET-1, ET-2 and ET-3 and from them ET-1 is the major isoform.

Endothelin-1 mediates its effects through two receptors, ETA, expressed on mesenchymal cells, and ETB, expressed on endothelial cells. In SSc ET-1 acts on fibroblasts, endothelial cells, smooth muscle cells, and macrophages. Endothelin-1 in SSc acts on the vascular smooth muscle cells to cause increased proliferation and altered vascular tone which in turn leads to vasoconstriction [5]. On endothelial cells it leads to increased proliferation and increased vascular permeability, while on fibroblasts it leads to increased cell proliferation, increased expression of α- smooth muscle actin, and transformation of fibroblasts to myofibroblasts with increased extracellular matrix deposition and decreased fibroblast apoptosis. Skin biopsies from SSc patients when stained with ET-1 reveal up-regulation in the microvessels and ET-1 levels in serum correlate with the extent of skin fibrosis [6]. In a study using bosentan, an ET-1 receptor blocker, 10 patients were treated in a prospective open-label, non-comparative trial for 24 weeks and both limited cutaneous systemic sclerosis (lcSSc) and dcSSc exhibited a statistical significant decrease in mRSS with a mean change in mRSS from baseline of 6.4 [7]. Randomized placebo controlled trials evaluating therapeutic agents for diffuse systemic sclerosis have been undertaken though often with negative results as these studies are often difficult to complete because of the rarity of the disease and the question if true placebo is an ethical option in such patients. Open label single center studies while inferior to the design of randomized controlled studies have in this particular disease helped establish certain agents as potential therapeutic agents in systemic sclerosis.

The hypothesis we based this study on is that endothelin receptor blockers in combination with disease modifying agents with antifibrotic properties will have additive influence on diminishing fibrosis, inhibiting cellular and humoral hyperactivity and interfering with smooth muscle proliferation in the vessel wall. Targeting the vasculopathic component of SSc and the potential overall disease modification effect this may have in the pathogenesis of the disease as a whole is an aspect that has as of yet not been clearly described in SSc but felt that it may influence disease progression based on the vasculopathic phenotype of the individual patient [8, 9] . The primary outcome measure of this study was to determine the benefit that ambrisentan in combination with an antifibrotic agent on the modified Rodnan skin score (mRSS) of early dcSSc patients.

Secondary outcome measures were to examine the effect of this combination therapy on the Medsger severity score [10] as well as quality of life measures as assessed by the SF-36 [11]. Safety parameters included clinical laboratory tests defining internal organ involvement, adverse events, physical examinations, vital signs and concomitant medications. Ambrisentan related adverse events such as anemia, fluid retention, peripheral edema, nasal congestion and flushing were of a primary focus.

Methods

We designed an open label, single center study to determine the efficacy and safety of ambrisentan in combination with an antifibrotic agent (which could include mycopheolate mofetil, mycophenolic acid, methotrexate or cyclophosphamide). The patients would have had to have a diagnosis of dcSSc and onset of skin sclerosis less than 48 months from study entry and would have to already be treated with one of the above antifibrotic agents. All patients received ambrisentan 5 mg per day for a total of 12 months in combination with the antifibrotic agent. Once we received ethical approval from the institutional review board of the University of Pennsylvania we recruited consecutive patients both from within our own Rheumatology clinic but also from outside referrals from the local region. Patients had an initial baseline evaluation to determine if they met inclusion criteria. Once they were enrolled in the study they had monthly follow ups to capture safety issues and efficacy of the combination therapy. A full physical exam was performed at screen, 1,3,5,6,7,9,11 and 12 months and the SF-36 at screen, 1,3,6,9,12 months, though for our analysis we compared the screen to month 12 questionnaires. The Medsger severity score was evaluated at the screen visit and at 12 months, while the modified Rodnan skin score (mRSS) at screen, 6 and 12 months. The physical exam, Medsger severity score, mRSS were performed by the same investigator (CTD) to avoid interrater variability. Temporary dose reduction of ambrisentan below 5 mg/day was allowed for no more than 14 days in total during the study period. Monthly liver enzymes were followed during the study period and if aminotransferases were > 5 x the upper limit of normal (ULN) or a bilirubin of > 2 x ULN the study agent was stopped. If the aminotransferase level was > 3× ULN but <5xULN ambrisentan was stopped until the levels were < 3xULN. Pregnancy testing was performed every 3 months in all women capable of conception while two forms of contraception were recommend in all such patients.

The recruited patients had to be at least 18 years of age, fulfill the American Rheumatism Association criteria for systemic sclerosis, and satisfy subset criteria for diffuse cutaneous involvement as published by LeRoy et al. [12, 13] as the study inception was before the development of the 2013 ACR/EULAR SSc classification criteria [14]. Inclusion criteria included skin sclerosis ongoing for less than 48 months from study entry and a current regimen consisting of a stable dose of an antifibrotic agent. Previous history of using an alternate antifibrotic agent was permitted. Subjects were excluded if they had previous exposure to an endothelin receptor antagonist or were diagnosed with pulmonary arterial hypertension (PAH) and were on a PAH targeted therapy. If the total duration of anti-fibrotic treatment prior to study entry exceeded 48 months, or if they required corticosteroids equivalent to a dose of more than 20 mg/day of prednisone. Prohibited medications were biologic agents such as tumor necrosis factor (TNF)-alpha inhibitors within 6 months from study entry or rituxan within 12 months from study entry. Other exclusions included pregnancy or nursing, other scleroderma like illness, or other concomitant autoimmune rheumatic disorder, major surgery in the past 1 month, history of gastrointestinal hemorrhage within 6 months of initiation of study, unhealed peptic ulcers, congenital or acquired immune deficiency, history of severe viral illness, history of severe cardiovascular disease, congestive heart failure, liver dysfunction, current intravenous antibiotics. For the sample size calculation, we assumed a difference in the mean skin score from maximum to study end at 0.45, a value based on data from a previous study [15]. Using an $\alpha = 0.05$, we calculated the sample size at $n = 19$ and we were able to recruit 15 patients into the study, all of whom agreed to the terms of participation and signed informed consent.

Results

Study population

A total of 15 patients were recruited for the study (Fig. 1), of which 10 were women and 5 were men. Fourteen of the patients were Caucasian and one was African American. The mean age was 47.6 ± 10.7 years old and 14 patients had a positive antinuclear antibody (ANA) with a median titer of 1:640. Ten patients had a speckled pattern and four a homogeneous pattern. One of our patients had a dual ANA pattern with both a speckled and a nucleolar pattern. The mean study entry white blood cell (WBC) count was 7907/μL blood, and mean erythrocyte sedimentation rate (ESR) 15.4 mm/h. At study entry, eight patients were taking a proton pump inhibitor, four a calcium channel blocker, five an

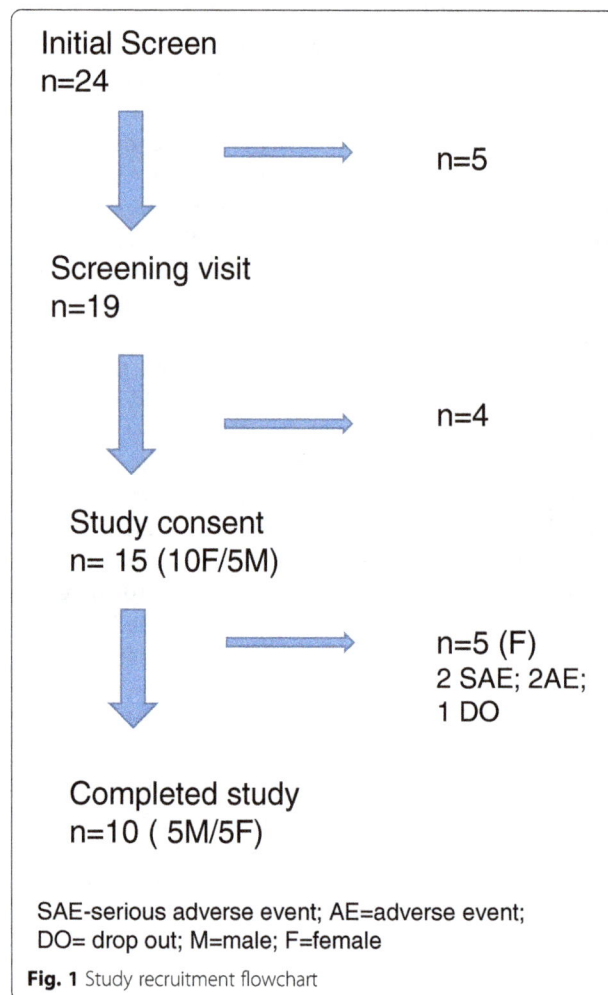

Fig. 1 Study recruitment flowchart

Initial Screen
n=24

n=5

Screening visit
n=19

n=4

Study consent
n= 15 (10F/5M)

n=5 (F)
2 SAE; 2AE;
1 DO

Completed study
n=10 (5M/5F)

SAE-serious adverse event; AE=adverse event; DO= drop out; M=male; F=female

angiotensin converting enzyme inhibitor, and four were taking daily aspirin. Six patients were taking daily prednisone (five patients were taking 5 mg per day and one was taking 10 mg per day) (Table 1).

The antifibrotic agents used included 12 patients on mycophenolate mofetil, two on mycophenolic acid and one on methotrexate. One of the patients on mycophenolate mofetil had also received cyclophosphamide prior to the initiation of the current antifibrotic agent. Five patients terminated the study early, two because of a serious adverse event (SAE) that required a hospitalization, two patients had an adverse event (AE) that caused them to terminate the study, while one patient was lost to follow-up. One patient had worsening anemia from gastric antral vascular ectasia (GAVE) at 6 months into the study and had to be hospitalized, one patient had anxiety, migraine headache, and adynamic ileus at 6 months which also required hospitalization. Another patient had lower extremity swelling at 1 month and one patient had pruritus, and tingling of the extremities and trunk also at 1 month. Finally, one patient was lost to follow up

Table 1 Study population characteristics (*n* = 15)

Age, mean (SD)	47.6 (10.7)
Race, n (%)	
White	14 (93)
Black or African American	1 (7)
Sex, n (%)	
female	10 (67)
male	5 (33)
Presence of ANA, n (%)	14 (93)
ANA Pattern[a], n (%)	
speckled	10 (67)
homogeneous	4 (27)
nucleolar	1 (7)
Scl-70	4 (27)
RNP	0
SSA/SSB	0
dsDNA	0
WBC (per μL), mean (SD)	7907 (2077)
ESR[b], mean (SD), mm/h	15.4 (8.8)
Medication use, n (%)	
Antifibrotic agent[c]	
mycophenolate mofetil	12 (80)
mycophenolic acid	2 (13)
methotrexate	1 (7)
cyclophosphamide	1 (7)
prednisone	
(none)	9 (60)
5 mg/d	3 (33)
10 mg/d	1 (7)
PPI	8 (53)
CCB	4 (27)
ACEi	5 (33)
ARB	0
statin	2 (13)
ASA	5 (34)
NSAID	1 (7)
Clinical symptoms, n (%)	
ILD	4 (27)
SIBO	1 (7)
GERD	9 (60)
Hypothyroidism	2 (13)
Raynaud's	15 (100)
DU	4 (27)
GAVE	1 (7)
Esophageal dysmotility	5 (33)
Pericardial effusion	1 (7)

Table 1 Study population characteristics (*n* = 15) *(Continued)*

SRC	1 (7)
HTN	1 (7)
Arthritis	2 (13)
Sicca	1 (7)
Calcinosis	1 (7)
Intestinal Pseudobstruction	1 (7)
Disease duration months(SD)	
Raynaud's	37 ± 40
Skin sclerosis	19 ± 15

ANA anti-nuclear antibody, *ESR* erythrocyte sedimentation rate, *PPI* proton pump inhibitor, *CCB* calcium channel blocker, *ACEi* angiotensin-converting enzyme inhibitor, *ARB* angiotensin receptor blocker, *NSAID* non-steroidal anti-inflammatory drug, *ILD* interstitial lung disease, *SIBO* small intestinal bacterial overgrowth, *GERD* gastroesophageal reflux disease, *DU* digital ulcer, *GAVE* gastric antral vascular ectasia, *SRC* scleroderma renal crisis, *HTN* hypertension
[a]1 patient had both a speckled and nucleolar pattern; 1 patient did not have the presence of an ANA detected; 1 patient's ANA status was unknown
[b]2 patients had unknown levels of ESR at study entry
[c]1 patient received both cyclophosphamide and mycophenolate mofetil

after the 6 month visit and on subsequent follow up communication the patient was well with no adverse events and did not follow up as he did not want to continue in the study.

mRSS

The primary outcome measure of the study was the mRSS. We used an intention-to-treat analysis for all patients who entered into the study and for missing data on patients who terminated the study early we imputed values based on the last observation carried forward. For the five patients who terminated early, in 2 the imputed values were collected at 1 month into the study and for 3 patients at 6 months into the study. The mean mRSS at study entry was 21 (standard deviation (SD) 7.4, range 13–36). At 6 months, the mean mRSS was 16 (SD 10.8) and at 12 months, 13 (SD 11.2) (Fig. 2). Using one-way ANOVA analysis, comparing the mean mRSS at the time of study entry and study end, we observed a mean difference in mRSS of − 8 ($t = − 5.08$, $p = 0.000167$).

Medsger severity score

The degree of visceral organ involvement was quantified using the Medsger severity score. The Medsger severity score includes nine categories (general, peripheral vascular, skin, joints, muscular, gastrointestinal, pulmonary, cardiac and renal) representing areas of potential organ involvement by SSc. Each category is rated on a scale from 0 to 4, with higher numbers signifying more severe organ disease. At study entry, the median Medsger severity score for the population studied (*n* = 15) was as follows: peripheral vascular 1 and skin 2. Median scores for all other categories were 0. At study end, the median peripheral vascular score was 1 and the median skin

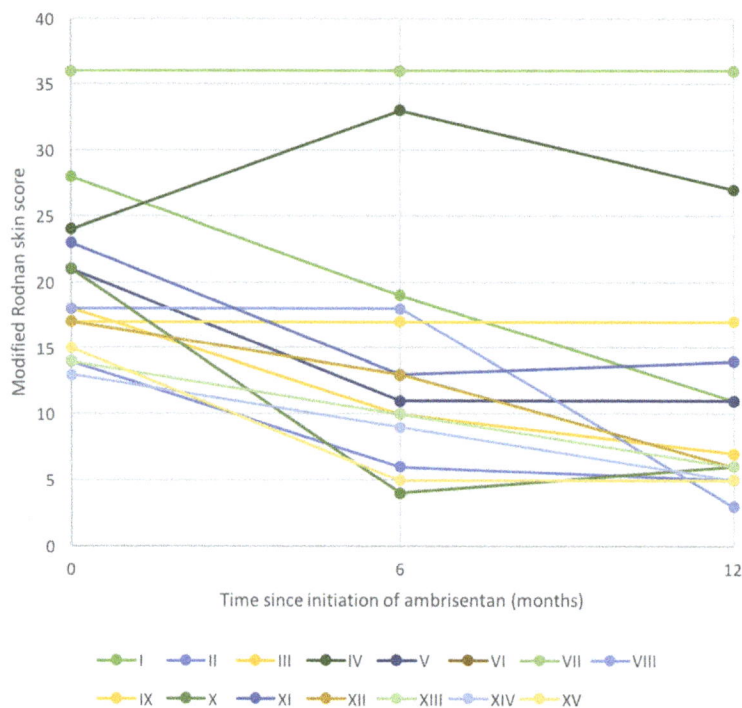

Fig. 2 Individual patient modified Rodnan skin scores at 0, 6 and 12 months of the study

score was 1. Median scores for all other categories remained 0.

Pulmonary function studies

All study patients were asked to have complete pulmonary function tests (PFT's) performed at study entry, 6 months and at the end of the study at 12 months. For the purpose of our study, we compared mean values for forced vital capacity (FVC), total lung capacity (TLC) and pulmonary diffusing capacity (DL_{CO}) for all patients ($n = 12$) at all three time points (Fig. 3). The mean FVC was 93.5% predicted at study entry, 88.2% predicted at 6 months, and 86.5% predicted at 12 months. The TLC was 93.7%

predicted at study entry, 87.3% predicted at 6 months, and 90.1% predicted at 12 months. The DL_{CO} was 85.7% predicted at study entry, 75% predicted at 6 months and 75.4% predicted at 1 2 months. Using a one-way ANOVA to analyze the data, there was no statistically significant change observed. All of our patients had echocardiograms at study entry and all patients had normal ejection fractions and no suggestions of elevated right ventricular systolic pressure, as such patients were excluded.

SF-36

Every 3 months each patient was asked to fill out the SF-36 questionnaire. For this study, we compared the

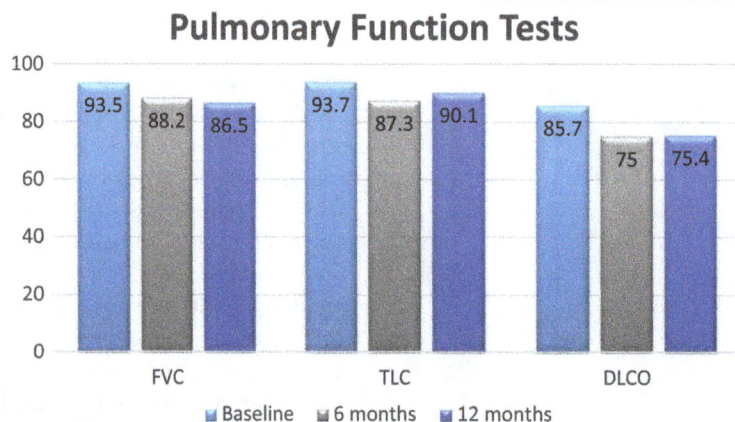

Fig. 3 Pulmonary Function Tests (PFTs) at 0, 6 and 12 months since initiation of ambrisentan

results at study entry with those at study end of the patients who completed all 12 months of therapy ($n = 10$). The SF-36 is a 36 item questionnaire which describes quality of life across eight different domains. Physical functioning; role limitations due to physical health; role limitations due to emotional problems; energy/fatigue; emotional wellbeing; social functioning; general health; and perceived change in health. The mean SF-36 score at study entry was 62 (23.3) and 65.9 (25.7) at study end, a difference that was not statistically significant ($p = 0.092$). However, the mean perceived change in health component at study entry was 37.5 (39.5) compared to 55 (38.7) at study end, a significant difference of 17.5 ($p = 0.025$). No statistically significant differences were detected among scores in the other 7 categories of the SF-36 questionnaire.

Discussion

Systemic Sclerosis continues to lack a universally acceptable therapy though consensus statements have recommended such agents as methotrexate and mycophenolate mofetil as acceptable therapies for dcSSc patients and this is based on open label studies, cases series and randomized controlled treatment trials [16]. Data from the two well designed randomized controlled trials for SSc related interstitial lung disease, the Scleroderma lung trial 1 and 2 have emphasized the statistical significant results on FVC in the group taking cyclophosphamide in the first study and the equivalent results of mycophenolate mofetil to cyclophosphamide in the second trial. While the absolute FVC changes are small, both studies also have suggested that these agents have significant skin results based on the mRSS [17, 18]. With the current study we attempt to look at the potential of combination therapy in dcSSc, targeting fibrosis, inflammation and the vasculopathy of this disease. Using a baseline antifibrotic agent such as methotrexate, mycophenolate mofetil or mycophenolic acid in combination with an ERA such as ambrisentan which may have a vascular modifying effect in SSc patients we attempted to see the tolerability of this regimen and its effect on the mRSS and other disease parameters and more specifically the SF-36 and Medger severity score. With the combination therapy in early dcSSc patients we attempted targeting fibrosis, inflammation and the vasculopathy of this disease. Patients who tolerated ambrisentan in combination with an antifibrotic agent showed an overall improvement in their mRSS and their perceived physical health, while over the 12 months of the study they did not have progression of their disease severity based on the Medsger severity scale. While the study has all of the limitations expected from an open label non-comparative study it does reveal that patients who tolerated the regimen had stability in their disease process and had improvement in their skin scores. Our inability to recruit the correct amount of patients to our study based on our power calculations may have also negatively affected some of our results where we observed some difference but not quiet statistically significant such as the total SF-36 score at study entry vs study end. Recruitment was hampered because many patients newly diagnosed with dcSSc at our institution are placed on antifibrotic agents as well as PAH related vasodilatory therapy either for PAH or Raynaud's. Another limitation is the fact that 5 patients did not complete the whole study based on SAEs, AEs and a single drop out. While the SAE's and AE's may have been related to the study agent patients who tolerated the study agent fared well as per our results and this can help future studies looking at this combination therapy to design based on such an estimated drop out from SAEs and AEs While our results don't clearly define if the improvement in the mRSS is based on delayed immunomodulatory effects from the antifibrotic agents the patients were already on at study entry, the natural course of the disease or specifically the combination therapy what we can conclude is that patients who tolerated the combination therapy and who had early dcSSc disease remained stable over the 12 months of the study among all of the Medsger severity domains and had an improvement in their skin scores and perceived changes in health. For this to be looked in more detail a randomized placebo controlled comparative study needs to be undertaken to decipher how much of this effect relates to the antifibrotic agent itself and how much from the combination of an antifibrotic and an ERA, and in addition to measures used in this study tissue and serum based biomarkers may also help us to better identify the potential of combination therapy for this disorder. Also more detailed measures of the individual organ involvement beyond the Medsger severity score will also give a better definition of organ involvement and treatment related changes. In the current study biomarkers were not explored as the inception of the study was previous to their more well defined description and use in clinical research [19]. While ERA's are only approved for pulmonary arterial hypertension in the US, bosentan has received approval in the EU for the reduction of the number of new digital ulcerations in SSc patients. As systemic sclerosis is a multifactorial illness characterized by early inflammation, immune dysregulation, vascular dysfunction and fibrosis, targeting just one of these components of the illness may not be a realistic way at looking at treating this autoimmune rheumatic disorder. Targeting all components that take part in the development of this disease may be a more realistic approach.

Conclusion

Combination therapy with an antifibrotic and an endothelin receptor antagonist in patients with dcSSc improved the mRSS and the patient's perceived physical health over a 12 month treatment period while disease severity did not worsen during the treatment period. A large randomized study is needed to further evaluate the utility of combination therapy in dcSSc.

Abbreviations

AE: Adverse event; ANA: Antinuclear antibody; CTGF: Connective tissue growth factor; dcSSc: Diffuse cutaneous systemic sclerosis; DLCO: Diffusing lung capacity; ESR: Erythrocyte sedimentation rate; ET: Endothelin; FVC: Forced vital capacity; GAVE: Gastric antral vascular ectasia; IL: Interleukin; lcSSc: Limited cutaneous systemic sclerosis; mRSS: Modified Rodnan skin score; PAH: Pulmonary arterial hypertension; PDGF: Platelet derived growth factor; PFT: Pulmonary function test; SAE: Serious adverse events; SD: Standard deviation; SF-36: Short form-36; SSc: Systemic sclerosis; TGF-β: Tissue growth factor beta; TLC: Total lung capacity; TNF: Tumor necrosis factor; ULN: Upper limit of normal; WBC: White blood cell

Funding

Funding and study drug for this study was provided by Gilead Pharmaceuticals. Gilead had no role in the design, collection, analysis, data interpretation or in writing of the manuscript.

Authors' contributions

AS: data collection, data analysis and manuscript preparation. MS: study design, institutional review application. RN: study implementation, data collection. CTD: study design, Institutional review application, study implementation, data collection, data analysis and manuscript preparation. All authors have read and approve the manuscript.

Competing interests

Schorpion A, Shenin M, Neubauer R: No conflicts.
Derk CT: Received research funding from Gilead.

Author details

[1]Hospital of the University of Pennsylvania, Philadelphia, USA. [2]Thomas Jefferson University Hospital, Philadelphia, USA. [3]Division of Rheumatology, University of Pennsylvania, 5th Floor White Building, 3400 Spruce Street, Philadelphia, PA 19107, USA.

References

1. Jimenez SA, Derk CT. Following the molecular pathways toward an understandingof the pathogenesis of systemic sclerosis. Ann Intern Med. 2004;140(1):37–50.
2. Allanore Y, Simms R, Distler O, Trojanowska M, Pope J, Denton CP, Varga J. Systemic sclerosis. Nat Rev Dis Primers. 2015;1:15002.
3. Elhai M, Avouac J, Kahan A, Allanore Y. Systemic sclerosis: recent insights. Joint Bone Spine. 2015;82:148–53.
4. Denton CP, Khanna D. Systemic sclerosis. Lancet. 2017;390(10103):1685–99.
5. La M, Reid JJ. Endothelin-1 and the regulation of vascular tone. Clin Exp Pharmacol Physiol. 1995;22(5):315–23.
6. Shetty N, Derk CT. Endothelin receptor antagonists as disease modifiers in systemic sclerosis. Inflamm Allergy Drug Targets. 2011;10(1):19–26.
7. Kuhn A, Haust M, Ruland V, Weber R, Verde P, Felder G, Ohmann C, Gensch K, Ruzicka T. Effect of bosentan on skin fibrosis in patients with systemic sclerosis: a prospective, open-label, non-comparative trial. Rheumatology. 2010;49(7):1336–45.
8. Allanore Y, Distler O, Matucci-Cerinic M, Denton CP. Defining a unified vascular phenotype in systemic sclerosis. Arthritis Rheum. 2018;70(2):162–70.
9. Mostmans Y, Cutolo M, Giddelo C, Decuman S, Melsens K, Declercq H, Vandecasteele E, De Keyser F, Distler O, Gutermuth J, Smith V. The role of endothelial cells in the vasculopathy of systemic sclerosis: a systematic review. Autoimmun Rev. 2017;16(8):774–86.
10. Medsger TA Jr, Silman AJ, Steen VD, Black CM, Akesson A, Bacon PA, Harris CA, Jablonska S, Jayson MI, Jimenez SA, Krieg T, Leroy EC, Maddison PJ, Russell ML, Schachter RK, Wollheim FA, Zacharaie H. A disease severity scale for systemic sclerosis: development and testing. J Rheumatol. 1999;26(10):2159 67.
11. Khanna D, Furst DE, Clements PJ, Park GS, Hays RD, Yoon J, Korn JH, Merkel PA, Rothfield N, Wigley FM, Moreland LW, Silver R, Steen VD, Weisman M, Mayes MD, Collier DH, Medsger TA, Seibold JR, Relaxin Study Group. Responsiveness of the SF-36 and the health assessment questionnaire disability index in systemic sclerosis clinical trial. J Rheumatol. 2005;32(5):832–40.
12. Subcommittee for scleroderma criteria of the American Rheumatism Association Diagnostic and Therapeutic Criteria Committee. Preliminary criteria for the classification of systemic sclerosis (scleroderma). Arthritis Rheum. 1980;23:581–90.
13. LeRoy EC, Black CM, Fleiscmajer R, et al. Scleroderma: classification, subsets and pathogenesis. J Rheumatol. 1988;15:202–5.
14. van den Hoogen F, Khanna D, Fransen J, Johnson SR, Baron M, Tyndall A, Mattuci-Cerinic M, Naden RP, Medsger TA, Carreira PE, Riemekasten G, Clements PJ, Denton CP, Distler O, Allanore Y, FUrst DE, Gabrielli A, Mayes MD, van Laar JM, Seibold JR, Czirjak L, Steen VD, Inanc M, KOwal-Bielecka O, Muller-Ladner U, Valentini G, Veale DJ, Vonk MC, Walker UA, Chung L, Collier DH, Ellen Csuka M, Fessler BJ, Guiducci S, Herrick A, Hsu VM, Jimenez S, Kahaleh B, Merkel PA, Sierakowski S, Silver RM, Simms RW, Varga J, Pope JE. 2013 classification criteria for systemic sclerosis; an American college of rheumatology/European league against rheumatism collaborative initiative. Ann Rheum Dis. 2013;72(11):1747–55.
15. Derk CT, Huaman G, Jimenez SA. A retrospective randomly selected cohort of D-penicillamine treatment in rapidly progressive diffuse cutaneous systemic sclerosis of recent onset. Br J Dermatol. 2008;158:1063–8.
16. Kowal-Bielecka O, Fransen J, Avouac J, Becker M, Kulak A, Allanore Y, Disteler O, Clements P, Cutolo M, Czirjak L, Damjanov N, Del Galdo F, Denton CP, Distler JHW, Foeldvari I, Figelstone K, Frerix M, Furst DE, Guiducci S, Hunzelmann N, Khanna D, Mattuci-Cerinic M, Herrick AL, van den Hoogen F, van Laar JM, Riemekasten G, Silver R, Smith V, Sulli A, Tarner I, Tyndall A, Welling J, Wigley F, Valentini G, Walker UA, Zulian F, Muller-Ladner U, EUSTAR Coauthors. Update of EULAR recommendations for the treatment of systemic sclerosis. Ann Rheum Dis. 2017;76(8):1327–39.
17. Goldin J, Elashoff R, Kim HJ, Yan X, Lynch D, Strollo D, Roth MD, Clements P, Furst DE, Khanna D, Vasunilashorn S, Li G, Tashkin DP. Treatment of scleroderma-interstitial lung disease with cyclophosphamide is associated with less progressive fibrosison serial thoracic high-resolution CT scan than placebo; findings from the scleroderma lung study. Chest. 2009;136(5):1333–40.
18. Tashkin DP, Roth MD, Clements PJ, Furst DE, Khanna D, Kleerup EC, Goldin J, Arriola E, Volkmann ER, Kafaja S, Silver R, Steen V, Strange C, Wise R, Wigley F, Mayes M, Riley DJ, Hussain S, Assassi S, Hsu VM, Patel B, Philips K, Martinez F, Golden J, Connolly MK, Varga J, Dematte J, Hitchcliff ME, Fischer A, Swirgis J, Meehan R, Theodore A, Simms R, Volkov S, Schraufnagel DE, Scholand MB, Frech T, Molitor JA, Highland K, Read CA, Dritzler MJ, Kim GHJ, Tseng CH, Scleroderma Lung Study II investigators. Mycophenolate mofetil versus oral cyclophosphamide in scleroderma-related interstitial lung disease (SLSII): a randomised controlled, double-blind, parallel group trial. Lancet Respir Med. 2016;4(9):708–19.
19. Ligon C, Hummers LK. Biomarkers in scleroderma: progressing from association to clinical utility. Curr Rheumatol Rep. 2016;18(3):17.

10

Network meta-analysis and cost per responder of targeted Immunomodulators in the treatment of active psoriatic arthritis

Vibeke Strand[1], M. Elaine Husni[2], Keith A. Betts[3*], Yan Song[4], Rakesh Singh[5], Jenny Griffith[5], Marci Beppu[5], Jing Zhao[4] and Arijit Ganguli[5]

Abstract

Background: Multiple targeted immunomodulators (TIMs) for psoriatic arthritis (PsA) treatment are available, but limited studies have directly compared these agents. This study indirectly compared the efficacy of TNF-α, interleukins, and phosphodiesterase-4 inhibitors for treatment of active PsA.

Methods: A systematic literature review was conducted to identify phase III randomized controlled trials (RCTs) for adalimumab, certolizumab pegol, etanercept, golimumab, infliximab, ustekinumab, secukinumab, and apremilast in active PsA. Joint (ACR20/50/70) and skin outcomes (PASI75/90) at Week 24 with each TIM were estimated via a Bayesian network meta-analysis, and the incremental cost per responder over the first 24 weeks of treatment was calculated. Similar analyses were conducted in a subgroup of biologic-naïve patients.

Results: Seventeen RCTs were identified; 13 included ACR and/or PASI responses at Week 24. Among the overall population, patients receiving adalimumab, golimumab, and infliximab showed higher ACR20/50/70 (adalimumab: 61.2/42.8/40.8%, golimumab: 61.6/39.8/27.4%, infliximab: 56.2/57.1/34.2%) and PASI75/90 (72.7/55.5%, 74.1/57.2%, and 77.1/61.0%, respectively) responses at Week 24 compared with other TIMs. In terms of cost-effectiveness, these treatments were also associated with the lowest incremental cost per responder for both skin and joint outcomes. Similar rankings of efficacy and incremental cost per responder were observed in the analysis among biologic-naive patients.

Conclusions: Adalimumab, golimumab, and infliximab were associated with higher efficacy and lower incremental costs per responder for both joint and skin responses in active PsA.

Keywords: Arthritis, psoriatic, Meta-analysis, Immunomodulators, Cost-benefit analysis

Background

Psoriatic arthritis (PsA) is a chronic inflammatory arthritis that occurs in up to 24% of psoriasis patients [1]. In the majority of PsA patients, skin symptoms precede the arthritis, and common manifestations of the disease may include synovitis, enthesitis, dactylitis, and anterior uveitis [2]. Similar to rheumatoid arthritis, PsA can be disabling and lead to erosive arthropathy in some patients [3]. A variety of therapeutic agents are available for the management of PsA, although the clinical heterogeneity of the disease poses a challenge to clinicians

in determining the best treatment [4]. PsA patients with moderate to severe symptoms typically require disease modifying anti-rheumatic drugs (DMARDs), non-steroidal anti-inflammatory drugs (NSAIDs), phototherapy, or a combination of the three [5]. Recent studies have shown that traditional DMARDs, such as methotrexate, are ineffective for preventing progression of joint damage and may have serious adverse effects [6–8].

Immunomodulators (TIMs) such as tumor necrosis factor-α (TNF) inhibitors, interleukin inhibitors, and phosphodiesterase-4 inhibitors have dramatically changed the therapeutic paradigm of PsA [9]. Although demonstrated to be more effective than traditional DMARDs, the relative efficacy and cost-effectiveness of these newly investigated agents remains uncertain. Reliable evidence

* Correspondence: Keith.Betts@analysisgroup.com
[3]Analysis Group Inc., 333 South Hope Street, 27th Floor, Los Angeles, CA 90071, USA
Full list of author information is available at the end of the article

regarding the comparative efficacy of these novel PsA agents is crucial for informing clinical and economic decisions about their most appropriate use.

The objective of this study was to determine the comparative efficacy of these TIMs, as well as the incremental cost per responder over the first 24 weeks of treatment in patients with active PsA in the US. Since few head-to-head studies of these therapies have been performed, a network meta-analysis was conducted to synthesize all available evidence from randomized trials and enable indirect comparisons among competing interventions [10]. Detailed methodological reviews and implementation guidelines for network meta-analyses have been published [11, 12], and network meta-analyses have become a preferred source of evidence among researchers, medical decision makers, and health technology assessment agencies [12–14].

Methods
Trial identification
A systematic literature review was conducted to identify Phase III randomized controlled trials (RCTs) of TNF inhibitors (adalimumab, certolizumab pegol, etanercept, golimumab, and infliximab), interleukin inhibitors (secukinumab and ustekinumab), and a phosphodiesterase-4 inhibitor (apremilast) for active PsA. Trials were conducted in adult patients (age ≥ 18) with active PsA, and included one of the TIMs listed above as active treatment versus placebo or versus another active comparator. RCTs were required to have reported clinical outcome measures for joint responses (by American College of Radiology [ACR] criteria) and/or skin responses (by Psoriasis Area and Severity Index [PASI]). ACR criteria is commonly used to assess the improvement in tender or swollen joint counts, acute phase reactant, patient and physician global assessments, pain scale, and disability/functionality questionnaire. PASI score evaluates the effectiveness of treatment through the assessment of psoriasis lesions in four body regions: head, upper extremities, trunk, and lower extremities. For inclusion, treatment arms were required to use the dose approved by the US Food and Drug Administration (FDA) for each TIM.

Efficacy measures
Joint responses were defined by the ACR20 (20% improvement in ACR criteria), ACR50, and ACR70 response criteria [15]. PASI75 (75% improvement in PASI) and PASI90 responses were used to define skin responses [16, 17]. Efficacy measures at Week 24 were used in the current study, as they were the primary outcome measures for newly investigated agents, including ustekinumab and secukinumab.

Costs
Unit drug costs in the US as of May 8, 2017 were based on wholesale acquisition costs (WAC) obtained from ReadyPrice®. Dosing schedules for each TIM were based on FDA labeling. Costs for infliximab were based on treatment costs of an 80-kg adult and administration costs (intravenous infusion) as of May 8, 2017 were obtained from the US Department of Health and Human Services (CPT code 96413 for the initial hour and 96415 for the subsequent 3 h) [18, 19]. Costs for each TIM over the first 24 weeks of treatment were calculated based on dosing schedules, acquisition costs, and infusion costs.

Statistical methods
A Bayesian network meta-analysis was conducted to assess the comparative efficacy (in terms of ACR20/50/70 and PASI75/90) of different TIMs in the treatment of active PsA. Using a fixed effect model, the number of patients achieving ACR20, ACR50, and ACR70 at Week 24 was assumed to follow a binomial distribution, with the corresponding probabilities linked to the treatment effects via a *logit* function. Non-informative priors were applied to the treatment effect parameter to ensure that treatment comparisons were driven by the observed data. Estimated ACR responses were summarized using posterior means and 95% credible intervals (CrI) for all treatments included in the network.

For the PASI outcomes, a fixed effect, ordinal model assumed that the number of patients achieving PASI50, PASI75, and PASI90 responses followed a multinomial distribution. A *probit* link was used to estimate the probability of each treatment achieving PASI responses based on all observed comparisons. This model allowed the three PASI outcomes to be analyzed jointly, and further assumed that each treatment had the same magnitude of additive effect versus placebo on subsequent levels of PASI responses on the inverse probit scale [20]. A non-informative prior was also specified for the response rates of the reference arm across all RCTs. Based on the model results, PASI75 and PASI90 responses for each therapy were estimated.

Numbers needed to treat (NNT) for each additional responder were calculated as the reciprocal of the difference in estimated response rate between active agent and placebo based on the network meta-analysis. Incremental cost per responder for each treatment relative to placebo was calculated as the product of the total costs over the first 24 weeks of treatment and the NNT. All analyses were conducted within a Bayesian framework and were estimated via Markov chain Monte Carlo using OpenBUGS 3.2.3. Analyses were repeated in the subset of patients without prior biologic treatment.

Results

The systematic literature review identified 17 RCTs that met the inclusion criteria. One trial [21] was excluded because it was only 12 weeks in duration and three other trials [22–24] were excluded because placebo patients crossed over to active treatment prior to Week 24. The remaining 13 trials reported ACR and/or PASI responses at Week 24 after initiation of treatment (Additional file 1: Table S1). Proportion of patients with conventional DMARDs use and with methotrexate (MTX) use at baseline was summarized. Evidence networks of ACR and PASI outcomes among the overall population are shown in Fig. 1a and b, respectively.

Across the selected RCTs, 11 provided stratified results for biologic-naive patients or were conducted in a biologic-naive population (Additional file 2: Table S2). Although Mease 2004 [25] did not explicitly indicate biologic treatment experience of participants, they were assumed to be all biologic-naïve given the era in which this trial was conducted. PASI responses in biologic-naive PsA patients were not available for apremilast and certolizumab pegol. Evidence networks of ACR and PASI outcomes among the biologic-naïve population are shown in Additional file 3: Figure S1A and S1B, respectively.

Network meta-analysis: ACR outcomes

Among the overall population, three TNF inhibitors – golimumab, adalimumab, and infliximab – demonstrated better ACR outcomes compared with other TIMs at Week 24. PsA patients treated with golimumab had the highest ACR20 responses (61.6%), followed by adalimumab (61.2%) and infliximab (56.2%). In terms of ACR50, infliximab had the highest efficacy (57.1%), followed by

etanercept (46.6%), adalimumab (42.8%), and golimumab (39.8%). In terms of ACR70, adalimumab (40.8%), infliximab (34.2%), and golimumab (27.4%) had higher efficacy compared with other TIMs (Table 1).

Similar rankings of ACR20/50/70 responses and NNTs for the different TIMs were observed in the analysis among biologic-naive patients (Additional file 4: Table S3). Biologic-naive patients treated with golimumab, adalimumab, secukinumab, or infliximab had higher ACR20 responses compared with other TIMs. Infliximab, etanercept, adalimumab, and golimumab had numerically higher ACR50 responses compared with other TIMs. In terms of ACR70, adalimumab, infliximab, golimumab, and secukinumab had higher efficacy than other TIMs among the biologic-naïve PsA population.

Network meta-analysis: PASI outcomes

PsA patients treated with infliximab had the highest PASI75 responses at Week 24 (77.1%), followed by golimumab (74.1%), adalimumab (72.7%), and secukinumab 300 mg (60.4%). In terms of PASI90, infliximab had the highest efficacy compared with other TIMs (61.0%), followed by golimumab (57.2%), adalimumab (55.5%), and secukinumab 300 mg (42.3%). Detailed results of the NMA of PASI75 and PASI90 for all TIMs among the overall PsA population are shown in Table 2.

Similar rankings of TIMs in PASI75 and PASI90 responses and NNTs among biologic-naive patients were observed. Among biologic-naive patients, infliximab, golimumab, and adalimumab showed higher PASI75 and PASI90 responses than other TIMs while etanercept had lower efficacy in PASI outcomes.

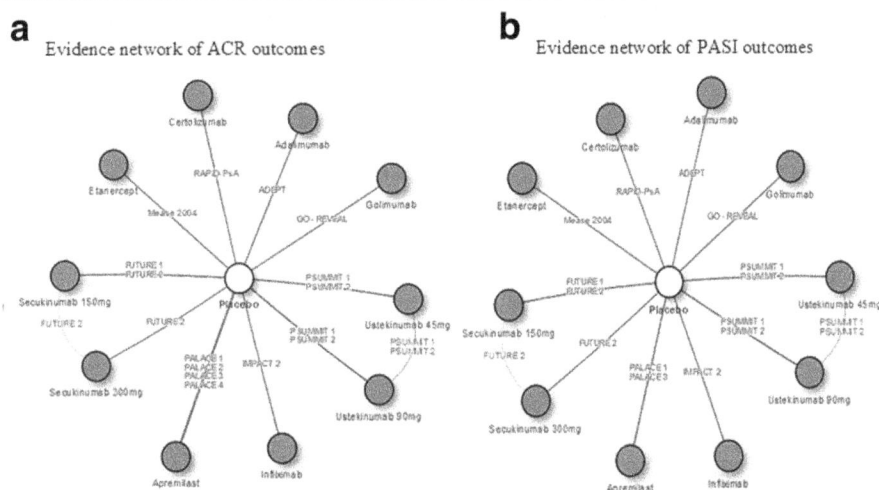

Fig. 1 Evidence network for ACR and PASI outcomes among the overall population. **a** Thirteen trials reported ACR responses at Week 24 were selected: ADEPT [34], PALACE 1 [39], PALACE 2 [40], PALACE 3 [41–43], PALACE 4 [44, 45], RAPID-PsA [46], Mease 2004 [25], GO-REVEAL [47], IMPACT 2 [48], FUTURE 1 [49], FUTURE 2 [50], PSUMMIT 1 [51], and PSUMMIT 2 [52]. (**b**) Eleven trials reported PASI responses at Week 24 were selected: ADEPT [34], PALACE 1 [39], PALACE 3 [41–43], RAPID-PsA [46], Mease 2004 [25], GO-REVEAL [47], IMPACT 2 [48], FUTURE 1 [49], FUTURE 2 [50], PSUMMIT 1 [51], and PSUMMIT 2 [52].

Table 1 ACR response rates and NNT at Week 24 among the overall population

Treatment	ACR20		ACR50		ACR70	
	Response rate (95% CrI)	NNT (95% CrI)	Response rate (95% CrI)	NNT (95% CrI)	Response rate (95% CrI)	NNT (95% CrI)
Placebo	17.0% (15.4%, 18.7%)	–	7.0% (5.9%, 8.2%)	–	2.5% (1.9%, 3.3%)	–
Adalimumab	61.2% (47.8%, 73.6%)	2.3 (1.8, 3.2)	42.8% (27.0%, 62.5%)	2.8 (1.8, 4.9)	40.8% (15.9%, 82.2%)	2.6 (1.3, 7.4)
Apremilast	33.4% (27.1%, 40.4%)	6.1 (4.4, 9.5)	15.5% (10.9%, 21.8%)	11.8 (7.0, 23.5)	5.0% (2.7%, 9.1%)	40.3 (15.8, 222.7)
Certolizumab pegol	50.2% (38.6%, 62.3%)	3.0 (2.2, 4.6)	27.9% (18.0%, 41.8%)	4.8 (2.9, 8.9)	16.7% (7.9%, 35.9%)	7.0 (3.0, 17.8)
Etanercept	50.1% (35.2%, 65.5%)	3.0 (2.1, 5.4)	46.6% (26.6%, 71.2%)	2.5 (1.6, 5.1)	9.1% (2.7%, 32.6%)	15.2 (3.3, 318.5)
Golimumab	61.6% (45.9%, 76.3%)	2.2 (1.7, 3.4)	39.8% (22.0%, 64.7%)	3.1 (1.7, 6.6)	27.4% (9.2%, 71.8%)	4.0 (1.4, 14.6)
Infliximab	56.2% (39.9%, 72.2%)	2.6 (1.8, 4.3)	57.1% (32.7%, 82.5%)	2.0 (1.3, 3.9)	34.2% (12.1%, 77.9%)	3.2 (1.3, 10.3)
Secukinumab 150 mg	51.1% (414%, 61.0%)	2.9 (2.3, 4.0)	33.8% (23.5%, 46.8%)	3.7 (2.5, 6.0)	27.3% (13.4%, 53.1%)	4.0 (2.0, 9.0)
Secukinumab 300 mg	55.2% (41.0%, 68.8%)	2.6 (1.9, 4.1)	34.0% (20.6%, 51.0%)	3.7 (2.3, 7.2)	27.0% (11.3%, 55.7%)	4.1 (1.9, 11.1)
Ustekinumab 45 mg	35.4% (27.5%, 44.4%)	5.4 (3.7, 9.2)	19.9% (13.0%, 29.9%)	7.7 (4.4, 15.8)	10.2% (4.8%, 21.9%)	13.0 (5.2, 39.7)
Ustekinumab 90 mg	39.9% (31.5%, 49.1%)	4.4 (3.2, 6.7)	23.5% (15.6%, 34.3%)	6.1 (3.7, 11.1)	12.1% (5.9%, 25.2%)	10.4 (4.4, 27.8)

CrI credible interval, *NNT* number needed to treat

Detailed results among the biologic-naïve population are shown in Additional file 5: Table S4.

Network meta-analysis: Incremental cost per responder over 24 weeks

From a cost-effectiveness perspective, infliximab, adalimumab, and golimumab have demonstrated lower incremental cost per responder in both joint and skin outcomes compared to other TIMs. Evaluation of the cost-effectiveness over 24 weeks revealed that infliximab ($48,859 for ACR50/$35,277 for PASI75), adalimumab ($74,438 for ACR50/$41,013 for PASI75), and golimumab ($75,966 for ACR50/$37,542 for PASI75) were associated with the lowest incremental costs per additional ACR50 responder and per additional PASI75 responder (Fig. 2a). Similar conclusions can be reached using incremental cost per responder for ACR70 and PASI90. Adalimumab ($69,641 for ACR70/$50,717 for PASI90), infliximab ($77,347 for ACR70/$42,171 for PASI90), and golimumab ($100,158 for ACR70/$45,926 for PASI90) were associated with the lowest incremental costs per responder over 24 weeks (Fig. 2b).

A similar ranking of these TIMs in terms of cost-effectiveness was observed in the biologic-naïve population. Infliximab, adalimumab, and golimumab were consistently associated with lower incremental cost per responder over 24 weeks in both joint and skin outcomes compared to other TIMs (Additional file 6: Figure S2A and S2B). Detailed results of incremental costs per responder for all ACR and PASI outcomes among overall and biologic-naïve populations are shown in Additional files 7 and 8: Tables S5 and S6, respectively.

Table 2 PASI response rates and NNT at Week 24 among the overall population

Treatment	PASI75		PASI90	
	Response (95% CrI)	NNT (95% CrI)	Response (95% CrI)	NNT (95% CrI)
Placebo	7.6% (5.2%, 10.8%)	–	2.9% (1.8%, 4.5%)	–
Adalimumab	72.7% (54.0%, 86.7%)	1.5 (1.3, 2.1)	55.5% (36.0%, 74.3%)	1.9 (1.4, 3.0)
Apremilast	23.9% (14.1%, 36.5%)	6.2 (3.6, 13.3)	12.0% (6.1%, 21.0%)	11.0 (5.7, 26.5)
Certolizumab pegol	45.6% (31.6%, 60.4%)	2.6 (1.9, 4.0)	28.4% (17.4%, 42.1%)	3.9 (2.6, 6.7)
Etanercept	26.0% (12.9%, 44.1%)	5.5 (2.8, 16.7)	13.4% (5.5%, 27.1%)	9.6 (4.2, 34.1)
Golimumab	74.1% (56.1%, 87.7%)	1.5 (1.3, 2.0)	57.2% (37.9%, 75.8%)	1.8 (1.4, 2.8)
Infliximab	77.1% (60.5%, 89.5%)	1.4 (1.2, 1.9)	61.0% (42.4%, 78.8%)	1.7 (1.3, 2.5)
Secukinumab 150 mg	50.3% (36.1%, 65.3%)	2.3 (1.8, 3.4)	32.4% (20.6%, 47.2%)	3.4 (2.3, 5.5)
Secukinumab 300 mg	60.4% (39.7%, 79.2%)	1.9 (1.4, 3.0)	42.3% (23.6%, 63.7%)	2.5 (1.7, 4.8)
Ustekinumab 45 mg	51.2% (37.5%, 64.8%)	2.3 (1.8, 3.2)	33.2% (21.8%, 46.6%)	3.3 (2.3, 5.1)
Ustekinumab 90 mg	58.2% (44.7%, 70.8%)	2.0 (1.6, 2.6)	39.9% (27.5%, 53.4%)	2.7 (2.0, 4.0)

CrI credible interval, *NNT* number needed to treat

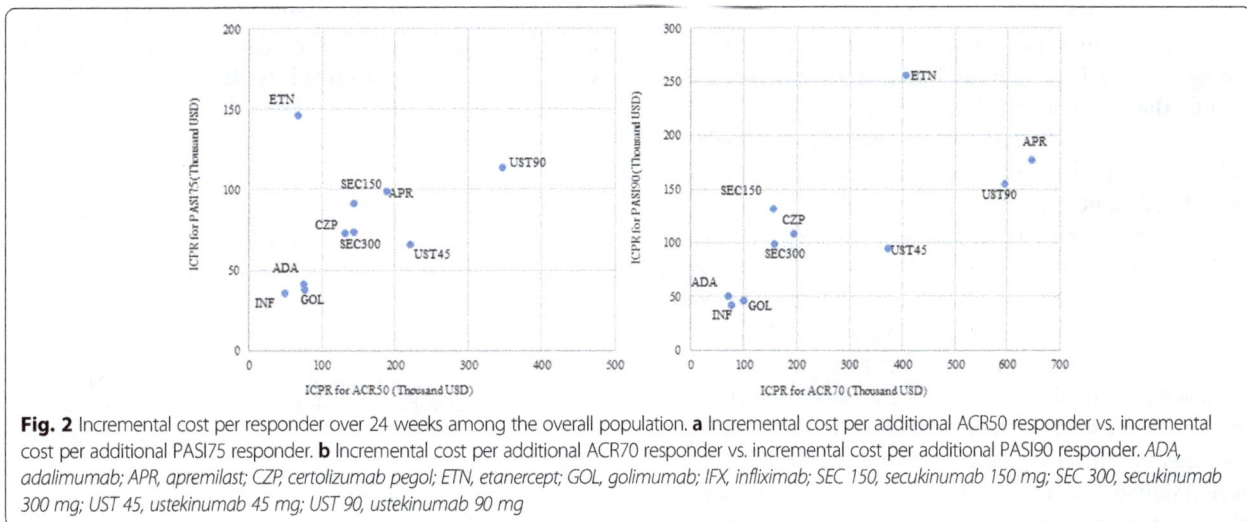

Fig. 2 Incremental cost per responder over 24 weeks among the overall population. **a** Incremental cost per additional ACR50 responder vs. incremental cost per additional PASI75 responder. **b** Incremental cost per additional ACR70 responder vs. incremental cost per additional PASI90 responder. *ADA, adalimumab; APR, apremilast; CZP, certolizumab pegol; ETN, etanercept; GOL, golimumab; IFX, infliximab; SEC 150, secukinumab 150 mg; SEC 300, secukinumab 300 mg; UST 45, ustekinumab 45 mg; UST 90, ustekinumab 90 mg*

Discussion

The treatment goal for PsA is to improve signs and symptoms of disease, including both peripheral arthritis (which is associated with radiographic progression and deterioration of physical function) and skin disease (which is associated with mental health and impaired quality of life) [26–28]. In this network meta-analysis, adalimumab, golimumab, and infliximab showed better efficacy and cost-effectiveness relative to other TIMs in both joint and skin outcomes. Specifically, these treatments had the lowest NNTs and incremental costs per additional responder over 24 weeks across all evaluated TIMs among the overall population as well as the biologic-naïve population. The rankings of other TIMs in terms of response rate, NNT, and incremental costs per additional responder were similar in the overall and biologic-naïve populations.

Several previous network meta-analyses / economic evaluations have investigated the efficacy and cost-effectiveness of TIMs for PsA. One conducted from the UK NHS perspective included adalimumab, etanercept, golimumab, and infliximab and concluded that etanercept was cost-effective – with similar joint responses by PsA response criteria (PsARC) despite lower PASI responses compared to adalimumab, golimumab, and infliximab [29, 30]. Another study, based on the same set of RCTs, concluded that golimumab and etanercept were associated with higher PsARC responses compared with adalimumab and infliximab [31]. Limitations of both analyses include inconsistent time points for outcome measurement. Thorlund et al. [31] used the last observed time point as the primary endpoint despite including some studies with only Week 12 endpoints [21, 23] and others with Week 24 endpoints. In the current systematic literature review, studies reporting only Week 12 outcomes were excluded from

analyses to facilitate a fair comparison across TIMs. In addition, a third study (McInnes 2016) concluded comparable response rates between secukinumab and TNF inhibitors across all ACR outcomes in the mixed population of biologic-naïve and biologic-experienced PsA patients [32]. A recent meta-analysis conducted by Dongze et al. evaluated efficacy and safety of anti-cytokine biologic agents including secukinumab, ustekinumab, clazakizumab, and ixekizumab for active PsA at Week 24 and concluded that secukinumab and ustekinumab were the most efficacious short-term treatments among assessed agents [33]. Clazakizumab and ixekizumab were not included in this study since neither was approved as treatment for PsA at the time of the analysis.

Previous studies focused on PsARC as the measure of articular response, defined by ≥30% improvement in tender or swollen joint counts and one-point improvement in patient or physician global assessment of disease activity on a five-point Likert scale. In contrast, ACR response criteria also include visual analogue scale (VAS) scores of patient reported pain, Health Assessment Questionnaire (HAQ), and acute phase reactants. ACR responses are considered more stringent and comprehensive, and have become the primary outcome measure in a majority of RCTs in PsA [34]. Consequently, the current analysis chose ACR over PsARC responses as the measure of joint responses in PsA.

Biologic-naïve PsA patients generally report higher absolute joint and skin responses; however, comparative efficacy and cost-effectiveness in this population has not been systematically reviewed. Two recent meta-analysis studies comparing the efficacy of TIMs in biologic-naïve PsA patients concluded that ACR responses were higher among TNF inhibitors (etanercept, infliximab, adalimumab, and golimumab) and secukinumab, compared with other TIMs such as apremilast and ustekinumab [32, 35]. Another meta-analysis study conducted in a biologic-naïve PsA population in a Taiwanese setting found that etanercept had lower annual costs per PsARC and ACR20 responders than adalimumab and golimumab [36]. The above-mentioned studies only considered joint outcomes from Week 12 to Week 16, whereas the current study assessed efficacy in terms of both joint and skin outcomes at Week 24, as well as the cost-effectiveness of these TIMs. The longer time frame, inclusion of additional clinically relevant endpoints, and the cost analysis attest to the greater strength of the evidence presented in our study. The current analyses are in fact the first to include the more recently approved treatments (including ustekinumab, certolizumab pegol, secukinumab, and apremilast) and comprehensively evaluate their comparative efficacy and cost-effectiveness.

This network meta-analysis is subject to limitations commonly present in indirect comparison studies, despite synthesizing data from RCTs. Network meta-analyses may be biased due to the heterogeneity of patient populations across different trials. Although they adjust for placebo treatment responses which may account for trial-specific factors likely to influence outcomes in the active treatment arms, such adjustment only reduces the between-study heterogeneity. Moreover, due to the relatively small numbers of eligible RCTs for each pairwise comparison in this network meta-analysis, it was not possible to adjust for baseline risks within each trial. One specific limitation was that biologic-naïve data were not available for apremilast or certolizumab, and biologic-naïve results for secukinumab were based on a small sample size, which limited potential comparative interpretation. In addition, due to the lack of published data on patients who achieve both responses in terms of both joint and skin outcomes, the efficacy and cost-effectiveness of dual responses could not be assessed. However, treatment decisions should be based upon comprehensive considerations of both aspects. Despite the above limitations, this network meta-analysis represents the best evidence available to assess the comparative efficacy of currently available TIMs among PsA patients to inform health technology assessments and other decision-making [20, 37, 38].

Conclusions

This study demonstrated the comparative efficacy and cost-effectiveness of TNF inhibitors, interleukin inhibitors, and phosphodiesterase-4 inhibitors for patients with active PsA in the US. Adalimumab, infliximab, and golimumab demonstrated better efficacy and lower incremental costs per responder by both joint and skin

responses across all PsA patients as well as biologic-naive PsA patients. In the absence of comparative evidence from head-to-head trials, these results can inform more cost-effective use of these TIMs.

Acknowledgements

The authors would like to thank Fan Wu from Analysis Group and Bill Reichmann, a former employee of Analysis Group, for significant contribution towards medical writing and analytical support. This support was funded by AbbVie.

Funding

The design, study conduct, and financial support for the study were provided by AbbVie. AbbVie participated in the interpretation of data, review, and approval of the publication.

Authors' contributions

VS and MH contributed to the data interpretation and revision of the manuscript. KB, YS, and JZ contributed to the conception or design of the work, data collection, data analysis, data interpretation, and writing and revision of the manuscript. RS, JG, MB, and AG contributed to the conception or design of the work, data interpretation, and revision of the manuscript. All named authors meet the International Committee of Medical Journal Editors (ICMJE) criteria for authorship for this manuscript, take responsibility for the integrity of the work as a whole, and have given final approval to the version to be published.

Competing interests

VS has served as consultant to AbbVie, Amgen, AstraZeneca, BMS, Boehringer Ingelheim, Celltrion, Genentech / Roche, GlaxoSmithKline, Janssen, Lilly, Merck, Novartis, Pfizer, Sandoz, UCB; MH, KB, YS, and JZ have served as consultants to AbbVie. RS, JG, MB, and AG are employees of AbbVie and may own company stock.

Author details

[1]Stanford University, Palo Alto, CA, USA. [2]Cleveland Clinic, Cleveland, OH, USA. [3]Analysis Group Inc., 333 South Hope Street, 27th Floor, Los Angeles, CA 90071, USA. [4]Analysis Group Inc., Boston, MA, USA. [5]AbbVie Inc., Mettawa, IL, USA.

References

1. Prey S, Paul C, Bronsard V, Puzenat E, Gourraud PA, Aractingi S, et al. Assessment of risk of psoriatic arthritis in patients with plaque psoriasis: a systematic review of the literature. J Eur Acad Dermatol Venereol. 2010;24(Suppl 2):31–5.
2. Huynh D, Kavanaugh A. Psoriatic arthritis: current therapy and future approaches. Rheumatology. 2015;54(1):20–8.
3. Lee S, Mendelsohn A, Sarnes E. The burden of psoriatic arthritis: a literature review from a global health systems perspective. P & T: a peer-reviewed journal for formulary management. 2010;35(12):680–9.
4. Cantini F, Niccoli L, Nannini C, Cassara E, Kaloudi O, Giulio Favalli E, et al. Tailored first-line biologic therapy in patients with rheumatoid arthritis, spondyloarthritis, and psoriatic arthritis. Semin Arthritis Rheum. 2016;45(5):519–32.
5. Gottlieb A, Korman NJ, Gordon KB, Feldman SR, Lebwohl M, Koo JY, et al. Guidelines of care for the management of psoriasis and psoriatic arthritis: section 2. Psoriatic arthritis: overview and guidelines of care for treatment with an emphasis on the biologics. J Am Acad Dermatol. 2008;58(5):851–64.
6. Soriano ER, McHugh NJ. Therapies for peripheral joint disease in psoriatic arthritis. A systematic review. J Rheumatol. 2006;33(7):1422–30.
7. Gottlieb AB. Psoriasis - enhanced epidermal differentiation and reduced cell-mediated inflammation are unexpected outcomes. Dis Manag Clin Outcomes. 1998;1(6):195–202.

8. Gottlieb AB. Novel immunotherapies for psoriasis: clinical research delivers new hope for patients and scientific advances. The journal of investigative dermatology Symposium proceedings / the Society for Investigative Dermatology, Inc [and] European Society for Dermatological Research. 2004;9(1):79–83.

9. Gottlieb AB. Psoriasis: emerging therapeutic strategies. Nat Rev Drug Discov. 2005;4(1):19 34.

10. Lu G, Ades AE. Combination of direct and indirect evidence in mixed treatment comparisons. Stat Med. 2004;23(20):3105–24.

11. Dias S, Welton NJ, Sutton AJ, Ades A. NICE DSU Technical Support Document 1: Introduction to evidence synthesis for decision making. University of Sheffield, Decision Support Unit 2011:1-24.

12. Jansen JP, Fleurence R, Devine B, Itzler R, Barrett A, Hawkins N, et al. Interpreting indirect treatment comparisons and network meta-analysis for health-care decision making: report of the ISPOR task force on indirect treatment comparisons good research practices: part 1. Value Health. 2011;14(4):417–28.

13. Sutton A, Ades A, Cooper N, Abrams K. Use of indirect and mixed treatment comparisons for technology assessment. PharmacoEconomics. 2008;26(9):753–

14. Ritchlin CT, Kavanaugh A, Gladman DD, Mease PJ, Helliwell P, Boehncke WH, et al. Treatment recommendations for psoriatic arthritis. Ann Rheum Dis. 2009;68(9):1387–94.

15. Felson DT, Anderson JJ, Boers M, Bombardier C, Chernoff M, Fried B, et al. The American College of Rheumatology preliminary core set of disease activity measures for rheumatoid arthritis clinical trials. The committee on outcome measures in rheumatoid arthritis clinical trials. Arthritis Rheum. 1993;36(6):729–40.

16. Langley RG, Ellis CN. Evaluating psoriasis with psoriasis area and severity index, psoriasis global assessment, and lattice system Physician's global assessment. J Am Acad Dermatol. 2004;51(4):563–9.

17. Louden BA, Pearce DJ, Lang W, Feldman SR. A simplified psoriasis area severity index (SPASI) for rating psoriasis severity in clinic patients. Dermatol Online J. 2004;10(2):7.

18. Johnson & Johnson Health Care Systems Inc. Reimbursement Resources (Remicade) 2017 [cited 2017 May 8]. Available from: https://www.janssencarepath.com/hcp/remicade/reimbursement.

19. Feldman SR, Garton R, Averett W, Balkrishnan R, Vallee J. Strategy to manage the treatment of severe psoriasis: considerations of efficacy, safety and cost. Expert Opin Pharmacother. 2003;4(9):1525–33.

20. Signorovitch JE, Betts KA, Yan YS, LeReun C, Sundaram M, Wu EQ, et al. Comparative efficacy of biological treatments for moderate-to-severe psoriasis: a network meta-analysis adjusting for cross-trial differences in reference arm response. Br J Dermatol. 2015;172(2):504–12.

21. Mease PJ, Goffe BS, Metz J, VanderStoep A, Finck B, Burge DJ. Etanercept in the treatment of psoriatic arthritis and psoriasis: a randomised trial. Lancet. 2000;356(9227):385–90.

22. Antoni CE, Kavanaugh A, Kirkham B, Tutuncu Z, Burmester GR, Schneider U, et al. Sustained benefits of infliximab therapy for dermatologic and articular manifestations of psoriatic arthritis: results from the infliximab multinational psoriatic arthritis controlled trial (IMPACT). Arthritis Rheum. 2005;52(4):1227–36.

23. Genovese MC, Mease PJ, Thomson GT, Kivitz AJ, Perdok RJ, Weinberg MA, et al. Safety and efficacy of adalimumab in treatment of patients with psoriatic arthritis who had failed disease modifying antirheumatic drug therapy. J Rheumatol. 2007;34(5):1040–50.

24. Gottlieb A, Menter A, Mendelsohn A, Shen YK, Li S, Guzzo C, et al. Ustekinumab, a human interleukin 12/23 monoclonal antibody, for psoriatic arthritis: randomised, double-blind, placebo-controlled, crossover trial. Lancet. 2009;373(9664):633–40.

25. Mease PJ, Kivitz AJ, Burch FX, Siegel EL, Cohen SB, Ory P, et al. Etanercept treatment of psoriatic arthritis: safety, efficacy, and effect on disease progression. Arthritis Rheum. 2004;50(7):2264–72.

26. Coates LC, Kavanaugh A, Ritchlin CT, Committee GTG. Systematic review of treatments for psoriatic arthritis: 2014 update for the GRAPPA. J Rheumatol. 2014;41(11):2273–6.

27. Kavanaugh AF, Ritchlin CT, Committee GTG. Systematic review of treatments for psoriatic arthritis: an evidence based approach and basis for treatment guidelines. J Rheumatol. 2006;33(7):1417–21.

28. Sampogna F, Tabolli S, Soderfeldt B, Axtelius B, Aparo U, Abeni D, et al. Measuring quality of life of patients with different clinical types of psoriasis using the SF-36. Br J Dermatol. 2006;154(5):844 9.

29. Cawson MR, Mitchell SA, Knight C, Wildey H, Spurden D, Bird A, et al. Systematic review, network meta-analysis and economic evaluation of biological therapy for the management of active psoriatic arthritis. BMC Musculoskelet Disord. 2014;15:26.

30. Lubrano E, Spadaro A. Pharmacoeconomic burden in the treatment of psoriatic arthritis: from systematic reviews to real clinical practice studies. BMC Musculoskelet Disord. 2014;15:25.

31. Thorlund K, Druyts E, Avina-Zubieta JA, Mills EJ. Anti-tumor necrosis factor (TNF) drugs for the treatment of psoriatic arthritis: an indirect comparison meta-analysis. Biologics. 2012;6:417–27.

32. McInnes IB, Nash P, Ritchlin C, Thom H, Kanters S, Palaka E, et al. THU0437 Secukinumab for the treatment of psoriatic arthritis: comparative effectiveness results versus licensed biologics and Apremilast from a network meta-analysis. Ann Rheum Dis. 2016;75(Suppl 2):348–9.

33. Dongze W, Jiang Y, Tam L. FRI0523 short-term efficacy and safety of new biological agents targeting the IL-6, IL-12/23 and IL-17 pathways for active psoriatic arthritis: a network meta-analysis of randomised controlled trials: BMJ Publishing Group Ltd; 2017.

34. Mease PJ, Gladman DD, Ritchlin CT, Ruderman EM, Steinfeld SD, Choy EH, et al. Adalimumab for the treatment of patients with moderately to severely active psoriatic arthritis: results of a double-blind, randomized, placebo-controlled trial. Arthritis Rheum. 2005;52(10):3279–89.

35. Ungprasert P, Thongprayoon C, Davis JM 3rd. Indirect comparisons of the efficacy of biological agents in patients with psoriatic arthritis with an inadequate response to traditional disease-modifying anti-rheumatic drugs or to non-steroidal anti-inflammatory drugs: a meta-analysis. Semin Arthritis Rheum. 2016;45(4):428–38.

36. Yang TS, Chi CC, Wang SH, Lin JC, Lin KM. Cost-efficacy of biologic therapies for psoriatic arthritis from the perspective of the Taiwanese healthcare system. International journal of rheumatic diseases. 2016;19(10):1002–9.

37. Singh JA, Christensen R, Wells GA, Suarez-Almazor ME, Buchbinder R, Lopez-Olivo MA, et al. A network meta-analysis of randomized controlled trials of biologics for rheumatoid arthritis: a Cochrane overview. Can Med Assoc J. 2009;181(11):787–96.

38. Wandel S, Juni P, Tendal B, Nuesch E, Villiger PM, Welton NJ, et al. Effects of glucosamine, chondroitin, or placebo in patients with osteoarthritis of hip or knee: network meta-analysis. BMJ. 2010;341:c4675.

39. Kavanaugh A, Mease PJ, Gomez-Reino JJ, Adebajo AO, Wollenhaupt J, Gladman DD, et al. Treatment of psoriatic arthritis in a phase 3 randomised, placebo-controlled trial with apremilast, an oral phosphodiesterase 4 inhibitor. Ann Rheum Dis. 2014;73(6):1020–6.

40. Cutolo M, Myerson GE, Fleischmann RM, Liote F, Diaz-Gonzalez F, Van den Bosch F, et al. Long-term (52-week) results of a phase 3, randomized, controlled trial of Apremilast, an oral Phosphodiesterase 4 inhibitor, in patients with psoriatic arthritis (PALACE 2). Arthritis Rheum. 2013;65(Suppl 10):815.

41. Edwards CJ, Blanco FJ, Crowley J, Hu C, Stevens RM, Birbara CA. Long-term 52-week results of Palace 3, a phase 3, randomized, controlled trial of Apremilast, an oral Phosphodiesterase 4 inhibitor, in patients with psoriatic arthritis and current skin involvement. Arthritis Rheum. 2014;53(Suppl 1):138–9.

42. Birbara C, Blanco FJ, Crowley JJ, Hu C, Stevens R, Edwards CJ. Efficacy of apremilast, an oral phosphodiesterase 4 inhibitor, on physical function and pain in patients with psoriatic arthritis, including current skin involvement: results of a phase 3, randomized, controlled trial. Ann Rheum Dis. 2013; 72(Suppl 3):678.

43. National Institutes of Health. PALACE 3: Efficacy and Safety Study of Apremilast to Treat Active Psoriatic Arthritis 2015 [cited 2015 August 3]. Available from: https://clinicaltrials.gov/ct2/show/results/NCT01212770.

44. Wells AF, Edwards CJ, Adebajo AO, Kivitz AJ, Bird P, Shah K, et al., editors. Apremilast in the treatment of DMARD-naïve psoriatic arthritis patients: results of a phase 3 randomized, controlled trial (PALACE 4). 2013 ACR/ARHP annual meeting late-breaking abstracts; 2013 October 25–30, 2013; San Diego, CA.

45. ClinicalTrials.gov. Efficacy and Safety Study of Apremilast to Treat Active Psoriatic Arthritis (PsA) (PALACE4) 2014 [cited 2015 July 6]. Available from: https://clinicaltrials.gov/ct2/show/results/NCT01307423.

46. Mease PJ, Fleischmann R, Deodhar AA, Wollenhaupt J, Khraishi M, Kielar D, et al. Effect of certolizumab pegol on signs and symptoms in patients with psoriatic arthritis: 24-week results of a phase 3 double-blind randomised placebo-controlled study (RAPID-PsA). Ann Rheum Dis. 2014;73(1):48–55.

47. Kavanaugh A, McInnes I, Mease P, Krueger GG, Gladman D, Gomez-Reino J, et al. Golimumab, a new human tumor necrosis factor alpha antibody, administered every four weeks as a subcutaneous injection in psoriatic arthritis: twenty-four-week efficacy and safety results of a randomized, placebo-controlled study. Arthritis Rheum. 2009;60(4):976–86.

48. Antoni C, Krueger GG, de Vlam K, Birbara C, Beutler A, Guzzo C, et al. Infliximab improves signs and symptoms of psoriatic arthritis: results of the IMPACT 2 trial. Ann Rheum Dis. 2005;64(8):1150–7.

49. Mease PJ, McInnes IB, Kirkham B, Kavanaugh A, Rahman P, van der Heijde D, et al. Secukinumab inhibition of interleukin-17A in patients with psoriatic arthritis. N Engl J Med. 2015;373(14):1329–39.

50. McInnes IB, Mease PJ, Kirkham B, Kavanaugh A, Ritchlin CT, Rahman P, et al. Secukinumab, a human anti-interleukin-17A monoclonal antibody, in patients with psoriatic arthritis (FUTURE 2): a randomised, double-blind, placebo-controlled, phase 3 trial. Lancet. 2015;386(9999):1137–46.

51. McInnes IB, Kavanaugh A, Gottlieb AB, Puig L, Rahman P, Ritchlin C, et al. Efficacy and safety of ustekinumab in patients with active psoriatic arthritis: 1 year results of the phase 3, multicentre, double-blind, placebo-controlled PSUMMIT 1 trial. Lancet. 2013;382(9894):780–9.

52. Ritchlin C, Rahman P, Kavanaugh A, McInnes IB, Puig L, Li S, et al. Efficacy and safety of the anti-IL-12/23 p40 monoclonal antibody, ustekinumab, in patients with active psoriatic arthritis despite conventional non-biological and biological anti-tumour necrosis factor therapy: 6-month and 1-year results of the phase 3, multicentre, double-blind, placebo-controlled, randomised PSUMMIT 2 trial. Ann Rheum Dis. 2014;73(6):990–9.

11

Patient-centred standards of care for adults with myositis

James B. Lilleker[1,2*], Patrick Gordon[3], Janine A. Lamb[4], Heidi Lempp[5], Robert G. Cooper[4,6], Mark E. Roberts[1], Paula Jordan[7], Hector Chinoy[2,8], On behalf of the UK Myositis Network (UKMYONET) and Myositis UK

Abstract

Background: The idiopathic inflammatory myopathies (IIM, myositis) are a heterogeneous group of chronic autoimmune disorders causing considerable physical and mental health impact. There is a lack of formalised guidance defining best practice for the management of myositis, contributing to inconsistent care provision and some patients feeling isolated and unsupported.

To address these issues, we evaluated the clinical services available to adults with myositis in the UK. We then created patient-centred standards of care using a structured process involving patients, their relatives and caregivers, physicians and allied healthcare professionals.

Methods: After an initial focus group, the clinical services available to patients with myositis were evaluated using a patient-completed questionnaire. Draft standards of care were created, each addressing deficits in care provision identified by patients. In response to feedback, including a two-stage modified Delphi exercise, these draft standards were iteratively improved until consensus was reached. Accompanying plain language versions of the standards of care and an audit tool were also created.

Results: We identified issues regarding diagnostic pathways, access to specialist services, advice and support regarding employment, medication-related adverse events and the treatment of extra-muscular manifestations. Fifteen standards of care were drafted. After modification, agreement was reached on eleven final standards of care.

Conclusion: These patient-centred standards of care for adults with myositis provide a benchmark for the evaluation of local practice. Their implementation will promote consistent good practice across care providers and empower patients when seeking access to local services.

Keywords: Myositis, Idiopathic inflammatory myopathy, Delphi process, Standards of care, Patient-centred care, Quality improvement

Background

The idiopathic inflammatory myopathies (IIM, myositis) are a heterogeneous group of long-term autoimmune inflammatory conditions. Myositis negatively impacts the quality of life of an estimated 250,000 patients worldwide [1]. A lack of formalised guidance defining best practice contributes to inconsistent care provision and may influence clinical outcomes.

In circumstances where evidence-based or data-driven approaches are not possible, or not yet available, the production of standards of care allows healthcare professionals to benchmark their service using a set of agreed 'minimum' or 'optimum' consensus standards. This contrasts with the definition of a guideline, which is generated through a systematic evaluation of the available evidence and usually assists with clinical decision making in a specific scenario [2]. The Arthritis and Musculoskeletal Alliance (ARMA) have defined standards of care for patients with connective tissue diseases, but nothing similar exists to address the specific needs of adults with myositis [3].

* Correspondence: james.lilleker@manchester.ac.uk
[1]Greater Manchester Neuroscience Centre, Salford Royal NHS Foundation Trust, Manchester Academic Health Science Centre, Stott Lane, Salford, UK
[2]NIHR Manchester Biomedical Research Centre, Central Manchester University Hospitals NHS Foundation Trust, The University of Manchester, Manchester, UK
Full list of author information is available at the end of the article

Polymyositis (PM), and other myositis subtypes, are classified as orphan diseases (ORPHA:98,482). The rarity and heterogeneity of myositis means that delayed diagnosis and misdiagnosis occur commonly [4]. Most clinicians are unfamiliar with the management of these chronic conditions and patients can feel isolated and unsupported [5]. To overcome some of these problems we surveyed the experiences of adults in the UK living with myositis and using a structured process have created patient-centred standards of care.

Methods

Six steps were undertaken to produce the final standards of care. These are summarised in Table 1.

Initial information gathering from patients, relatives and caregivers

An initial focus-group of 30 participants (approximately 50% patients, 50% relatives/caregivers) was held at the Myositis UK (www.myositis.org.uk) Annual General Meeting (AGM) in July 2014. Information regarding the physical implications of disease and the social and emotional difficulties faced was gathered. These findings contributed to the development of a service evaluation questionnaire which was distributed by email and posted to all adult patient members of Myositis UK ($n = 485$) (Additional file 1 – Section One).

Statement drafting and initial feedback

Responses to the service evaluation questionnaire were analysed and 15 draft statements produced by agreement of the steering team (JBL, HC, JAL). Each reflected an *optimum* expected standard of care to address a matter highlighted by patients in the service evaluation questionnaire. These draft statements were then presented to attendees at the Myositis UK AGM in July 2015 and to members of the UK Myositis Network (UKMYONET) by email. Updating the statements in response to oral and written feedback received was overseen and agreed amongst the steering team.

Modified Delphi exercise

A modified, two-round Delphi consensus building exercise using a website-based survey system was then performed according to a pre-specified protocol. Briefly, the statements were sent to a multidisciplinary Delphi panel who were asked to indicate their level of agreement with each one using a ten point Likert scale, and to provide suggestions for improvement. A predetermined consensus level was agreed by the steering team (a mean agreement score ≥ 8.5 out of 10, unknown to the Delphi panel). Statements reaching this consensus level passed through to the final stage of the process. Where this level was not reached, suggestions for improvement were

Table 1 Steps taken to produce the patient-centred standards of care for adults with myositis

Step 1 - Initial information gathering from patients, relatives and caregivers

• Focus group at Myositis UK AGM, July 2014 (30 participants)
• Patient completed service evaluation questionnaire, March 2015
  o 151 responses obtained

Step 2 - Statement drafting

• 15 draft statements reflecting *optimum* standards of care created by steering team.
• Each statement addressed perceived deficits in current care arrangements as identified by patients

Step 3 - Initial feedback

• Feedback on draft statements sought from:
  o Myositis UK AGM, July 2015 (75 participants)
  o Members of the UK Myositis Network (UKMYONET) (responses from 12 individuals received)
• Statements updated. One statement removed from process

Step 4 - Modified Delphi exercise - Round one

• 14 updated draft statements presented electronically to the Delphi panel (December 2015). Responses from 25 individuals received.
• Level of agreement and suggestions for improvement analysed:
  o Eight statements met predetermined consensus level (mean level of agreement ≥8.5)
  o Six statements failed to meet predetermined consensus level. These were updated based on 40 individual items of feedback

Step 5 - Modified Delphi exercise - Round two

• Updated statements ($n = 6$) re-presented to panel (April 2016)
• Three statements reached predetermined consensus level.
• Remaining three statements were removed from the process

Step 6 - Final production of the patient-centred Standard of Care

• Approved updated statements arranged into three themes (December 2016)
• Minor changes to grammar and readability of three statements
• Creation of suggested audit standards to accompany each statement
• Creation of plain language versions of each statement (January 2017)

AGM = annual general meeting

examined and incorporated into an updated version of the statements, which were then sent back to the panel. Those not reaching consensus at this point were removed from the list of standards. Twenty-eight patient representatives and healthcare professionals (including Allied Health Professionals, Rheumatologists and Neurologists) were invited to take part on the panel.

Final production

The final standards of care were grouped into domains. Suggested audit standards were produced, and plain language versions of the standards in a checklist format were agreed after a teleconference focus-group with patients, caregivers and Myositis UK charity representatives.

Statistics

A descriptive statistical analysis of the service evaluation questionnaire was performed (JBL). The mean and standard deviation (SD) were calculated where data were normally distributed, whereas medians and interquartile ranges (IQR) were calculated for non-normally distributed data. For hypothesis testing Fisher's exact test or Mann Whitney rank-sum test were used where applicable. A p-value of <0.05 was considered as significant.

Results

Initial information gathering from patients, relatives and caregivers

In total, 151 responses (31% [151/485] return rate, 145 online and 6 by post) to the service evaluation questionnaire were obtained. Patients with dermatomyositis (DM) (37%), PM (27%) and inclusion body myositis (36%) participated. The mean age of respondents was 59 years (SD 14) and 33% were male. Diagnostic delays were common, particularly between presentation to the general practitioner and onwards referral to secondary care (median interval 2 months [IQR 0–4]). The majority of patients (58%) had been given at least one incorrect diagnosis prior to their final accurate diagnosis.

Satisfaction levels regarding access to Allied Healthcare Professionals were low to moderate (19% satisfied with access to rehabilitation services, 51% to physiotherapy and 55% to occupational therapy). Most respondents (83%) were unaware of any local support groups for patients with myositis. In addition, low levels of satisfaction were reported regarding the management of extramuscular and non-medical aspects of the disease. For example, only 23% of patients were satisfied that they had received sufficient support relating to employment issues, and only 24% stated that psychological aspects had being adequately addressed.

Overall, 54% of patients reported that they had received satisfactory counselling about potential adverse effects of treatments and 64% were confident that they could obtain urgent medical advice regarding their myositis, e.g. in the event of a disease flare. Furthermore, 69% of those with IBM were reviewed by a specialist less than once annually. Only 33% of patients indicated that they had been invited to participate in myositis research studies.

Statement drafting, feedback and updating

Fifteen draft statements were created, of which 13 were changed after feedback from attendees at the Myositis UK AGM 2015 ($n = 75$) and UKMYONET (12 responses, 57 individual items of feedback). One statement was removed from the process at this stage due to overwhelmingly negative feedback from both sources (Additional file 1 – Section Two).

Full results of the modified Delphi exercise are detailed in the Additional file 1 (Section Three). In the first round, responses were received from 24 of the 28 (86%) invited panel members. Eight of the 14

statements met the pre-determined consensus agreement level (a mean agreement score $\geq$ 8.5 out of 10). Forty items of feedback were received regarding the statements not reaching this consensus level. Analysis of this feedback informed statement updates, agreed amongst the steering team. During this process, one deviation from the protocol occurred where a statement was slightly refocussed by the steering team, to ensure that a key area of concern from the service evaluation questionnaire (the low levels of satisfaction regarding management of psychological aspects) was addressed.

In the second round of the Delphi exercise, 21 responses from 28 invitations (75%) were obtained. Despite the modifications, three statements failed to reach the pre-determined consensus level (mean agreement levels: 6.9, 8.1, 8.2) and were therefore removed from the process. The three remaining ones (mean agreement levels: 8.7, 9.1, 9.3) passed to the final stage.

Final production

The final eleven statements underwent minor modifications to improve readability and accessibility (Table 2). A log of all such changes to the statements is included in the Additional file 1 (Section Four). These were then arranged in to three emerging themes: (i) presentation, referral and diagnosis; (ii) care arrangements and the interaction between myositis specialists and other healthcare professionals; (iii) disease management and holistic care. An audit tool with suggested audit standards (Additional file 1 - Section Five) and plain language versions of the statements were also created (Table 2).

Discussion

Our patient-centred approach has helped to create a set of unique standards of care for adults with myositis. By specifically addressing deficiencies in care highlighted by patients and then using an iterative process that considered feedback from patients, relatives, caregivers and healthcare professionals, we have produced standards of care tailored to the individual healthcare needs of patients with myositis.

The service evaluation questionnaire involved a wide variety of patients with myositis living in England, Scotland and Wales, thus capturing a variety of experiences and views. In addition to patient representatives, the Delphi panel also represented a range of healthcare professionals from diverse geographic locations, minimising bias from one professional group or location. However, there is the possibility that not all relevant stakeholders have been included and we have not included feedback or approval from those with juvenile-onset myositis (i.e. Juvenile-onset DM). It is acknowledged that some

Table 2 Final patient-centred standards of care for adults with myositis and accompanying plain language versions of the standards

Patient-centred standards of care	Plain language version of standards
Domain 1: Presentation, referral and diagnosis	
Myositis should be considered in patients with *unexplained weakness, fatigue, rash, myalgia or arthralgia* • Testing of serum *CK is a useful screening tool*, but can be normal in some scenarios	9.1 When I first developed symptoms of myositis, was the correct diagnosis considered early?
GPs should identify patients presenting with features of myositis (e.g. muscle weakness, raised CK +/– rash) and refer to a specialist *as soon as this diagnosis is considered*	8.8 Was I referred to an appropriate specialist quickly?
Domain 2: Care arrangements and the interaction between myositis specialists and other healthcare professionals	
Patients with myositis should be *under the care of a specialist with specific expertise and experience in managing myositis* • This could be either directly or as part of a formal shared-care agreement with a local physician	9.5 Am I under the care of a specialist (either directly or under shared-care) who is experienced and competent in the management of patients with myositis?
Patients with myositis should continue to be *periodically reviewed by a myositis specialist* for as long their disease is active or muscle strength continues to deteriorate • This could be either directly or as part of a formal shared-care agreement with a local physician	9.1 Do I see my specialist with sufficient frequency to meet my needs?
The services for patients with myositis should include access to *ongoing specialist* physiotherapy, occupational therapy and speech and language therapy • This could be integrated in to the specialist clinic or via a formal shared-care agreement between specialist and non-specialist (local) therapists	9.2 Do I have adequate support from other health professionals (including physiotherapists, occupational therapists and speech and language therapists) that have experience in managing patients with myositis?
There should be *clear protocols defining how* patients with myositis should *seek urgent advice.* • For example, the specialist centre might provide a *dedicated telephone advice line* for patients and other healthcare professionals	8.9 Should the need arise, am I able to obtain appropriate urgent medical advice regarding my myositis or its treatment?
Domain 3: Disease management and holistic care	
When considering starting patients with myositis on immunosuppression, *detailed discussion regarding the potential benefits and possible side effects must take place.* • This could be reinforced by other members of the multidisciplinary team (e.g. pharmacist) • Formal shared-care agreements with GPs should also be in place	8.8 Before I am offered treatments for my myositis, do I understand the relevant benefits and potential risks?
Healthcare professionals should specifically address *extra-muscular symptoms* such as pain, fatigue and depression at each consultation	8.7 Are issues such as pain, fatigue or low mood addressed in addition to my muscle weakness during consultations with my specialist?
Services for patients with myositis should provide *holistic care* that addresses *physical and psychological aspects* of disease and its *social implications* • For example, this may include difficulties with employment	8.7 If required, do I have access to support with how myositis affects my day-to-day life (for example, the effect on my job)?
Patients with myositis should be *signposted to appropriate information resources and patient groups*	9.3 Have I been made aware of relevant myositis information resources and patient groups?
Patients with myositis should be *offered participation in clinical trials* as part of routine practice	8.8 Have I been offered participation in clinical trials for myositis?

Mean level of agreement is shown adjacent to each standard of care and is derived from responses on a ten point Likert scale. GPs = general practitioners

aspects of the produced standards may apply more to certain subgroups of myositis patient than others. Similarly, our work is derived from views regarding the UK healthcare system, and may therefore not be applicable or relevant in other locales.

Implementation of the standards would require additional resources, e.g. to improve access to Allied Healthcare Professionals, such as physiotherapists who have experience in caring for and managing patients with myositis. However, other standards could be quickly implemented, e.g. an

up-to-date list of ongoing myositis clinical trials and the production of patient information resources that can be kept in clinics for access during consultations.

Despite the potential to improve the quality of healthcare, there is often inconsistent implementation of new research findings or practice recommendations [6]. Several barriers to implementation have been identified and various solutions offered [7, 8]. The process undertaken to create these standards of care is consistent with several of these recommendations. Importantly, there has been prominent patient and caregiver involvement throughout to ensure acceptability and appropriateness of the standards. We have also created plain language statements in collaboration with patient charity representatives. These will be disseminated by Myositis UK and via the active myositis social media community. From the perspective of the clinician we have facilitated dissemination and implementation of the standards of care by publishing this manuscript Open Access and have minimised the volume of information by presenting the standards as a single accessible table. Implementation measures, including an assessment of adoption and coverage of the standards of care, will be assessed after 12 months and reported through UKMYONET and Myositis UK.

We anticipate that these standards of care for adults with myositis will support clinicians, benefit patients and reduce variation by providing a benchmark of good practice that local services can be assessed against. As a consequence, we seek to mirror the improvements in practice seen in the management of stroke and epilepsy observed since the commencement of national audit programmes for these conditions [9, 10].

Conclusion

Healthcare provision for patients with myositis is inconsistent. Consequently, many patients feel isolated and unsupported. Our service evaluation questionnaire identified common issues relating to diagnostic delays, poor access to specialists and allied healthcare professionals with experience in the care of patients with myositis, difficulties obtaining urgent medical advice, inadequate counselling regarding the risks of medications and poor management of extramuscular symptoms.

To address these issues, we have created patient-centred standards of care for adults with myositis. To facilitate implementation, plain language versions of the standards and an audit tool have been created. Implementation of these standards of care in the UK will promote consistent good practice and improve healthcare quality for patients with myositis.

Abbreviations

AGM: Annual General Meeting; ARMA: Arthritis and Musculoskeletal Alliance; DM: Dermatomyositis; GP: General practitioner; IIM: Idiopathic inflammatory myopathies; IQR: Interquartile range; PM: Polymyositis; SD: Standard deviation; UKMYONET: UK Myositis Network

Acknowledgements

The authors thank all patients, families and healthcare professionals contributing to this study. The authors also thank the Myositis UK Executive Committee and all members of Myositis UK for allowing presentation at their annual general meeting and facilitating completion of the service evaluation questionnaire.

Myositis UK is a registered charity providing information and support to individuals and their families affected by Dermatomyositis, Polymyositis, Inclusion Body Myositis and Juvenile Dermatomyositis.

UK Myositis Network (UKMYONET) members providing feedback:
Robert G Cooper, *Professor of Rheumatology, MRC-ARUK Institute for Ageing and Chronic Disease, University of Liverpool.*
Christopher Edwards, *Professor of Rheumatology, University Hospital Southampton NHS Foundation Trust.*
David Hilton-Jones, *Consultant Neurologist, Oxford University Hospitals NHS Foundation Trust.*
David Isenberg, *Professor of Rheumatology, University College London Hospitals NHS Foundation Trust.*
Patrick Kiely, *Consultant Rheumatologist, St George's University Hospitals NHS Foundation Trust.*
Heidi Lempp, *Senior Lecturer in Medical Sociology, Kings College London.*
Neil McHugh, *Professor of Pharmacoepidemiology, University of Bath.*
Pedro Machado, *NIHR RD TRC Postdoctoral Fellow & Honorary Consultant in Rheumatology and Muscle Diseases, MRC Centre for Neuromuscular Diseases & Centre for Rheumatology, University College London.*
John Pauling, *Senior Lecturer and Consultant Rheumatologist, Royal National Hospital for Rheumatic Diseases.*
Sarah Tansley, *Clinical Research Fellow, Royal National Hospital for Rheumatic Diseases.*
John Winer, *Consultant Neurologist, University Hospitals Birmingham NHS Foundation Trust.*
Delphi panel participants:
Shirley Caldwell, *Senior Rheumatology Research Coordinator, Salford Royal NHS Foundation Trust.*
Robert G Cooper, *Professor of Rheumatology, MRC-ARUK Institute for Ageing and Chronic Disease, University of Liverpool.*
Shouma Dutta, *Consultant Rheumatologist, Staffordshire and Stoke-on-Trent Partnership NHS Trust.*
Christopher Edwards, *Professor of Rheumatology, University Hospital Southampton NHS Foundation Trust.*
Nagui Gendi, *Consultant Rheumatologist, Basildon and Thurrock University Hospitals NHS Foundation Trust.*
Joanne Goode, *Patient representative and Myositis UK Treasurer.*
Patrick Gordon, *Consultant Rheumatologist, King's College Hospital NHS Foundation Trust.*
Will Gregory, *Specialist Rheumatology Physiotherapist and Advanced MSK Practitioner, Salford Royal NHS Foundation Trust.*
David Hilton-Jones, *Consultant Neurologist, Oxford University Hospitals NHS Foundation Trust.*
Patrick Kiely, *Consultant Rheumatologist, St George's University Hospitals NHS Foundation Trust.*
Heidi Lempp, *Senior Lecturer in Medical Sociology, Kings College London.*
Pedro Machado, *NIHR RD TRC Postdoctoral Fellow & Honorary Consultant in Rheumatology and Muscle Diseases, MRC Centre for Neuromuscular Diseases & Centre for Rheumatology, University College London.*
Neil McHugh, *Professor of Rheumatology, Royal National Hospital for Rheumatic Diseases.*
James Miller, *Consultant Neurologist, The Newcastle upon Tyne Hospitals NHS Foundation Trust.*
Paula Jordan, *Patient representative and Myositis UK General Secretary.*
John Pauling, *Senior Lecturer and Consultant Rheumatologist, Royal National Hospital for Rheumatic Diseases.*
Fiona Pearce, *Clinical Lecturer in Rheumatology, University of Nottingham.*
Michael Rose, *Consultant Neurologist King's College Hospital NHS Foundation Trust.*
Jade Skeates, *Specialist Rheumatology Physiotherapist, Royal National Hospital for Rheumatic Diseases.*
Sarah Tansley, *Clinical Research Fellow, Royal National Hospital for Rheumatic Diseases.*
Paul Truepenny, *Patient representative.*
Yvonne Truepenny, *Relative/caregiver.*

David Tucker, *Patient representative.*
John Winer, *Consultant Neurologist, University Hospitals Birmingham NHS Foundation Trust.*
Participants in focus group to create plain language versions of statements:
Paul Truepenny, *Patient representative.*
Yvonne Truepenny, *Relative/caregiver.*
David Tucker, *Patient representative.*
Irene Oakley, *Patient representative (relative/caregiver) and Myositis UK Group Coordinator.*
Joanne Goode, *Patient representative and Myositis UK Treasurer.*
Steering team.
James B Lilleker, *Clinical Research Fellow, The University of Manchester.*
Hector Chinoy, *Senior Lecturer and Consultant Rheumatologist, The University of Manchester.*
Janine Lamb, *Reader, The University of Manchester.*
We wish to thank those who reviewed the manuscript for their constructive comments (Additional file 2).

Funding
This study was supported in part by Arthritis Research UK (18474), the Medical Research Council (MR/N003322/1) and the UK Myositis Network (UKMYONET). UKMYONET is supported by the Manchester Academic Health Science Centre (MAHSC).
This report includes independent research supported by the NIHR Biomedical Research Unit Funding Scheme. The views expressed in this publication are those of the authors and not necessarily those of the NHS, the National Institute for Health Research or the Department of Health.

Authors' contributions
HC, PG and PJ had the original idea for this project. JBL, JAL and HC formed the steering committee and agreed on the draft statements and any changes made in response to feedback. JBL organised and analysed the service evaluation questionnaire and modified Delphi process and facilitated the final focus group to create plain language versions of the statements and the audit tool. JBL drafted the manuscript. HL, MER and RGC critically reviewed the intellectual content of the draft manuscript. All authors critically reviewed the draft manuscript, approved the final version and agree to be accountable for all aspects of the work.

Competing interests
The authors declare that they have no competing interests.

Author details
[1]Greater Manchester Neuroscience Centre, Salford Royal NHS Foundation Trust, Manchester Academic Health Science Centre, Stott Lane, Salford, UK. [2]NIHR Manchester Biomedical Research Centre, Central Manchester University Hospitals NHS Foundation Trust, The University of Manchester, Manchester, UK. [3]King's College Hospital NHS Foundation Trust, London, UK. [4]Centre for Integrated Genomic Medical Research, School of Health Sciences, Faculty of Biology Medicine and Health, The University of Manchester, Manchester, UK. [5]Academic Rheumatology, Faculty of Life Sciences & Medicine, King's College London, London, UK. [6]MRC-ARUK Institute for Ageing and Chronic Disease, University of Liverpool, Liverpool, UK. [7]Myositis UK, Southampton, UK. [8]Rheumatology Department, Salford Royal NHS Foundation Trust, Manchester Academic Health Science Centre, Stott Lane, Salford, UK.

References
1.   Furst DE, Amato AA, Iorga ŞR, Gajria K, Fernandes AW. Epidemiology of adult idiopathic inflammatory myopathies in a U.S. managed care plan. *Muscle Nerve.* 2012;**45**:676–83.
2.   Stoffer MA, Smolen JS, Woolf A, et al. Development of patient-centred standards of care for osteoarthritis in Europe: the eumusc.net-project. *Ann Rheum Dis.* 2015;**74**:1145–9.
3.   Arthritis and Musculoskeletal Alliance. *Standards of Care for people with Connective Tissue. Diseases.* 2007;
4.   Meyer A, Meyer N, Schaeffer M, Gottenberg J-EJ-E, Geny B, Sibilia J. Incidence and prevalence of inflammatory myopathies: a systematic review. *Rheumatology.* 2015;**54**:50–63.
5.   Truepenny P, Kaushik V, Lempp H. Polymyositis. *BMJ.* 2012;**344**:e1181.
6.   Flodgren G, Hall AM, Goulding L, et al. Tools developed and disseminated by guideline producers to promote the uptake of their guidelines. *Cochrane database Syst Rev.* 2016:CD010669.
7.   Schipper K, Bakker M, De Wit M, Ket JCF, Abma TA. Strategies for disseminating recommendations or guidelines to patients: a systematic review. *Implement Sci.* 2015;**11**:82.
8.   Cabana MD, Rand CS, Powe NR, et al. Why Don't Physicians Follow Clinical Practice Guidelines? *JAMA.* 1999;**282**:1458.
9.   Dixon PA, Kirkham JJ, Marson AG, Pearson MG. National Audit of Seizure management in Hospitals (NASH): results of the national audit of adult epilepsy in the UK. *BMJ Open.* 2015;**5**:e007325.
10. Rudd AG, Irwin P, Rutledge Z, et al. The national sentinel audit for stroke: a tool for raising standards of care. *J R Coll Physicians Lond.* 1999;**33**:460–4.

12

Living with osteoarthritis is a balancing act: an exploration of patients' beliefs about knee pain

Ben Darlow[1]* , Melanie Brown[1], Bronwyn Thompson[2], Ben Hudson[3], Rebecca Grainger[4], Eileen McKinlay[1] and J. Haxby Abbott[5]

Abstract

Background: This study aimed to explore the beliefs of people with knee osteoarthritis (OA) about the disease, and how these beliefs had formed and what impact these beliefs had on activity participation, health behaviour, and self-management.

Methods: Semi-structured interviews were conducted with 13 people with knee OA recruited from general practices, community physiotherapy clinics, and public advertisements in two provinces of New Zealand. Data were analysed using Interpretive Description.

Results: Two key themes emerged. 1) *Knowledge: certainty and uncertainty* described participants' strong beliefs about anatomical changes in their knee. Participants' beliefs in a biomechanical model of progressive joint degradation often appeared to originate within clinical encounters and from literal interpretation of the term 'wear and tear'. These beliefs led to uncertainty regarding interpretation of daily symptoms and participants' ability to influence the rate of decline and certainty that joint replacement surgery represented the only effective solution to fix the damaged knee. 2) *Living with OA* described broader perspectives of living with OA and the perceived need to balance competing values and risks when making decisions about activity participation, medication, attentional focus, accessing care, and making the most of today without sabotaging tomorrow. Misunderstandings about knee OA negatively impacted on activity participation, health behaviours, and self-management decisions.

Conclusion: Biomechanical models of OA reduced participant exploration of management options and underpinned a perceived need to balance competing values. Improved information provision to people with knee OA could help guide positive health behaviour and self-management decisions and ensure these decisions are grounded in current evidence.

Keywords: Osteoarthritis, Knee, Patient perceptions, Health knowledge, attitudes, practice, Qualitative research

Background

Osteoarthritis (OA) is a common condition that causes considerable disability and high levels of health expenditure [1, 2]. Knee OA accounts for over 80% of the total OA disease burden [3] and its prevalence is rapidly increasing [4]. This will have considerable social and economic consequences, particularly as people with OA are twice as likely to be absent from work or retire early due to ill-health [5, 6].

People's beliefs about knee OA have an important impact on their lived experience of the disease, influencing activity levels, social and leisure participation, and emotional wellbeing [7, 8]. Beliefs about knee OA aetiology have been explored in a number of qualitative studies, indicating that many people consider OA to be an inevitable part of ageing that is influenced by wear and tear due to joint use and obesity [9–12]. There is a commonly held mechanical view of OA that focuses on loss of cartilage and bone abutting directly on bone [10, 13].

* Correspondence: ben.darlow@otago.ac.nz
[1]Department of Primary Health Care and General Practice, University of Otago - Wellington, Wellington, New Zealand
Full list of author information is available at the end of the article

Physical inactivity may predispose to knee OA [4, 14] and physical activity is a key tenet of OA management recommendations [15]. Beliefs about physical activity among people with knee OA have been explored in the context of general physical activity [16] and adherence to exercise-based OA self-management programmes [9, 17]. Beliefs that OA is caused by wear and tear result in worry that weight bearing exercise will exacerbate joint damage [17] and these concerns may cause people to reduce activity levels or avoid activities [16].

There is currently inadequate understanding of how people's beliefs about knee OA are informed. Given the discordance between evidence-based physical activity recommendations for knee OA and consumer beliefs about OA aetiology and the role of activity, it is important to address the gap in the literature regarding *how* people's beliefs about knee OA and activity are formed and *what specific impact* these beliefs have on activity participation and self-management. Improved understanding of how beliefs are formed and factors that influence this process may enable clinicians to positively influence beliefs about knee OA and improve people's experience of living with this condition.

This qualitative study aimed to explore the beliefs of New Zealanders with knee OA about the disease, and in particular, how these beliefs had formed and what specific impact these beliefs had on activity participation, health behaviour, and self-management.

Methods

This study adhered to the Consolidated criteria for reporting qualitative studies (COREQ; Additional file 1).

Research design

Qualitative data were gathered and analysed using Interpretive Description [18, 19]. This methodology aims to inform clinical understanding by identifying themes and patterns within participant perspectives [18, 19]. The study complied with the Declaration of Helsinki. The University of Otago Human Ethics Committee (Health) (H15/081) approved the study and participants gave written informed consent.

Recruitment

Participants were recruited in two provinces of New Zealand from general practices and community physiotherapy clinics, and from advertisements to Arthritis New Zealand members and in public areas such as libraries, swimming pools, and supermarkets.

Participants were included in the study if they had been told by a health care professional that they had knee OA. Participants were excluded if they had received a total knee replacement or could not speak English. There was no age limitation. Purposive sampling

maximised the range of viewpoints in terms of gender, age, cultural backgrounds, disease severity, and level of functional limitation [20].

Data collection

Participants were interviewed by experienced qualitative researchers (MB or BT) in a location of their choice; for most, this was the participant's home. Participants were unknown to interviewers prior to recruitment and were asked to speak to interviewers as lay people. Interviews were conducted in person; face-to-face or by web-based video-conferencing. Participants were able to have a support person present, but all chose to be interviewed alone. A semi-structured interview schedule was developed using questions framed around research aims, but kept flexible to allow participants to focus on what they deemed important (Table 1). Interviews consisted of open-ended questions to elicit the participants' views on their experiences and perceptions of knee OA, including activity. Afterward, participants completed a demographic questionnaire including self-reported duration of knee pain and clinicians consulted, the Oxford Knee Scale [21] to indicate functional limitation, and the Pain Self-Efficacy Questionnaire [22] to indicate confidence in performing activities despite pain. Interviews were audio-recorded and transcribed verbatim; field notes were also kept.

Data analysis

Recruitment, data collection, and data analysis occurred concurrently to enable collected data to inform subsequent interviews and to cease recruitment once theme saturation was achieved. Data were managed using NVivo 11 software (QSR International Pty Ltd).

Initial transcript coding was undertaken independently by MB and BT on a line-by-line basis using 'open coding' to allow multiple codes to be applied to single segments of data. These researchers subsequently discussed and agreed on codes and categories within each transcript. The relationships between and within categories emerging from this process were explored with increasingly higher levels of conceptualisation. Negative case analysis was used to broaden

Table 1 Semi-structured interview guide

1. Please tell me about your knee problem from the beginning?

2. How would you describe your pain?

3. What do you think is happening in or around your knee

4. Can you tell me about the things that affect your knee problem?

5. Is there anything that concerns you about your knee problem?

6. How have you found out about what is wrong with your knee?

7. What do you think is the best way to manage your knee problem?

8. What are your expectations for the future with regards to your knee problem?

understandings and challenge initial interpretations of the data [20]. Transcripts and coding were crosschecked by another researcher (BD), with all disagreements resolved through regular discussions. Theme documentation was checked and discussed with other authors (BH/RG/JHA/ EM) following eight interviews and again following thirteen interviews to further develop the emerging analysis, ensure themes represented participants' reported experiences and views, and test assumptions related to theme saturation. Consistent with Interpretive Description, participants did not review transcripts or validate findings [19] and there were no repeat interviews.

Research team

The research team consisted of academics and clinicians with backgrounds in family medicine (BH), health coaching (MB), nursing (EM), occupational therapy (BT), physiotherapy (BD/JHA), and rheumatology (RG). Several researchers (BD/MB/BT/JHA/RG/EM) had experience with qualitative research in musculoskeletal pain.

Results

Thirteen participants were interviewed (Table 2). Ten further eligible respondents were not interviewed because their characteristics were similar to previous participants

($n = 7$), they changed their mind ($n = 1$), or were unable to schedule time for the interview ($n = 2$). Interviews lasted 60 to 90 min. Data saturation was achieved after eight interviews. Five further participants were purposively recruited and interviewed, but no further themes or significant variations on existing themes emerged.

Two overarching themes emerged from the data;, *Knowledge: certainty and uncertainty* and *Living with osteoarthritis*. Findings are presented with illustrative extracts from participants' interviews; additional quotes are in Additional files 2 and 3. An additional theme emerged around *Health System Support*; as this large theme was conceptually distinct and unrelated to the primary aims of this study, it will be presented in a future publication.

Knowledge: certainty and uncertainty

This theme described participants' beliefs about OA and how it should be managed, describing how these beliefs have been formed and influenced as well as the impact of these beliefs.

Structural model of progressive degeneration

Participants used descriptive language and imagery to express their strong beliefs about anatomical and

Table 2 Participant characteristics

Pseudonym Gender	Age	Ethnicity	Occupational category	Knee pain duration	Clinical consultation for knee pain	OKS[a]	PSEQ[b]
Geoff, Male	60–64	NZE	Community & personal service worker	14–16 years	Family doctor	26	35
James, Male	70–74	NZE	Retired professional	4–6 years	Family doctor, orthopaedic surgeon,	18	17
Anne, Female	60–64	NZE	Clerical & administrative worker	10–12 years	Family doctor, orthopaedic surgeon	25	49
George, Male	80–84	NZE	Retired professional	8–10 years	Orthopaedic surgeon	25	54
John, Male	65–69	NZE	Professional	4–6 years	Family doctor, orthopaedic surgeon, physiotherapist	42	17
Iosefo, Male	70–74	Samoan	Labourer	4–6 years	Family doctor	22	60
Tui, Female	60–64	Māori	Retired professional	6–12 months	Family doctor, nurse, orthopaedic surgeon,	57	32
Linda, Female	50–54	Danish	Professional	20+ years	Family doctor, orthopaedic surgeon	34	16
Karen, Female	60–64	NZE	Clerical & administrative worker	18–20 years	Family doctor, orthopaedic surgeon, physiotherapist	24	52
Susan,Female	60–64	NZE	Professional	1–2 years	Bowen therapist, family doctor, Reiki practitioner	32	40
Mary, Female	70–74	NZE	Retired	14–16 years	Family doctor, orthopaedic surgeon, physiotherapist	36	35
Brenda, Female	55–59	NZE	Professional	0–6 months	Acupuncturist, family doctor, homeopath, homeopathic chemist, naturopath, physiotherapist	40	27
William, Male	60–64	NZE	Community & personal service worker	4–6 years	Acupuncturist; chiropractor, family doctor; orthopaedic surgeon, osteopath,, physiotherapist	22	56

NZE New Zealand European, *OKS* Oxford Knee Scale, *PSEQ* Pain Self Efficacy Questionnaire
[a]Scored on a range from 12 to 60 with higher scores indicating greater functional limitation
[b]Scored on a range from 0 to 60 with higher scores indicating greater confidence in performing activities despite pain

pathological changes in their knees. The phrases 'wear and tear', 'bone-on-bone', and 'missing cartilage' were used frequently to explain their understanding of OA:

"It doesn't take a rocket scientist to work out that [it's bone-on-bone]. If the fluid between the ball-bearing and the thing has all gone, you know, it's like a car situation."

–Tui

For many, certainty about this biomechanical model of structural deterioration led to a matter-of-fact attitude, and often a lack of curiosity about seeking information or exploring management options:

"It's sort of like a pound of butter. That's what it is! It's butter. Arthritis is arthritis."

–George

Despite the sense of certainty around the biomechanical model, participants often had no explanations for the variability of symptoms, the speed of potential degradation, or the best ways to optimise function and slow deterioration. This model of progressive deterioration was in conflict with some participants' experiences of stable or improving symptoms. Participants appeared not to recognise this discordance.

Participants saw 'wear and tear' as synonymous with OA and interpreted the concept literally. Consequently, participants felt that they needed to protect their joint to prevent further wear and tear. These concepts were often reported as originating with, or being reinforced by, health professionals:

"They always say same thing: wear and tear, you know, you're getting older."

–Iosefo

Many participants had been shown X-rays that provided graphic evidence of the loss of space between bone ends. Participants expressed shock at seeing these changes; several explained that the X-rays led them to believe that they needed to protect their knee from further damage. These concepts were reinforced by what participants saw, heard, and felt from their knee (such as a bowed appearance, grinding, or knocking):

"It's really obvious I have no cushioning in that knee."

–John

Approaches to osteoarthritis management

The strongly-held model of ongoing structural deterioration led to participants using strategies such as: avoiding, reducing, or pacing activities to limit wear and tear; participating in activities they considered not to cause joint impact; and taking natural supplements to lubricate the joints (e.g. fish oil) or feed the cartilage (e.g. glucosamine or gelatine). Two participants ('Linda' and 'William') attributed their successes in managing OA to specific weight-loss management or strength-based exercise regimes.

Pain or stiffness guided activity participation or avoidance, but participants were often uncertain about these choices. Some participants interpreted pain that lasted after they stopped exercise as a sign of further damage, whereas pain that abated was a reminder to be careful. Participants' understandings of helpful and unhelpful strategies were strongly influenced by their structural model of what was happening to, and beliefs about what might be safe or good for, the knee:

"[Biking] there's no load on your knees… it's keeping you in motion, keeping you active, and it's not stress or anything on your knees."

–Anne

Participants often spoke about stages of management related to the degree of joint degeneration. These included things they had done in the past and things they may try in future. Participants planned to continue with their current strategies until these were no longer effective, indicating progression to another stage. Differing stages helped explain why certain remedies might work for some people but not others:

"All that sort of stuff [like glucosamine] is supposed to help your cartilage and protect it. But once it's not there, it's not going to make more of it … once it's gone it's gone."

–Karen

Although participants expressed hope that they may be able to maintain the status quo or slow the rate of deterioration, they were generally resigned to progressive degradation over which they had little control. The inevitability of further deterioration was supported by the beliefs that OA is part of ageing and the joint is worn away by movement.

"I don't think it would improve. It may stay the same, but I would expect it to get worse… you can't change osteoarthritis."

–Karen

Participants anticipated increasing pain and activity limitation, which would reduce their quality of life:

"It worries me that one day I won't be able to do the things I can do today."

–Linda

Participants believed joint replacement surgery is inevitable and represents the only effective solution to fix OA (albeit a temporary fix, as they expected the joint replacement would also wear out). This belief was expressed most participants including those with early-stage OA and those who expressed positive expectations around managing day-to-day.

Living with osteoarthritis
This theme described broader perspectives of living with OA and the decisions and trade-offs that participants made based on their beliefs about OA.

The big picture
When discussing the meaning of symptoms and symptom fluctuation participants did not usually talk about structural changes within their knee. Rather, they talked about how pain and symptoms limited activity and day-to-day life, and OA's broader effects on, and interactions with, mood, wellbeing, and sleep.

Participants often downplayed OA and used minimising language to discuss the condition and its effects. Regardless of age of onset, participants saw OA as part of getting older. Participants perceived OA was not as serious as other health conditions, such as cancer, and a topic that would bore their peers or health professionals. Some participants explicitly downplayed the condition to reduce OA's place in their lives, or avoid being perceived as a moaner or identifying as 'someone with arthritis'.

"I decided I don't want this to define me, I'm much more than my knee."

–Susan

Similarly, many perceived OA was downplayed by clinicians; some commented that this was harmful:

"I've made a decision not to use that [term 'wear and tear']... the implication is that it's not unusual and everybody gets it and, you know, it's not something we need to take any notice of."

–Brenda

Participants knew that they could not keep playing it down forever. They anticipated a time when OA would

affect more than day-to-day activities and begin to affect their core identity and sense of self. Loss of satisfaction or identity were key indicators that it was time for surgery.

Participants discussed benefits of exercise for general physical and mental health and for managing comorbidities. Some participants reported exercising despite concerns about further wear and tear:

"I'm prepared to face up with a bit of further degeneration in my right knee if everything else benefits."

–George

Living with osteoarthritis is a balancing act
Participants saw living with OA as a 'balancing act'. Participants' understandings of OA and expectations of future decline, combined with uncertainty about the meaning of fluctuating symptoms and effects of exercise or movement, led to balancing competing values and risks (Fig. 1). On the one hand, participants identified benefits of activity for their knee and general health, but on the other hand they were concerned about increasing pain or further joint degradation:

"Am I strengthening it or am I sort of destroying the cartilage? I don't know."

–William

Participants considered the safety of an exercise for the knee when weighing benefits against costs or risks. However, 'safe' activities were not always activities participants liked, felt comfortable with, or were able to do. There was also tension between the notion of the knee needing rest, pacing, and protection versus the need to keep moving, to keep one's identity, and to get on with things.

"It's the balance between activity and rest for the joint... I'm probably wearing it more, but weighing that up against not doing anything then everything else will fall apart."

–Susan

Participants spoke about the importance of putting OA out of their minds and not letting it define their identity but simultaneously balancing this with the need to plan and choose activities.

"It's not always at the front of my mind, but it's probably always in the back of my mind... because it has to be."

–Karen

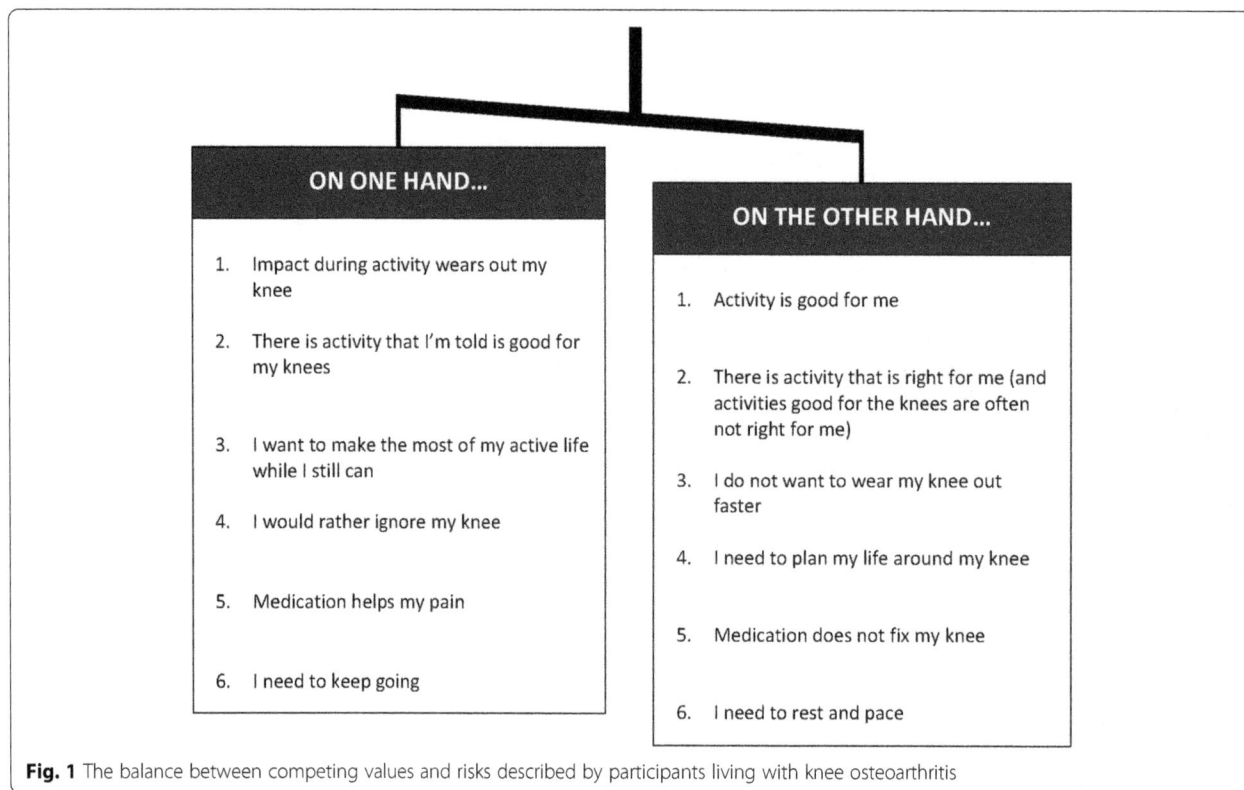

Fig. 1 The balance between competing values and risks described by participants living with knee osteoarthritis

Expectation of progressive decline meant participants wanted to be active while still able, but equally they were concerned that activity would accelerate their joint degradation:

"I've got a window of time to do all these things in. But then, at the same time, I've got to do this in a way that doesn't impact that window of time, make it shorter than it otherwise would be. So it's really, yeah, finding that balance."

–Linda

Many participants mentioned the cost-benefit payoff between medication and side effects, especially as analgesics were not addressing the perceived inevitable degeneration:

"All it's really doing is taking the pain away a little bit. But the joint continues to deteriorate, the pain gets worse."

–James

Many participants wanted to delay surgery as long as possible due to concerns about surgery, recovery times, and uncertainty about how long the new joint would last. However, they were also concerned about the impact of increasing age or disability on joint replacement outcomes.

Discussion

This study explored beliefs about the OA disease process and impact in people with knee OA. In particular, and not fully explored in previous literature, it also explored belief formation and influence on decisions about activity participation, health behaviours, and self-management. Irrespective of duration or severity of knee symptoms, all participants viewed OA as progressive joint degradation due to wear and tear and ageing. Participants' biomechanical explanation of symptoms and expectations of inevitable decline appeared to be derived from, or perpetuated by, clinicians' language and explanations. Despite the limited correlation between X-ray findings and symptoms or disability [23], participants considered that their symptoms directly reflected their joint surface condition as seen on X-ray. Previous studies have indicated that clinicians may trivialise or minimise OA and associate it with old age and these findings were supported by the current study [9, 11, 24, 25]. This may influence a fatalistic attitude amongst people with knee OA and pessimism about engaging in care [9–11].

Participants preferred to discuss the impact of knee OA on their daily lives rather than explain their understanding of the biological mechanisms involved, which they saw as straightforward. Consistent with findings from people with rheumatoid arthritis, participants sought a balance between managing OA and living their daily lives, and matched management strategies to their perceived stage of disease [26]. Pouli et al. [10] found that people with knee OA weigh the pain relieving benefits of medication against the negative side effects or risk of dependence. The current study expands understanding of the range of factors people with knee OA balance in their daily lives. These include balancing benefits of physical activity against risks, 'safe' activities against activities they enjoyed, putting OA out of their mind while also planning lives around it, not being perceived as a moaner while also accessing necessary care, and making the most of their current function without jeopardising the future.

This study confirms that those with knee OA are often cautious of physical activity due to fear of accelerating joint degradation [12, 16, 17], and that some people engage in activity despite concerns or expectations of damage because of perceived benefits related to their general health and well-being [17]. These beliefs conflict with research demonstrating that exercise improves cartilage volumes, is safe for people with OA, and improves pain and function [27–31].

A number of studies have reported ambivalent views about joint replacement surgery in people with knee OA as a result of concerns about the surgery effectiveness, surgical risk, recovery times, and a compromised sense of internal control [10, 11, 24]. These concerns were discussed by participants in the current study, however, they strongly believed that joint replacement surgery was the only way to fix their knee joint and an inevitable part of their clinical journey. Reasons for this discrepancy could be explored with future research. Expectations of inevitable decline and ultimate joint replacement surgery decreased exploration of, and engagement in, strategies to improve joint function and health.

Strengths and limitations

The qualitative methodology allowed in-depth exploration of participants' beliefs about knee OA. Transcripts were independently analysed by two researchers to increase rigour and all findings were reviewed and debated by the entire interdisciplinary research team. Participants were recruited from two geographically separate provinces of New Zealand and the sampling frame enabled inclusion of participants with a range of characteristics. There was no age restriction, however, no participants under 50 years of age volunteered to participate. Consequently, this study does not represent the views of younger people with knee OA, however, it does represent the main age group affected. Recruitment continued until

no new themes emerged from the data. Saturation was achieved after eight interviews, demonstrating strong commonalities in language and beliefs despite differences in background, disease severity, and functional limitation. This study was not designed to explore differences between subgroups with different characteristics (e.g. length of symptoms or disease severity), however, beliefs and conceptual frameworks were surprisingly consistent. Information provided to participants may have been different from what they reported, however, the use of 'wear and tear' and minimisation of OA by clinicians has been directly observed in consultations [25]. Although these findings are consistent with those found with other populations [13, 16, 17], caution is advised when applying these findings to other settings. The inclusion of consumers as part of the research team could have added insights to the analysis.

Implications for clinical practice and future research

People with OA make difficult decisions on a daily basis, but many decisions are premised on inaccurate information or beliefs that are often not addressed, and may even be promulgated, by clinicians. Clinicians' use of the term 'wear and tear' may represent an attempt to present the diagnosis of OA in a less threatening way or an effort to shift focus from the diagnosis of 'osteoarthritis' to strategies for managing symptoms and improving function [25, 32]. However, participants saw 'wear and tear' as being synonymous with 'osteoarthritis', so it did not reduce the threat associated with diagnosis. Literal interpretation of 'wear and tear' established inaccurate biomechanical models that reinforced the perceived need to limit activity to protect the joint and thereby prevented engagement in positive self-management. Minimisation associated with 'it's just wear and tear' may also limit access to appropriate care and reduce the perceived need to engage in proactive self-management and behaviour change.

Information provided to people with OA should focus on living with OA rather than biomedical aspects of the disease [33]. The current study highlights a need to address unhelpful or inaccurate language and beliefs. Participants' universal adoption of a biomedical model limited activity participation, increased uncertainty, negatively influenced expectations for the future, and forced people with knee OA to make unnecessary decisions and trade-offs. These findings will be used to inform the development of novel information resources. Future research should explore the impact of information resources on modifying patients' beliefs about knee OA and empowering increased participation in activities and behaviours known to improve pain, function, and experiences of living with OA.

Conclusions

Participants' biomechanical models of OA and expectations of inevitable decline were influenced by clinicians' language and explanations. These beliefs reduced participant exploration of management options and underpinned a perceived need to balance competing values. Improved information provision to people with knee OA could help guide positive health behaviour and self-management decisions and ensure these decisions are grounded in current evidence.

Abbreviation

OA: Osteoarthritis

Acknowledgements

The authors gratefully acknowledge the contribution of the research participants.

Funding

This work was supported by an Otago Medical School Collaborative Research Grant. The funder played no role in the design of the study and collection, analysis, or interpretation of data, or in writing the manuscript.

Authors' contributions

BD, BH, and BT developed the concept for the study and obtained ethical approval. BD, BH, BT, RG, EM and JHA obtained funding. BD, MB, BH, BT, RG, EM and JHA contributed to study design. MB and BT recruited participants, conducted the interviews, and undertook primary analysis with support from BD. All authors contributed to interpretation of results. MB and BD wrote the first draft of the manuscript. BD, MB, BH, BT, RG, EM and JHA edited and revised the draft manuscript. All authors read and approved the final manuscript.

Competing interests

Rebecca Grainger is a member of the editorial board of BMC Rheumatology. All other authors declare that they have no competing interests.

Author details

[1]Department of Primary Health Care and General Practice, University of Otago - Wellington, Wellington, New Zealand. [2]Department Orthopaedic Surgery & Musculoskeletal Medicine, University of Otago - Christchurch, Christchurch, New Zealand. [3]Department of General Practice, University of Otago - Christchurch, Christchurch, New Zealand. [4]Department of Medicine, University of Otago - Wellington, Wellington, New Zealand. [5]Department of Surgical Sciences, University of Otago, Dunedin, New Zealand.

References

1. Vos T, Allen C, Arora M, Barber RM, Bhutta ZA, Brown A, Carter A, Casey DC, Charlson FJ, Chen AZ, et al. Global, regional, and national incidence, prevalence, and years lived with disability for 310 diseases and injuries, 1990–2015: a systematic analysis for the Global Burden of Disease Study 2015. Lancet. 2016;388(10053):1545–602.
2. Dieleman JL, Baral R, Birger M, Bui AL, Bulchis A, Chapin A, Hamavid H, Horst C, Johnson EK, Joseph J. US spending on personal health care and public health, 1996–2013. JAMA. 2016;316(24):2627–46.
3. Vos T, Flaxman AD, Naghavi M, Lozano R, Michaud C, Ezzati M, Shibuya K, Salomon JA, Abdalla S, Aboyans V, et al. Years lived with disability (YLDs) for 1160 sequelae of 289 diseases and injuries 1990–2010: a systematic analysis for the global burden of disease study 2010. Lancet. 2012; 380(9859):2163–96.
4. Wallace IJ, Worthington S, Felson DT, Jurmain RD, Wren KT, Maijanen H, Woods RJ, Lieberman DE. Knee osteoarthritis has doubled in prevalence since the mid-20th century. Proc Natl Acad Sci U S A. 2017;114(35):9332–6.
5. Pit SW, Shrestha R, Schofield D, Passey M. Health problems and retirement due to ill-health among Australian retirees aged 45–64 years. Health Policy. 2010;94(2):175–81.
6. Hunter DJ, Schofield D, Callander E. The individual and socioeconomic impact of osteoarthritis. Nat Rev Rheumatol. 2014;10(7):437–41.
7. Hall M, Migay AM, Persad T, Smith J, Yoshida K, Kennedy D, Pagura S. Individuals' experience of living with osteoarthritis of the knee and perceptions of total knee arthroplasty. Physiother Theory Pract. 2008;24(3):167–81.
8. Holden DM, Nicholls ME, Young MJ, Hay PE, Foster PN. The role of exercise for knee pain: what do older adults in the community think? Arthritis Care Res. 2012;64(10):1554–64.
9. Campbell R, Evans M, Tucker M, Quilty B, Dieppe P, Donovan J. Why don't patients do their exercises? Understanding non-compliance with physiotherapy in patients with osteoarthritis of the knee. J Epidemiol Community Health. 2001;55(2):132–8.
10. Pouli N, Das Nair R, Lincoln NB, Walsh D. The experience of living with knee osteoarthritis: exploring illness and treatment beliefs through thematic analysis. Disabil Rehabil. 2014;36(7):600–7.
11. Sanders C, Donovan J, Dieppe P. Unmet need for joint replacement: a qualitative investigation of barriers to treatment among individuals with severe pain and disability of the hip and knee. Rheumatology. 2003;43(3): 353–7.
12. Turner A, Barlow J, Buszewicz M, Atkinson A, Rait G. Beliefs about the causes of osteoarthritis among primary care patients. Arthritis Care Res. 2007;57(2):267–71.
13. Leov J, Barrett E, Gallagher S, Swain N. A qualitative study of pain experiences in patients requiring hip and knee arthroplasty. J Health Psychol. 2017;22(2):186–96.
14. Manninen P, Riihimaki H, Heliovaara M, Suomalainen O. Physical exercise and risk of severe knee osteoarthritis requiring arthroplasty. Rheumatology. 2001;40(4):432–7.
15. Nelson AE, Allen KD, Golightly YM, Goode AP, Jordan JM. A systematic review of recommendations and guidelines for the management of osteoarthritis: The Chronic Osteoarthritis Management Initiative of the US Bone and Joint Initiative. Semin Arthritis Rheum. 2014; 43(6):701–12.
16. MacKay C, Jaglal SB, Sale J, Badley EM, Davis AM. A qualitative study of the consequences of knee symptoms: 'It's like you're an athlete and you go to a couch potato'. BMJ Open. 2014;4(10):e006006.
17. Hendry M, Williams NH, Markland D, Wilkinson C, Maddison P. Why should we exercise when our knees hurt? A qualitative study of primary care patients with osteoarthritis of the knee. Fam Pract. 2006; 23(5):558–67.
18. Thorne S, Kirkham SR, MacDonald-Emes J. Interpretive description: a noncategorical qualitative alternative for developing nursing knowledge. Res Nurs Health. 1997;20(2):169–77.
19. Thorne S, Kirkham SR, O'Flynn-Magee K. The analytic challenge of Interpretative Description. Int J Qual Methods. 2004;3(1):Article 1.
20. Braun V, Clarke V. Successful qualitative research: a practical guide for beginners. Los Angeles: SAGE; 2013.
21. Dawson J, Fitzpatrick R, Murray D, Carr A. Questionnaire on the perceptions of patients about total knee replacement. J Bone Joint Surg Br. 1998;80(1): 63–9.
22. Nicholas MK. The pain self-efficacy questionnaire: taking pain into account. Eur J Pain. 2007;11(2):153–63.
23. Hannan MT, Felson DT, Pincus T. Analysis of the discordance between radiographic changes and knee pain in osteoarthritis of the knee. J Rheumatol. 2000;27(6):1513–7.
24. Alami S, Boutron I, Desjeux D, Hirschhorn M, Meric G, Rannou F, Poiraudeau S. Patients' and practitioners' views of knee osteoarthritis and its management: a qualitative interview study. PLoS One. 2011;6(5):e19634.
25. Paskins Z, Sanders T, Croft PR, Hassell AB. The identity crisis of osteoarthritis in general practice: a qualitative study using video-stimulated recall. Ann Fam Med. 2015;13(6):537–44.

26. Flurey CA, Morris M, Richards P, Hughes R, Hewlett S. It's like a juggling act: rheumatoid arthritis patient perspectives on daily life and flare while on current treatment regimes. Rheumatology. 2014;53(4):696–703.

27. Urquhart DM, Tobing JF, Hanna FS, Berry P, Wluka AE, Ding C, Cicuttini FM. What is the effect of physical activity on the knee joint? A systematic review. Med Sci Sports Exerc. 2011;43(3):432–42.

28. Abbott J, Robertson M, Chapple C, Pinto D, Wright A, de la Barra SL, Baxter G, Theis J-C, Campbell A, team MT. Manual therapy, exercise therapy, or both, in addition to usual care, for osteoarthritis of the hip or knee: a randomized controlled trial. 1: clinical effectiveness. Osteoarthr Cartil. 2013;21(4):525–34.

29. Fransen M, McConnell S, Harmer AR, Van der Esch M, Simic M, Bennell KL. Exercise for osteoarthritis of the knee. Cochrane Database Syst Rev. 2015;1: Cd004376.

30. Juhl C, Christensen R, Roos EM, Zhang W, Lund H. Impact of exercise type and dose on pain and disability in knee osteoarthritis: a systematic review and meta-regression analysis of randomized controlled trials. Arthritis Rheum. 2014;66(3):622–36.

31. Roddy E, Zhang W, Doherty M, Arden N, Barlow J, Birrell F, Carr A, Chakravarty K, Dickson J, Hay E. Evidence-based recommendations for the role of exercise in the management of osteoarthritis of the hip or knee—the MOVE consensus. Rheumatology. 2005;44(1):67–73.

32. Bedson J, McCarney R, Croft P. Labelling chronic illness in primary care: a good or a bad thing? Br J Gen Pract. 2004;54(509):932–8.

33. Grime JC, Ong BN. Constructing osteoarthritis through discourse–a qualitative analysis of six patient information leaflets on osteoarthritis. BMC Musculoskelet Disord. 2007;8:34.

13

Methotrexate therapy impacts on red cell distribution width and its predictive value for cardiovascular events in patients with rheumatoid arthritis

Julia Held[1], Birgit Mosheimer-Feistritzer[1], Johann Gruber[1], Erich Mur[2] and Günter Weiss[1,3]*

Abstract

Background: Methotrexate (MTX) is well known to affect folic acid metabolism, so MTX treatment can result in alterations of mean corpuscular volume (MCV), which may impact on red cell distribution width (RDW), as MCV levels feed into RDW calculation. We thus questioned whether RDW levels and subsequently its diagnostic utility in RA subjects, as reported before, are influenced by ongoing MTX therapy.

We assessed the impact of disease modifying drug (DMARD) treatment, especially MTX, on RDW and evaluated their influence on the predictive value of RDW for cardiovascular (CV) events in patients with rheumatoid arthritis (RA). As far as we know, this is the first study evaluating the influence of MTX on RDW.

Methods: Medical treatment, disease activity, laboratory parameters and history of CV events were retrospectively analysed in 385 RA patients at disease onset and at last follow up at our clinic. Additionally, in patients with CV event, data were recorded at last follow up prior the CV event.

Results: Disease parameters and laboratory findings associated with a serious vascular event were older age ($p < 0,001$), longer disease duration ($p = 0,002$) and a higher RDW at diagnosis ($p = 0,025$). No differences in RDW levels became evident with any other treatment regimen beside MTX. MTX treated patients had significantly higher RDW compared to subjects without this drug ($p < 0,001$). In RA patients without MTX treatment, we found RDW level significantly different between those with versus without a CV event, whereas this difference disappeared in subjects receiving MTX.

Conclusion: MTX impacts on RDW and might therefor reduce its prognostic value for CV events in patients taking MTX, whereas an increased RDW at diagnosis remains an early risk predictor for myocardial infarction and stroke in RA patients.

Keywords: Rheumatoid arthritis, Red cell distribution width, Methotrexate, Cardiovascular events

Background

Rheumatoid arthritis (RA) is one of the most prevalent systemic inflammatory diseases which involve joints and extra-articular tissues, thereby causing organ damage. Based on the chronic inflammation and immune dysregulation, the presence of RA has been associated with cardiovascular (CV) disease and an increased CV associated mortality [1, 2]. Classical risk factors for CV disease have been investigated in RA patients, however, epidemiological studies indicate that they cannot provide a sufficient explanation for the poorer CV prognosis of RA patients as compared to non-RA subjects [3, 4]. Therefore, a combination of yet not fully elucidated factors and regulatory mechanisms may contribute to CV morbidity in RA subjects. However, it is of clinical importance to identify markers which indicate an increased CV risk or predict CV mortality in RA patients. In this regard, recent studies reported an association of elevated red cell distribution width (RDW) with CV disease in

* Correspondence: guenter.weiss@i-med.ac.at
[1]Department of Internal Medicine II, Infectious Diseases, Immunology, Rheumatology, Pneumology, Medical University of Innsbruck, Anichstr. 35, A-6020 Innsbruck, Austria
[3]Christian Doppler Laboratory for Iron Metabolism and Anemia Research, Innsbruck, Austria
Full list of author information is available at the end of the article

the general population [5] but also in patients with RA [6, 7].

RDW is an automated measure of the range of variation of red blood cell (RBC) volume and is calculated as the standard deviation (SD) in red blood cell size divided by the mean corpuscular volume (MCV) (RDW (%) = 1 SD of RBC volume/MCV × 100). RDW is part of the complete blood count and has traditionally been used in anemia diagnosis [8–10] and to predict the response to iron treatment [11]. A retrospective analysis of > 20.000 patients with RA indicated that higher RDW, as well as increased levels of markers of inflammation, like C-reactive protein (CRP) or erythrocyte sedimentation rate (ESR), were associated with an increased risk of a subsequent CV event in RA-patients [12].

The mechanism behind the association of elevated RDW and CV risk in RA is yet incompletely understood. Possible explanations include that RDW reflects endothelial damage and impaired vascular repair, but also that RDW mirrors vascular inflammation underlying atherosclerosis and thereby effects myocardial infarction and stroke [13]. The described positive association between IFN-alpha, a cytokine contributing to endothelial damage, and RDW would be in agreement with this concept [14].

Of note, RDW is influenced by multiple factors related to erythropoiesis, such as iron, vitamin B12 or folic acid availability, as well as by hemolysis [9]. Moreover, RDW is also affected by organ dysfunctions (e.g. liver or renal dysfunction), inflammatory activity and some specific medications [15–17]. The latter might also affect the diagnostic potential of RDW in RA patients, as these subjects are treated with numerous disease modifying antirheumatic drugs (csDMARDs), like Methotrexate (MTX), or biological DMARDs (bDMARDs), including several cytokine antibodies [18]. According to EULAR recommendations, treatment of RA should be initiated with csDMARDs, most notably MTX in combination with low dose glucocorticoids. Although low dose MTX therapy is regarded as an anchor therapy in RA, full details of its mechanism of action and off target effects are still incompletely understood [19].

Because, MTX is well known to affect folic acid metabolism, MTX treatment can result in alterations of MCV, which may impact on RDW, as MCV levels feed into RDW calculation [6]. We thus questioned, whether RDW levels and subsequently its diagnostic utility and potential in RA subjects, as reported before [7, 11, 19, 20], are influenced by ongoing MTX therapy.

Methods

Patients

We evaluated a total of number of 385 patients with RA. These patients were either consecutively registered in the database for evaluating iron homeostasis in RA patients ($n = 261$), or were evaluated retrospectively following their clinical examination at our outpatient clinics ($n = 124$). All patients fulfilled the 2010 ACR classification criteria for the diagnosis of RA [21]. At inclusion in the database, clinical and laboratory parameters were collected of these 261 patients. The 124 patients, who consulted the outpatients' clinic in 2014, were retrospectively evaluated. Full blood count, disease activity parameters and medication were available from that appointment. Additionally, we retrospectively evaluated clinical and laboratory findings at last visit before a CV event occurred, this visit was defined as last follow up in these patients. In patients without a CV event, either the date the patients were included in the database or the routine follow up at our outpatient clinic was defined as last follow up. The study was approved by the Ethics committee at Medical University Innsbruck, Austria (study number AN2014-0277).

CV-Event

The medical history was examined until Nov. 2016. A severe CV-Event was defined as myocardial infarction with or without ST-wave elevation or as an ischemic stroke. According to previous studies, CV events were clustered together [7, 22].

RDW

RDW is mathematically calculated based on the results of a routine blood count as the one SD of RBC volume/MCV × 100 [23]. The laboratory analyses were all performed by the Central Institute of Medical and Chemical Laboratory Diagnostics, University Hospital, Innsbruck. RDW was evaluated at initial diagnosis, during follow up between 2009 and 2016 and prior to a CV event. ΔRDW showed the change between the RDW at diagnosis and prior to CV event or at last follow up in patients without CV event.

Statistical analysis

Statistical analysis was performed using IBM SPSS Statistics 24 software. Normal distribution of laboratory parameters was assessed and retained by Kolmogorov-Smirnov-Test and One-Sample Chi-Square Test, respectively. Correlation among parameters was determined using Spearman-Rank-analysis. For comparative analysis between groups we applied Mann-Whitney-U-test, respectively cross tables. Linear regression model was applied to evaluate effects of medical treatment and laboratory findings on RDW.

Results

We retrospectively analysed 385 RA-outpatients, of whom 77 (20%) were male and 308 (80%) female. The mean duration of RA was 14,5 years (SD 11,9), 77,2% of patients were positive for anti-citrullinated-peptide-anti-bodies (ACPA) and 73,5% of patients had a positive rheumatoid factor (RF) test, both parameters linked to disease severity in RA [24]. Upon evaluation of their medical history, we found that 23/385 (6%) had a documented severe CV event during the observation period (17 patients with myocardial infarction, six patients with stroke). We could not find an association between ACPA and/or RF positivity and the risk for a CV event. Disease parameters and laboratory findings associated with a vascular event were older age ($p < 0,001$) and a longer disease duration ($p = 0,002$). Patients with a cardiovascular event during follow up had a higher RDW at the date of initial diagnosis of RA as compared to subjects without a subsequent cardiovascular event ($p = 0,025$; Table 1).

We then studied for associations between disease activity, measured by DAS-28-CRP, haematological parameters (RDW and MCV at last visit or last visit before a CV event) and csDMARDs therapy in patients with or without a CV event. While no significant difference was seen for laboratory parameters, disease activity and all other medications including biological DMARDs between patients with and without a subsequent CV event, we found that leflunomid was administrated more frequently in patients with CV events, however, the total number of patients receiving leflunomid was very low ($p = 0,05$; Table 2) .

Out of 385 RA patient included in the evaluation 284/385 (73,8%) were under treatment with csDMARDs and 83/284 (29,2%) patients were under combination therapy with biological DMARDs and csDMARDs. Because certain csDMARDs may impact on erythropoiesis or modulate the availability of factors involved in erythropoiesis, such as folic acid [25], we next studied for differences in RDW according to underlying therapy. Whereas no

differences in RDW levels became evident with any other DMARD treatment, patients receiving MTX therapy had significantly higher RDW as compared to subjects without this drug ($p < 0,001$), although all patients under MTX treatment had folic acid supplementation prescribed (Table 3).

We then studied whether or not MTX treatment had an effect on the predictive value of RDW for severe CV events. The last routine follow up of patients with evaluation of laboratory parameters prior to the CV events was 82 days (mean) prior to such a CV complication. No significant differences in RDW, hemoglobin levels, CRP or ΔRDW (change in RDW between initial diagnosis and follow up prior to the CV event/last patient visit)

Table 2 Clinical and laboratory findings during follow up

	CV-Event		P
	Yes ($n = 23$)	No ($n = 362$)	
DAS 28 at follow up, mean (SD)	3,12 (0,93)	2,82 (1,37)	0,252
MCV at follow up, mean (SD)	86,6 (5,97)	87,2 (5,7)	0,533
RDW at follow up, mean (SD)	15,1 (2,2)	14,3 (1,5)	0,130
DMARDs at follow up, n (%)			
Methotrexate	15 (65,2%)	207 (57,2%)	0,451
Sulfasalazine	0	9 (2,5%)	0,445
Hydroxychloroquine	2 (8,7%)	27 (7,5%)	0,868
Leflunomide	3 (13%)	15 (4,1%)	0,050
Azathioprine	0	6 (1,7%)	0,533
Glucocorticoids	8 (34,8%)	133 (37,5%)	0,810
bDMARD	8 (34,8%)	130 (36%)	0,892

Clinical and laboratory findings during follow up associated with CV event, significance level at p level ≤ 0,05 –see legend to Table 1, *DAS 28* disease activity score 28, *MCV* mean corpuscular volume, *(b)DMARD* (biological) disease modifying antirheumatic drug

Table 1 Demographics and laboratory parameters at initial diagnosis of RA

	CV-Event		P
	Yes ($n = 23$)	No ($n = 362$)	
Gender Female, n (%)	15 (65,2)	293 (80,9)	0,068
Age, mean (SD), years	74,1 (7,1)	61,8 (13,2)	< 0,001
Disease duration, mean (SD), years	23,7 (13,2)	14,1 (11,7)	0,002
RF positive, n (%)	17 (73,9)	268 (74)	0,990
ACPA positive, n (%)	18 (78,3)	279 (77,1)	0,896
RDW, mean (SD)	15,6 (0,78)	13,6 (1,28)	0,025

Demographics and laboratory parameters at initial diagnosis of RA according to a CV event during follow up, p values for statistical significances between the two groups are given by Mann Whitney U test, respectively cross tables, significance level at p level ≤ 0,05, *SD* standard deviation, *n* sample size, *RF* rheumatoid factor, *ACPA* anti citrullinated peptide antibodies, *RDW* red cell distribution width

Table 3 RDW distribution as a function of underlying DMARD therapy

DMARD	Intake	n	RDW, mean (SD)	p
Methotrexate	Yes	222	14,5 (1,44)	< 0,001
	No	163	14,0 (1,55)	
Sulfasalazine	Yes	9	13,7 (1,56)	0,119
	No	376	14,3 (1,5)	
Hydroxychloroquine	Yes	30	13,9 (1,19)	0,085
	No	355	14,4 (1,52)	
Leflunomide	Yes	18	14,7 (2,06)	0,429
	No	367	14,3 (1,47)	
Azathioprine	Yes	6	14,7 (1,23)	0,273
	No	379	14,3 (1,51)	
bDMARDs	Yes	139	14,2 (1,45)	0,381
	No	246	14,4 (1,53)	

RDW distribution as a function of underlying DMARD therapy, significance level at p level ≤ 0,05, *bDMARDs* biological DMARDs, see tables above, *n* number of patients in respective groups were found in our cohort between patients incurring a CV event or not. Of note, we found a highly significant difference in RDW levels at last follow up, see definition above, in subjects without MTX treatment which was absent in subjects under MTX treatment comparing patients with and without a CV event (Fig. 1). Moreover, MTX-treated patients had significantly higher RDW levels than patients without MTX therapy (Table 4).

In patients without MTX therapy RDW was significantly higher in those with a subsequent CV event. ($p = 0,006$; Fig. 1). This predictive value of RDW was abolished in patients taking MTX ($p = 0,448$, Fig. 1).

Multiple linear regression analysis confirmed the relationship between RDW prior to the CV event and MTX treatment as well as associations of haemoglobin levels and age with RDW (Table 5A).

When performing binary regression for the risk of a CV event, we found that MTX naïve patients had a significant correlation between RDW and a CV event (Table 5B) which was not true for patients receiving MTX.

Discussion

As far as we know, this is the first study evaluating the influence of csDMARDs on RDW. MTX impacts on

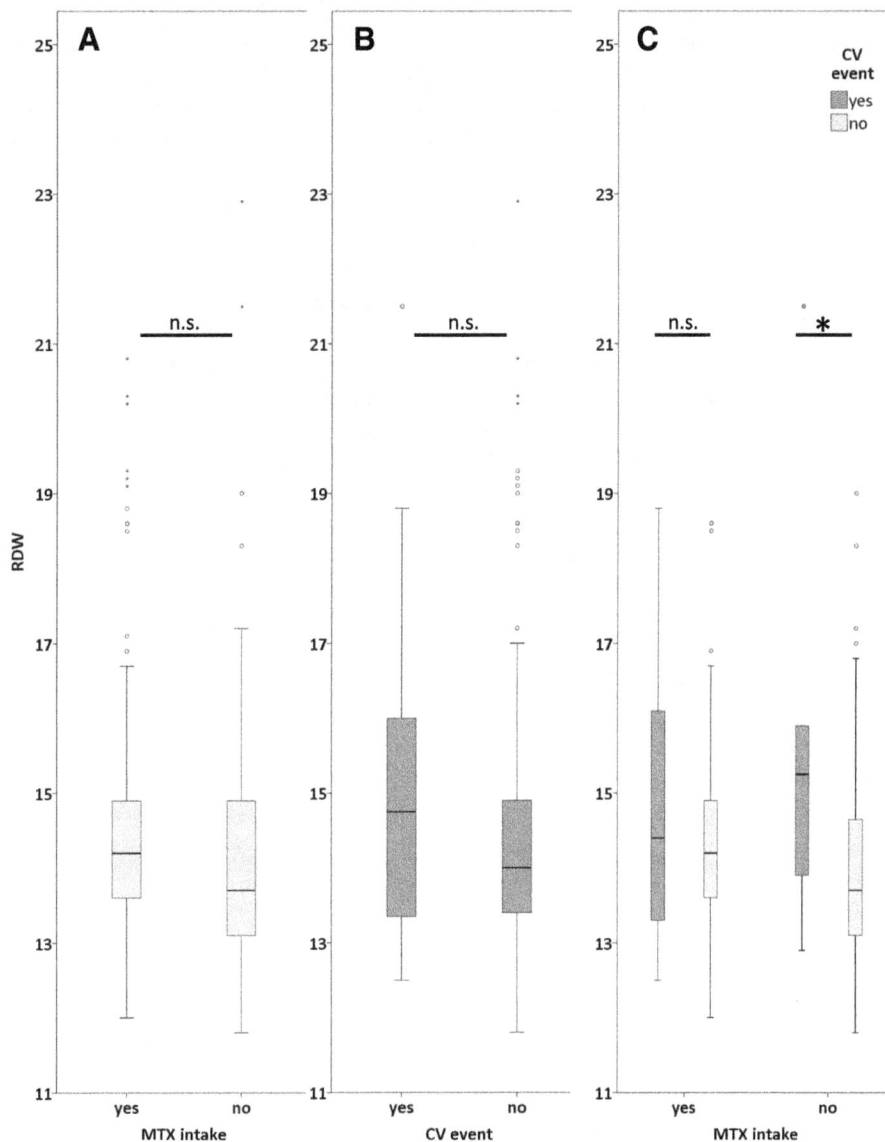

Fig. 1 Differences in RDW levels in patients with CV events and with/without MTX; **a** RDW at last follow up in all RA patients notwithstanding concomitant treatment, depending on CV-events (yes: $n = 23$, no: $n = 362$). **b** RDW in all patients independent of CV events, depending on MTX-treatment (yes: $n = 222$, no: $n = 163$). **c** RDW in patients with and without MTX intake conditional to CV events. (MTX yes+CV yes: $n = 15$, MTX yes+CV no: $n = 207$, MTX no+CV yes: $n = 8$, MTX no+CV no: $n = 155$), n.s. not significant at p-level 0,05, *: $p = 0,006$ as determined by Mann Whitney U test

Table 4 Effects of MTX intake on laboratory parameters at last follow up

	MTX-use		p	CV-Event		p
	Yes (n = 222)	No (n = 163)		Yes (n = 23)	No (n = 362)	
RDW, mean(SD), %	14,5 (1,4)	14,1 (1,6)	< 0,001	15,05 (2,2)	14,25 (1,4)	0,116
Hb, mean(SD), g/l	134,8 (14,5)	132,9 (14)	0,101	130,2 (14,4)	134,2 (14,3)	0,058
CRP, mean(SD), mg/dl	0,65 (0,97)	1,03 (2,1)	0,559	0,99 (1,1)	0,8 (1,6)	0,060
ΔRDW, mean(SD)	0,53 (1,24)	0,23 (1,0)	0,057	0,45 (0,6)	0,43 (1,2)	0,809

Effects of MTX intake on laboratory parameters at last visit prior to the CV event/last follow up. *ΔRDW* Change in RDW between initial diagnosis and follow up prior to the CV event/last follow up in patients without CV event. *Hb* hemoglobin level. In the overall cohort RDW at established disease was not applicable as predictive marker for a CV event. A tendency with lower hemoglobin levels and higher CRP was shown. MTX intake significantly affected RDW

RDW hence on the predictive value of RDW for CV events. Previous studies suggest that RDW is a good prognostic marker for CV disease and survival, but none of them evaluated concomitant treatment [6, 7, 12, 17]. This was also confirmed in our study indicating that an enhanced RDW at initial diagnosis, but neither ACPA nor RF positivity, is associated with an increased risk of a severe CV event [26].

However, we found that the predictive potential of RDW during follow up largely depends on the treatment of patients. Specifically, we identified that the diagnostic value of RDW as a risk indicator for subsequent CV disease is abolished in RA patients receiving MTX therapy. Although MTX is regarded as the anchor drug in RA, the mechanism of action is incompletely understood and it has been associated with negative effects on hematopoiesis, mainly via its impact on folic acid pathways, but also via direct toxic effects on hematopoietic progenitors. Accordingly, MTX but neither other csDMARDs nor bDMARD treatment resulted in alterations of red blood cell volume (MCV) and haemoglobin content of erythrocytes [27, 28]. To avoid such negative effects, patients under MTX therapy are supplemented with folic acid which was also the case in our subjects under MTX treatment [29]. However, RA patients under MTX treatment had increased RDW and MCV levels as compared to RA patients without MTX. It remains to be clarified, whether this can be referred to effects of MTX not linked to folic acid deficiency, or a reduced compliance of patients in regard to folic acid supplementation, which we could not study, because incomplete results of folic acid determination in blood were available in our study cohort. However, while MTX treatment resulted in a loss of the predictive value of RDW for subsequent CV events, higher RDW at initial diagnosis of all patients, at follow up prior to a CV event in patients without MTX treatment were significantly associated with an increased risk for a CV event.

Our study has limitations because of the retrospective design, the low number of patients with CV events and the fact that we had only insufficient data to evaluate the association of RDW, MTX therapy and CV events with other important variables including classical CV factors, the implication of a genetic component, or iron homeostasis [11, 30, 31]. In this regard, patients with RA who carried the methylene tetrahydrofolate reductase (MTHFR) 1298 allele C frequency were previously found to have an increased frequency of CV events after 5 and 10 years of follow-up. Moreover, patients carrying the MTHFR 1298 AC and CC genotypes had a significantly decreased flow-mediated endothelium-dependent vasodilatation, a marker of endothelial dysfunction that is an early indicator of atherogenesis, when compared with those carrying the MTHFR 1298 AA genotype [32]. More recent results also indicate that MTHFR expression is significantly reduced in patients with RA compared to controls. It was found to be especially true for RA patients with ischemic heart disease [33]. Taken these considerations together, these

Table 5 A) multiple linear regression modelling the relationship with RDW. B) Binary regression relationship between CV events and RDW

A: Multiple linear regression			B: Binary regression			
Dependent variable: RDW at follow up			CV-Event			
	p	95% CI	MTX		p	95%CI
MTX	< 0,001	0,290–0,818	no	RDW follow up	0,018	0,491–0,935
Age, y follow up	< 0,001	0,011–0,031	yes	RDW follow up	0,511	0,624–1,247
Hb, g/l follow up	< 0,001	−0,057––0,039				

A) Multiple linear regression modelling the relationship with RDW at follow up, B) Binary regression, relationship between CV events and RDW at follow up according to MTX intake, *y* years, *Hb* hemoglobine level, *MTX* methotrexate, *CV* cardiovascular, *CI* confidence interval results indicate that MTHFR gene may influence the risk of subclinical atherosclerosis and CV disease in patients with RA.

Therefore, we need prospective evaluations of such risk markers and profiles to gain further insights into the functional and diagnostic role of RDW and alterations of hematological parameters as risk predicators for CV events in patients with RA. Accordingly, such confirmation may also translate into clinical practice, because patients at a higher risk, based on increased RDW may deserve an intensified clinical follow up with an improved control of classical CV risk factors, such as lipid status, hypertension, smoking status or hyperuricemia.

Conclusion
Our study approves RDW at initial diagnosis of RA as a risk predictor for serious CV events but also indicates that its predictive value is lost during follow up in patients receiving MTX therapy, whereas it remains valid in subjects receiving non-MTX containing treatments.

Abbreviations
ACR: American College of Rheumatology; CRP: C-reactive protein; CV: Cardiovascular; DAS-28: Disease activity score 28; DMARD: Disease modifying drugs; ESR: Erythrocyte sedimentation rate; EULAR: European League against Rheumatism; MCV: Mean corpuscular volume; MTHFR: Methylene tetrahydrofolate reductase; MTX: Methotrexate; RA: Rheumatoid arthritis; RDW: Red cell distribution width; SD: Standard deviation

Acknowledgements
Support by the Christian Doppler Society, Austria is gratefully acknowledged.

Funding
This work was supported by the Austrian research funds, project FWF-TRP-188 to GW.

Authors' contributions
JH: acquisition of data, analysis and interpretation of data; drafting the manuscript, given final approval of the version to be published, agreed to be accountable for all aspects of the work. BM: acquisition and analysis of data, given final approval of the version to be published, agreed to be accountable for all aspects of the work. JG: acquisition and analysis of data, given final approval of the version to be published, agreed to be accountable for all aspects of the work. EM: acquisition and analysis of data, given final approval of the version to be published, agreed to be accountable for all aspects of the work. GW: analysis and interpretation of data; drafting the manuscript, given final approval of the version to be published, agreed to be accountable for all aspects of the work.

Competing interests
The authors declare that they have no competing interests.

Author details
Department of Internal Medicine II, Infectious Diseases, Immunology, Rheumatology, Pneumology, Medical University of Innsbruck, Anichstr. 35, A-6020 Innsbruck, Austria. 2Department for Physical Medicine and Rehabilitation, University of Innsbruck, Innsbruck, Austria. 3Christian Doppler Laboratory for Iron Metabolism and Anemia Research, Innsbruck, Austria.

References
1. Smolen JS, Aletaha D, McInnes IB. Rheumatoid arthritis. Lancet. 2016;388: 2023–38.
2. Maradit-Kremers H, Crowson CS, Nicola PJ, Ballman KV, Roger VL, Jacobsen SJ, et al. Increased unrecognized coronary heart disease and sudden deaths in rheumatoid arthritis: a population-based cohort study. Arthritis Rheum. 2005;52:402–11.
3. del Rincón ID, Williams K, Stern MP, Freeman GL, Escalante A. High incidence of cardiovascular events in a rheumatoid arthritis cohort not explained by traditional cardiac risk factors. Arthritis Rheum. 2001;44: 2737–45.
4. Gonzalez A, Maradit Kremers H, Crowson CS, Ballman KV, Roger VL, Jacobsen SJ, et al. Do cardiovascular risk factors confer the same risk for cardiovascular outcomes in rheumatoid arthritis patients as in non-rheumatoid arthritis patients? Ann Rheum Dis. 2008;67:64–9.
5. Patel KV, Semba RD, Ferrucci L, Newman AB, Fried LP, Wallace RB, et al. Red cell distribution width and mortality in older adults: a meta-analysis. J Gerontol A Biol Sci Med Sci. 2010;65:258–65.
6. Felker GM, Allen LA, Pocock SJ, Shaw LK, McMurray JJV, Pfeffer MA, et al. Red cell distribution width as a novel prognostic marker in heart failure: data from the CHARM Program and the Duke Databank. J Am Coll Cardiol. 2007;50:40–7.
7. Rodríguez-Carrio J, Alperi-López M, López P, Alonso-Castro S, Ballina-García FJ, Suárez A. Red cell distribution width is associated with cardiovascular risk and disease parameters in rheumatoid arthritis. Rheumatology (Oxford). 2015;54(4): 641–6.
8. Demir A, Yarali N, Fisgin T, Duru F, Kara A. Most reliable indices in differentiation between thalassemia trait and iron deficiency anemia. Pediatr Int. 2002;44:612–6.
9. Thomas C, Thomas L. Biochemical markers and hematologic indices in the diagnosis of functional iron deficiency. Clin Chem. 2002;48:1066–76.
10. Bessman JD, Gilmer PR, Gardner FH. Improved classification of anemias by MCV and RDW. Am J Clin Pathol. 1983;80:322–6.
11. Weiss G. Monitoring iron therapy in chronic heart failure. Eur J Heart Fail. 2013;15:711–2.
12. Hassan S, Antonelli M, Ballou S. Red cell distribution width: a measure of cardiovascular risk in rheumatoid arthritis patients? Clin Rheumatol. 2015; 34(6):1053–7.
13. Iadecola C, Anrather J. The immunology of stroke: from mechanisms to translation. Nat Med. 2011;17:796–808.
14. Rodríguez-Carrio J, Alperi-López M, López P, Alonso-Castro S, Carro-Esteban SR, Ballina-García FJ, et al. Red cell distribution width is associated with endothelial progenitor cell depletion and vascular-related mediators in rheumatoid arthritis. Atherosclerosis. 2015;240:131–6.
15. Balta S, Demirkol S, Cakar M, Aydogan M, Akhan M. The red cell distribution width may be affected by many factors in the clinical practice. J Clin Diagn Res. 2013;7:1830.
16. Mori S, Hidaka M, Kawakita T, Hidaka T, Tsuda H, Yoshitama T, et al. Factors associated with myelosuppression related to low-dose methotrexate therapy for inflammatory rheumatic diseases. PLoS One. 2016;11:e0154744.
17. Luo R, Hu J, Jiang L, Zhang M. Prognostic value of red blood cell distribution width in non-cardiovascular critically or acutely patients: a systematic review. PLoS One. 2016;11:e0167000.
18. Smolen JS, Landewé R, Bijlsma J, Burmester G, Chatzidionysiou K, Dougados M, et al. EULAR recommendations for the management of rheumatoid arthritis with synthetic and biological disease-modifying antirheumatic drugs: 2016 update. Ann Rheum Dis. 2017;76:960–77.
19. Brown PM, Pratt AG, Isaacs JD. Mechanism of action of methotrexate in rheumatoid arthritis, and the search for biomarkers. Nat Rev Rheumatol. 2016;12:731–42.
20. Al Taii H, Yaqoob Z, Al-Kindi SG. Red cell distribution width (RDW) is associated with cardiovascular disease risk in Crohn's disease. Clin Res Hepatol Gastroenterol. 2017;41(4):490–492.
21. Aletaha D, Neogi T, Silman AJ, Funovits J, Felson DT, Bingham CO, et al. 2010 rheumatoid arthritis classification criteria: an American College of Rheumatology/European League Against Rheumatism collaborative initiative. Arthritis Rheum. 2010;62:2569–81.
22. Gonzalez-Gay MA, Gonzalez-Juanatey C, Lopez-Diaz MJ, Piñeiro A, Garcia-Porrua C, Miranda-Filloy JA, et al. HLA-DRB1 and persistent chronic inflammation contribute to cardiovascular events and cardiovascular mortality in patients with rheumatoid arthritis. Arthritis

Rheum. 2007;57:125–32.

23. Lippi G, Mattiuzzi C, Cervellin G. Learning more and spending less with neglected laboratory parameters: the paradigmatic case of red blood cell distribution width. Acta Biomed. 2017;87:323–8.

24. Song YW, Kang EH. Autoantibodies in rheumatoid arthritis: rheumatoid factors and anticitrullinated protein antibodies. QJM. 2010;103:139–46.

25. Leeb BF, Witzmann G, Ogris E, Studnicka-Benke A, Andel I, Schweitzer H, et al. Folic acid and cyanocobalamin levels in serum and erythrocytes during low-dose methotrexate therapy of rheumatoid arthritis and psoriatic arthritis patients. Clin Exp Rheumatol. 1995;13:459–63.

26. Berendsen MLT, van Maaren MC, Arts EEA, den Broeder AA, Popa CD, Fransen J. Anticyclic citrullinated peptide antibodies and rheumatoid factor as risk factors for 10-year cardiovascular morbidity in patients with rheumatoid arthritis: a large inception cohort study. J Rheumatol. 2017; https://doi.org/10.3899/jrheum.160670.

27. Gilani STA, Khan DA, Khan FA, Ahmed M. Adverse effects of low dose methotrexate in rheumatoid arthritis patients. J Coll Physicians Surg Pak. 2012;22:101–4.

28. Dubey L, Chatterjee S, Ghosh A. Hepatic and hematological adverse effects of long-term low-dose methotrexate therapy in rheumatoid arthritis: an observational study. Indian J Pharmacol. 2016;48:591.

29. McInnes IB, Schett G. Pathogenetic insights from the treatment of rheumatoid arthritis. Lancet. 2017;389:2328–37.

30. Fernández-Gutiérrez B, Perrotti PP, Gisbert JP, Domènech E, Fernández-Nebro A, Cañete JD, et al. Cardiovascular disease in immune-mediated inflammatory diseases. Medicine (Baltimore). 2017;96:e7308.

31. López-Mejías R, Castañeda S, González-Juanatey C, Corrales A, Ferraz-Amaro I, Genre F, et al. Cardiovascular risk assessment in patients with rheumatoid arthritis: the relevance of clinical, genetic and serological markers. Autoimmun Rev. 2016;15:1013–30.

32. Palomino-Morales R, Gonzalez-Juanatey C, Vazquez-Rodriguez TR, Rodriguez L, Miranda-Filloy JA, Fernandez-Gutierrez B, et al. A1298C polymorphism in the MTHFR gene predisposes to cardiovascular risk in rheumatoid arthritis. Arthritis Res Ther. 2010;12(2):R71.

33. Remuzgo-Martínez S, Genre F, López-Mejías R, Ubilla B, Mijares V, Pina T, et al. Decreased expression of methylene tetrahydrofolate reductase (MTHFR) gene in patients with rheumatoid arthritis. Clin Exp Rheumatol. 2016;34:106–10.

14

Giant cell arteritis: pathogenic mechanisms and new potential therapeutic targets

Matthew J. Koster* and Kenneth J. Warrington

Abstract

Giant cell arteritis (GCA) is the most common idiopathic systemic vasculitis in persons aged 50 years or greater. Treatment options for GCA, to-date, have been limited and have consisted primarily of glucocorticoids. Significant advances in the understanding of the genetic and cellular mechanisms in GCA are leading to identification of potential pathogenic targets. The recent success of interleukin-6 blockade in the treatment of GCA has opened the landscape to targeted biologic therapy. T cells, particularly T helper 1 and T helper 17 cell lineages have been identified as key inflammatory cells in both active and chronic vascular inflammatory lesions. Therapeutic agents, including abatacept and ustekinumab, which can impede both vasculitogenic cell lines are of particular interest. Inhibition of signalling pathways, including the janus kinase-signal tranducers and activation of transcription (JAK-STAT) and Notch pathways are evolving options. Tocilizumab has shown clear benefit in both newly diagnosed and relapsing patients with GCA and approval of this medication for treatment of GCA has led to rapid incorporation into treatment regimens. More information is required to understand the long-term outcomes of tocilizumab and other investigational targeted therapeutics in the treatment of GCA.

Keywords: Vasculitis, Giant cell arteritis, Pathogenesis, Therapeutics, Biologics

Background

Giant cell arteritis (GCA) is the most common idiopathic systemic vasculitis in persons aged 50 years or older [1] and demonstrates a predilection for involvement of the aorta and its primary branches. The clinical presentation of GCA is variable and is based on the distribution of vascular involvement with most patients demonstrating classical cranial manifestations (headache, scalp tenderness, jaw claudication, vision loss) while others present primarily with constitutional and/or musculoskeletal symptoms. Less commonly, arterial occlusive disease of the extremities leads to symptoms of vascular claudication. Histopathologic examination of a temporal artery biopsy (TAB) specimen remains the gold-standard method of diagnosis, although vascular imaging studies are increasingly used in conjunction with, or instead of, an invasive biopsy. The aetiology and pathogenesis underscoring the development of GCA are still incompletely understood. Nevertheless, several advances in genetic and immunology research have led to a greater insight into the pathomechanisms that initiate and sustain vascular inflammation in GCA. Despite the availability of effective biologic agents for other autoimmune conditions, the treatment options for GCA, to-date, have been limited. Although glucocorticoids (GC) have been the standard-of-care for over six decades, treatment is not curative and is associated with significant morbidity. Therefore, the ongoing identification of key immune mediators in disease pathogenesis is encouraging the pursuit of clinical trials with targeted therapeutic agents. The aim of this article is to summarize the fundamental pathogenic mechanisms and new potential therapeutic options for the treatment of GCA. In order to accomplish this, we searched PubMed for the following search terms: "giant cell arteritis", "large vessel vasculitis", "temporal arteritis", "arteritis" and "vasculitis". Publications from the past 10 years were analyzed for pathogenic and therapeutic studies. Case reports were not included, unless providing unique insights into pathogenic pathways. The date of the last search was 1 July 2017.

* Correspondence: koster.matthew@mayo.edu
Division of Rheumatology, Mayo Clinic College of Medicine and Science, 200 1st St SW, Rochester, MN 55905, USA

Main text

Genetic associations

Several independent studies have implicated associations between GCA susceptibility and certain human leukocyte antigen (HLA) class I and class II alleles. In particular, carriage of HLA-DRB1*0401 and DRB1*0404 haplotypes have been consistently identified in multiple GCA cohorts [2–7]. A large-scale, international, genome-wide association study has further reinforced the importance of the HLA class II region [8]. Comparison of 2134 patients with GCA to 9125 controls demonstrated strong independent signals associated with conferring predisposition to GCA located in the HLA regions between HLA-DRA and HLA-DRB1 as well as between HLA-DQA1 and HLA-DQA2 [8]. Over-representation of these HLA class II genes strongly suggests that GCA is mediated by an antigen-driven immune response.

While HLA class II genetic factors have demonstrated the strongest association with risk of GCA development, several single nucleotide polymorphism risk signals in loci among non-HLA regions have also been recognized (Table 1). However, it should be noted that most studies evaluating genetic associations in GCA have included small groups of patients and will require validation in larger patient cohorts. Nevertheless, the wide array of potentially involved cellular pathways associated with GCA susceptibility underscores the polygenic nature and complex immunopathogenesis employing both the innate and adaptive immune response in this condition.

Infection

Isolation of identical T cell clones from different vasculitic sites suggests a response to a specific antigenic stimulus [9] and studies have proposed that arterial wall dendritic cells may be activated by environmental infectious agents or autoantigens [10]. Several microorganisms have been suggested as a possible infectious trigger including *Chlamydia pneumoniae* [11, 12], *Mycoplasma pneumoniae* [13], *Burkholderia pseudomallei* [14], parvovirus B19 [15, 16], herpes simplex virus [17] and Ebstein-Barr virus [18]. Although infection-induced autoimmunity leading to loss of self-tolerance through mechanisms of molecular mimicry, bystander T-cell activation and epitope spreading is plausible, direct evidence of such remains elusive. Indeed, attempts to identify pathologic organisms in temporal artery biopsy specimens have produced inconsistent results for any specific causal infectious agent [15, 19–21].

Varicella zoster virus (VZV) has received recent focus as a potential associated infectious aetiology. The presence of VZV antigen by immunohistochemistry was identified in 68 of 93 (73%) patients with histologically confirmed GCA and 45 of 70 (64%) patients with biopsy-negative GCA, compared to only 11 of 49 (22%)

Table 1 Non-HLA genetic loci associated with giant cell arteritis

Non-HLA Locus	Function
Sample size ≥ 1000[a]	
Plasminogen (PLG) [8]	Lymphocyte recruitment, wound healing, fibrinolysis, angiogenesis
Prolyl 4-hydroxylase subunit alpha 2 (P4HA2) [8]	Collagen biosynthesis, folding of procollagen chains, hypoxia response
Tyrosine phosphatase non-receptor type 22 (PTPN22) [102]	Regulation of T and B cell receptor signaling
Interleukin-12B [8]	Th1 differentiation
Interleukin-17A ([103]; [104])	Th17 lymphocyte differentiation and maintenance
Interleukin-33 [105]	Th2 lymphocyte and mast cell activation, endothelial cell activation
Sample size ≥ 500	
NLR family pyrin domain containing 1 (NLRP1) [106]	Inflammasome assembly, activation of proinflammatory cytokines IL-1β, IL-18, IL-33
Sample size ≥ 250	
CC chemokine receptor 5 (CCR5) [107]	Proinflammatory chemokine activating cellular chemotaxis of macrophages, T lymphocytes, dendritic cells
Vascular endothelial growth factor (VEGF) ([108]; [109]; [110])	Neoangiogenesis, vascular remodeling
Interleukin-6 ([110]; [111]; [112])	Pleotropic pro-inflammatory cytokine
Sample size < 250	
Endothelial nitric oxide synthase (eNOS) ([113]; [114])	Synthesis of nitric oxide; regulation of endothelial cell vascular tone, cellular proliferation, platelet aggregation, and leukocyte adhesion
Tumor necrosis factor-a2 (TNFa2) [115]	Pleotropic pro-inflammatory cytokine
Interleukin-10 [116]	Regulation of Th1 and Th2 immunity, skews immune response to Th2 phenotype by inhibition of IL-12 production
Interleukin-18 [117]	Th1 differentiation

[a]If more than one study listed, then the sample size refers to the combined total of patients evaluated

normal controls [22]. The same investigators identified VZV DNA by PCR amplification in a blinded analysis in 3 of 3 TAB-positive GCA patients and 4 of 6 TAB-negative GCA patients [23]. These investigators have proposed that the VZV is transported along the afferent nerves to the temporal artery inciting an inflammatory process resulting in arteritis. Consequently, Gilden et al. have advocated for use of the antiviral medication acyclovir in the treatment of patients with active or refractory GCA [24]. The presence of VZV as a causative agent for GCA, however, has not been substantiated by other groups. Muratore and colleagues evaluated 79 formalin-fixed and fresh-frozen temporal artery biopsies (34 TAB-positive GCA, 15 TAB-negative GCA, and 30 controls) by immunohistochemistry and PCR analysis [25]. Only 1 of 34 patients with TAB-positive GCA had evidence of VZV antigen whereas VZV antigen was not detected among any of the TAB-negative GCA patients or controls. Furthermore, VZV DNA was not found in any of the formalin-fixed or fresh-frozen TAB samples. In a recent prospective study, Procop and colleagues similarly did not identify VZV DNA from surgically sterile temporal artery and thoracic aortic samples from patients with large-vessel vasculitis [26].

In addition to histopathology evaluations, population level studies have failed to show a causal role of VZV in GCA. In comparing 204 cases of incident GCA diagnosed between 1950 and 2004 to 408 matched controls from the same geographic location, Schäfer and colleagues found no associated risk of incident VZV among patients with GCA compared to the general population [27]. Rhee et al. performed a population-based case-control study evaluating a larger sample of patients with GCA ($n = 4559$) and controls ($n = 22,795$) and similarly concluded there was minimal-to-no association of clinically overt VZV with GCA [28]. At current, conclusive evidence does not support direct infection with VZV as a causal process for the development of GCA and the use of acyclovir as an adjunct to, or in lieu of, immunosuppression is unsubstantiated and not recommended.

Innate immune system
Vascular dendritic cells
Although the specific immunostimulatory trigger(s) is unknown, the immunopathology of GCA appears to originate from a dysregulated interaction between the vessel wall and both the innate and adaptive immune systems [29, 30]. Unlike small vessels which rely primarily on oxygen through luminal diffusion, large vessels require a microvascular network (vasa vasorum) to distribute oxygen to the media-adventia vascular cell layers. Arteries with vasa vasorum contain vascular dendritic cells (vasDCs) at the media-advential border where they are thought to participate in immune surveillance. In normal arteries, vasDCs are immature and lack the capacity to stimulate T cells [31] allowing arteries to maintain immune privilege and self-tolerance. In vasculitic lesions immune privilege is lost and vasDCs become activated via Toll-like receptors (TLRs), redistributing throughout the vessel wall [32]. Activated vasDCs are able to attract and activate T lymphocytes and macrophages through production of specific chemokine and cytokine signatures, providing a microenvironment necessary for initiating and sustaining arterial inflammation

and granuloma formation [29]. This central role of vasDCs in arteritis has been demonstrated using a model in which human temporal arteries were engrafted into immunodeficient mice, following which targeted depletion of CD83+ vasDCs resulted in marked reduction of observed vasculitis. Due to their role early in the disease process, prevention of initial vasDCs activation is an unlikely therapeutic target. However therapies addressing persistently activated vasDCs remain a viable option.

Macrophages
GCA is a granulomatous vasculitis and multinucleated giant cells, a key feature of macrophage involvement, are a considered a pathognomonic hallmark of arterial lesions. Giant cell formation is present in approximately 50% of positive temporal artery biopsies. Macrophages recruited by activated vasDCs and T lymphocytes infiltrate the arterial wall through the vasa vasorum and further differentiate into M1 and M2 phenotypes according to the arterial microenvironment. In the adventitia, activated M1 macrophages primarily secrete proinflammatory cytokines (IL-1 and IL-6) [33] while M1 macrophages in the medial layer degrade the arterial matrix through secretion of matrix metalloproteinases and damage vascular smooth muscle cells (VSMCs) and endothelial cells (ECs) through local oxidative stress mechanisms [34]. On the contrary, M2 macrophages colocalize to the intima-media border and produce proangiogenic growth factors (vascular endothelial growth factor, fibroblast growth factor and platelet-derived growth factor) which results in myofibroblast proliferation, relocation, and the marked thickening of the arterial intima.

The emerging paradigm of personalized medicine is encouraging development of nanoparticle-based theranostic agents, which integrate therapeutic and imaging functionalities. These molecules are being explored in cancer and inflammatory diseases [35]. Selective targeting of specific macrophage phenotypes may overcome the toxicity associated with macrophage inhibition through non-selective cytotoxic drugs. Preclinical models for imaging and treatment of pathogenic macrophages have shown initial promise [36]; however, further advances in this evolving field will be needed prior to consideration of selective macrophage ablation, inhibition, or phenotype modulation in GCA.

Adaptive immune system
T lymphocytes
Normal arteries are devoid of CD4+ T cell infiltration. In GCA, T cells are recruited via chemokines secreted by activated vasDCs, enter the arterial layer initially through the vasa vasorum, polarize into effector cell types and infiltrate the arterial layers. Two distinct

CD4+ T effector cell subtypes have been identified as key regulators in vasculitic lesions of GCA; type 17 helper T cells (Th17) and type 1 helper T cells (Th1) [37]. These T cell lineages are likely to be stimulated by independent signals from distinct antigen presenting cells (APC) with Th17 cells dependent on IL-1β, IL-6, IL-21 and IL-23, while the Th1 pathway requires APCs secreting IL-12 and IL-18 [30, 37].

Studies conducted in patients with active, untreated GCA show that both Th1 and Th17 lineages are present in the inflammatory arterial infiltrates and are expanded in the peripheral circulation [38, 39]. The Th17 pathway appears to be very responsive to treatment and glucocorticoids (GCs) rapidly reduce the Th17 effector cytokine production of IL-1, IL-6, IL-17 and IL-23 [30, 38] with simultaneous depletion of both circulating and tissue infiltrative Th17 cells.

The rapid decline in these cytokines upon GC initiation contributes to the prompt decrease of systemic inflammatory features. Despite the effective reduction of the Th17 pathway, a Th1 cell response persists, both in blood samples and arterial specimens from patients treated with high-dose GC [38]. The Th1 cytokine signature identified in chronic vasculitis in GCA is associated with production of IL-2 and interferon-gamma (IFN- γ) and is poorly susceptible to GCs. It is likely that persistence of vascular Th1 cellular infiltrates despite prolonged courses of GCs is responsible for the chronicity and relapsing nature observed in GCA [30].

In addition to Th1/Th17 effector T cells, regulatory T cells (Tregs) appears to have an important role in GCA pathogenesis. Tregs, which are tasked with maintaining tolerance and prevention of autoimmunity, are decreased in the blood and arterial lesions of patients with GCA [39]. Compared to healthy controls, Tregs in patients with GCA appear to be defective and potentially pathogenic, exhibiting decreased proliferation and increased production of IL-17 [40]. While GC appear to be ineffective in modifying Treg dysfunction in GCA [39], IL-6 blockade was recently shown to revert the Treg abnormalities detected in active GCA [40].

Further confirmation that T cells are implicated in the development of large-vessel vasculitis is provided by the demonstration of T cell immune check point dysregulation in GCA. Checkpoint molecules, particularly cytotoxic T-lymphocyte-associated protein 4 (CTLA-4) and programmed death-1 (PD-1), play a key role in downregulating T cell activation, maintaining self-tolerance and limiting autoimmunity. T cell activation requires antigen recognition through the T-cell receptor as well as a second signal delivered by co-stimulatory molecules. CTLA-4 and its homologous protein, cluster of differentiation 28 (CD28), are expressed on activated T cells and participate in the co-stimulatory check point. Binding of

CD28 to the CD80/86 molecules on APCs results in T cell activation and clonal expansion. On the contrary, down regulation of the immune response occurs through binding of CTLA4 to CD80/86, which results in T cell anergy. Checkpoint blockade immunotherapy is now being utilized in cancer treatments [41, 42]. Competitive inhibition of CTLA-4 by the immunostimulatory medication, ipilimumab, increases cytokine production, leads to persistent T cell activation and enhances T cell mediated immune responses to tumors [43]. However, use of ipilimumab has been associated with development of autoimmune conditions and organ-specific inflammation, including drug-induced giant cell arteritis [44].

The receptor molecule PD-1 provides inhibitory signals by binding to programmed cell death ligand 1 and 2 (PD-L1 and PD-L2), resulting in T cell anergy, apoptosis, or polarization to Tregs [45]. Recent transcriptome analysis of temporal arteries positive for GCA has demonstrated an inefficiency of the PD-1/PD-L1 checkpoint. Specifically, inflamed arteries of patients with GCA lack the inhibitory ligand PD-L1 and are enriched for PD-1–expressing T cells [46]. PD-1 blockade in a mouse model with engrafted temporal arteries worsened vascular inflammation, promoted PD-1+ effector T cells and increased effector T cell cytokines IL-17, IL-21, and IFN-γ [46]. These pre-clinical findings have been corroborated with recent reports of GCA developing in patients treated with pembrolizumab, a monoclonal antibody directed against PD-1 [47, 48].

B cells

Currently, the role of B cells in GCA is not fully understood. While plasma cells have been observed in positive temporal artery specimens in up to 83% of cases, the functional role of these cells remains indeterminate [49]. Associations with humoral immunity have been suggested by the presence of auto-antibodies directed against cardiolipin [50], ferritin [51, 52], endothelial cells [53] and recently 14–3-3 proteins [54]. However detection of auto-antibodies overall lacks specificity, has not been universally replicated, and is of unknown significance in the pathogenesis of GCA.

Although a major immunologic role of B cells is the production of antibodies, B cells can also regulate T cell responses in auto-immunity through the secretion of both pro-inflammatory (TNF-α and IL-6) and anti-inflammatory (IL-10) cytokines [55]. In a prospective study, patients with active GCA were observed to have low levels of circulating B cells, particularly IL-6 secreting effector B cells, with a return to near normal levels during GC-induced remission [55]. It is hypothesized that the B cells are distributed into secondary lymphoid organs and/or inflamed tissues and then on normalization of the inflammatory process return to the peripheral blood. However, the reservoir for B cells during active disease is incompletely known and remains an area of ongoing research.

One potential location for B cell redistribution during disease is within artery tertiary lymphoid organs (ATLO). Ciccia and colleagues evaluated temporal artery biopsies from fifty patients with active, untreated GCA and found distinct artery tertiary lymphoid organ structures in the medial layer among 60% of patients with biopsies positive for GCA [56]. These structures were organized into specific T cell areas, B cell follicles and associated with a network of follicular dendritic cells. Compared to patients without ATLOs and healthy controls, arteries with ATLOs had a high level of B cell activating factor (BAFF) and a proliferation inducing ligand (APRIL), proteins which are strongly correlated with the differentiation and proliferation of B cells. Production of these proteins was primarily driven by endothelial cells and vascular smooth muscle cells highlighting an interaction between myointimal cells and B cells, an area that requires further exploration and confirmation [56].

Although a potential role of B cells exists in the pathogenesis of GCA, the efficacy of B cell depletion is largely unknown. Rituximab, an anti-CD20 monoclonal antibody, has only been reported in two patients with GCA with observed benefit [57, 58]. Further investigation of this agent in prospective trials is needed before considering as a viable treatment option in GCA.

Endothelial cells

Endothelial cells, the interface between the circulating blood and vessel wall, are active participants in the regulation of inflammation and angiogenesis. The intercellular adhesion molecules expressed on endothelial cells mediate leukocyte trafficking, migration, and development of inflammatory infiltrates. Increased expression of endothelin-1 and endothelin-B receptor immunoreactivity has been seen in higher concentration in the medial layer of temporal arteries from patients with GCA compared to controls and this immunoreactivity has been observed to correlate with the degree of systemic inflammation [59]. In addition, the endothelin system is increased at the protein level in temporal artery lesions in patients with GCA, creating a microvascular environment that is predisposed to develop ischemic complications, which is not immediately abrogated by glucocorticoid administration [60]. Indeed, upregulation of endothelin-1 in GCA lesions promotes migration of vascular smooth muscle cells to migrate towards the intima, leading to development of intimal hyperplasia and resulting in vascular occlusion [61]. Blockade of endothelin receptors using macitentan, a dual endothelin-A/endothelin-B receptor

antagonist, has been shown to reduce vascular smooth muscle proliferation in biopsy-proven GCA and may prove to be a promising future adjunct in the treatment of GCA [62].

Novel treatments

For over six decades, treatment with high-dose GCs has been the mainstay for both induction to remission and maintenance therapy in GCA. Unfortunately, GCs contribute substantial toxicity and GC-associated adverse events are nearly universal [63, 64]. In addition, despite adequate treatment with GCs, relapses are frequent [65] and chronic arterial inflammation can persist despite clinical and biochemical remission [38, 49]. Therefore, a great unmet need has existed for safe and effective GC-sparing agents for both induction and maintenance therapy in GCA.

Methotrexate was evaluated in 3 small clinical trials for treatment of GCA, and results were variable. According to expert consensus, methotrexate has been generally recommended as a second-line agent after GC in patients with relapsing or severely active disease or in patients with high-risk for GC-associated adverse events [66]. However, an individual patient data meta-analysis of the three clinical trials evaluating methotrexate found only a modest benefit in decreasing relapse risk and reducing GC exposure. Moreover, the effect of methotrexate on reducing relapse risk only became significant after about 48 weeks of treatment, and GC-related adverse effects were not diminished [67]. Limited to no benefit has been observed among other oral conventional immunosuppressive agents including azathioprine [68], leflunomide [69, 70] and mycophenolate mofetil [71].

Due to the limited success of conventional immunosuppressive agents, targeted therapeutics have gained greater interest and investigation for control of GCA. Early reports of increased expression of tumor necrosis factor (TNF)-alpha in temporal artery specimens among patients with GCA [72] and dramatic benefit of TNF-inhibitors in other autoimmune diseases (e.g. rheumatoid arthritis) led to evaluation of TNF-alpha blockade in this condition. Unfortunately placebo-controlled trials utilizing TNF-inhibition with infliximab [73], etanercept [74], and adalimumab [75] have failed to show significant therapeutic efficacy in patients with GCA and did not result in significant reduction of GC use or adverse events. Despite the inadequate results of TNF-alpha inhibition, several other targeted therapeutics are being investigated (Fig. 1).

Interleukin-6 inhibitors

IL-6 is produced locally in the arterial vasculitic lesion [9], and is expressed in circulating monocytes from patients with GCA [33]. IL-6 is known to be a critical

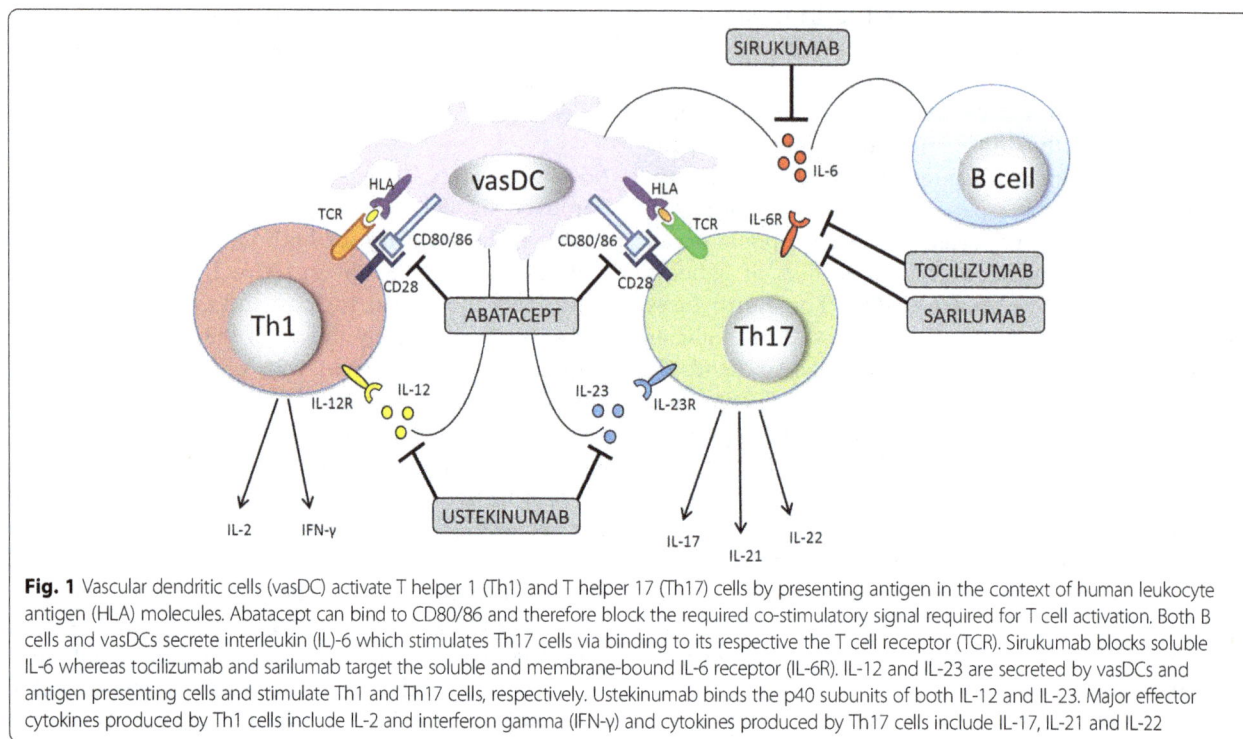

Fig. 1 Vascular dendritic cells (vasDC) activate T helper 1 (Th1) and T helper 17 (Th17) cells by presenting antigen in the context of human leukocyte antigen (HLA) molecules. Abatacept can bind to CD80/86 and therefore block the required co-stimulatory signal required for T cell activation. Both B cells and vasDCs secrete interleukin (IL)-6 which stimulates Th17 cells via binding to its respective the T cell receptor (TCR). Sirukumab blocks soluble IL-6 whereas tocilizumab and sarilumab target the soluble and membrane-bound IL-6 receptor (IL-6R). IL-12 and IL-23 are secreted by vasDCs and antigen presenting cells and stimulate Th1 and Th17 cells, respectively. Ustekinumab binds the p40 subunits of both IL-12 and IL-23. Major effector cytokines produced by Th1 cells include IL-2 and interferon gamma (IFN-γ) and cytokines produced by Th17 cells include IL-17, IL-21 and IL-22

factor in the induction of acute-phase proteins, which are typically markedly elevated in patients with GCA and are used in clinical practice to monitor disease activity. Moreover, although IL-6 is highly elevated in untreated GCA, levels drop promptly with GC therapy. Indeed, IL-6 levels correlate with disease activity and can be a useful biomarker in evaluating disease activity [76, 77]. Tocilizumab (TCZ), a humanized anti IL-6 receptor antibody has shown efficacy in both newly diagnosed and relapsing patients in several small observational series [78–85] and two double-blind, placebo-controlled trials [86, 87].

In the first reported double-blind, placebo-controlled phase 2 trial evaluating TCZ in GCA, Villiger and colleagues randomized 30 patients with GCA (23 newly diagnosed, 7 relapsing) to receive prednisolone taper with intravenous tocilizumab (8 mg/kg/4 weeks) or prednisolone taper with placebo infusions [87]. Among the 20 patients receiving TCZ, complete remission at 12 weeks (85% vs. 40%) and relapse-free survival at 1 year (85% vs 20%) were significantly higher in the treatment group compared to placebo. On the contrary, serious adverse events were less frequent in the TCZ group (35% vs. 50%). Only one relapse was observed in the TCZ group and no relapses occurred after discontinuation of prednisolone in patients receiving TCZ.

The benefit and safety profile of TCZ has further been confirmed in the tocilizumab in GCA (GiACTA) trial [86]. GiACTA constitutes the largest international, multi-center, placebo-controlled trial in GCA to-date and the first to employ a blinded prednisone taper and a dual-assessor strategy to avoid bias created by knowledge of inflammatory markers [86]. In this phase 3 trial, Stone and colleagues recruited 251 patients (119 newly diagnosed, 132 relapsing) to one of four arms: weekly TCZ (162 mg, subcutaneous) plus a 26-week prednisone taper, every other week TCZ plus a 26-week prednisone taper, weekly placebo plus a 26-week prednisone taper, or weekly placebo plus a 52-week prednisone taper. Patients were diagnosed based on modifications to the 1990 American College of Rheumatology criteria for classification of GCA [88], which permitted inclusion of patients based on evidence of large-vessel vasculitis (LVV) on cross-sectional imaging. Whereas 62% of patients had a positive temporal biopsy, 37% of patients were ultimately enrolled on the basis of radiographic findings of LVV, regardless of temporal artery biopsy results.

The primary outcome, sustained remission at 52-weeks, was significantly higher among patients receiving weekly TCZ (56%) and every other week TCZ (53%) compared to the placebo groups (placebo plus 26-week prednisone taper, 14%; placebo plus 52-week prednisone taper, 18%; respectively). Disease flares occurred less frequently in patients receiving weekly TCZ (23%) and every other week TCZ (26%) compared to the 26-week (68%) and 52-week (49%) placebo arms. Over the 12-month trial, GC exposure in the treatment arms was approximately half compared to the placebo arms. Overall adverse events were frequent in all groups (92–98%);

however, serious adverse events were lower among patients receiving weekly TCZ (15%) and every other week TCZ (14%) compared to placebo plus 26-week prednisone taper (22%) or 52-week prednisone taper (25%). Despite the accelerated GC taper, permanent vision loss did not occur in any arm and only one patient receiving every other week TCZ had transient visual loss, which recovered with glucocorticoids.

The landmark findings of TCZ safety and efficacy reported in GiACTA have led to the United States Food and Drug Administration to approve TCZ 162 mg administered subcutaneously weekly for the treatment of GCA; the first-ever medication to receive such distinction. The successful results of TCZ have prompted further investigation into additional novel anti-IL-6 molecules in this disease. A phase 3 trial utilizing sirukumab (human anti-IL-6 monoclonal antibody) is currently in progress (Clinical Trials.gov Identifier NCT02531633) and an upcoming trial of sarilumab (anti-IL-6 receptor monoclonal antibody), is planned. The results of these studies will strongly influence whether additional candidate IL-6 blockers will be evaluated in GCA; including clazakizumab, olokizumab, and vobarilizumab. While the benefit of IL-6 blockade in treatment of GCA is apparent, 44–47% of patients receiving TCZ in GiACTA were still unable to reach sustained remission at 52 weeks [86]. In an earlier report, a patient with GCA who achieved apparent clinical remission on TCZ was noted to have evidence of persistent and active vascular inflammation at autopsy, despite normalization of inflammatory markers [85]. Active disease despite IL-6 blockade highlights that other immunologic pathomechanisms are present in ongoing inflammatory states in GCA and further investigation into other novel therapeutics is still needed.

Abatacept

Whereas the checkpoint inhibitor ipilimumab has led to the generation of arterial inflammation, inhibition of co-stimulatory T cell signalling via CTLA-4 is a possible target for controlling GCA. Abatacept is a fusion protein composed of the Fc region of the immunoglobulin IgG1 fused to the extracellular domain of CTLA-4 and blocks the co-stimulatory signal required for T cell activation. Langford and colleagues investigated the safety and efficacy of intravenous abatacept (10 mg/kg) in patients with newly diagnosed or relapsing GCA [89]. Following a remission induction phase, 41 patients in remission at week 12 were randomized to receive either placebo infusions or monthly abatacept. Relapse-free survival at 12 months, the primary outcome, was achieved by 48% on abatacept and 31% receiving placebo (p = 0.049). In addition, the duration of remission was on average 6 months longer in patients receiving abatacept compared to placebo. No difference in adverse events was

observed. Although considered statistically and clinically significant findings, the effectiveness of abatacept in GCA needs to be confirmed in larger cohorts prior to incorporation of this agent in routine clinical care.

Ustekinumab

Tocilizumab, through blockade of IL-6R, mediates its effect largely on the Th17/Treg imbalance, without significant impact on the Th1 cellular pathway. On the contrary, ustekinumab, a monoclonal antibody directed against IL-12/23p40 has the potential to disrupt both Th1 (IL-12) and Th17 (IL-23) pathways. The effect of modulating the Th1/Th17/Treg imbalance has been demonstrated by Samson and colleagues in a refractory GCA patient treated with ustekinumab [90]. Compared to baseline, peripheral blood mononuclear cells evaluated after three injections of ustekinumab (45 mg weeks 0, 4, 16) demonstrated that Th1 and Th17 cells each fell by 50%, cytotoxic T lymphocytes reduced by 64%, and Tregs increased 5-fold. This dramatic improvement in T cell homeostasis is promising and the benefit of ustekinumab has been observed in a small open-label study. Conway and colleagues studied 12 patients with relapsing GCA and administered ustekinumab 90 mg at weeks 0, 4, and then every 12 weeks for a median of 8 months [91]. During the course of treatment GC requirements were noticeably reduced (median 23 mg prior, 5 mg after). Three patients were able to discontinue GC and eight patients were able to stop additional baseline immunosuppressives. No relapses were observed during treatment with ustekinumab but two of three patients experienced a flare following cessation of therapy. These findings demonstrate the potential efficacy of ustekinumab as a treatment option for GCA and a phase 2 trial to confirm these results is ongoing (ClinicalTrials.gov Identifier NCT02955147).

Janus kinase / signal transducers and activators of transcription inhibitors

The Janus kinase–signal transducers and activators of transcription (JAK-STAT) signalling pathway is involved in cellular regulation and has been implicated in the pathogenesis of several inflammatory and autoimmune conditions, including rheumatoid arthritis, inflammatory bowel disease, and psoriasis [92]. Ligand binding of immune relevant mediators (e.g. IL-2, IL-4, IL-6, IL-7, IL-9, IL-12, IL-15, IL-21, IL-23, IL-27, type 1 interferon, interferon-gamma) to their cell surface receptors leads to activation of associated JAKs [93]. The activated JAKs increase their kinase activity, recruit, bind and activate STATs. The STAT molecules then form hetero- or homo-dimers which translocate to the nucleus and induce transcription and expression of target genes, which in the context of pro-inflammatory cytokines can lead to increased inflammation and autoimmunity [94]. As a result, targeted intervention of the JAK-STAT signalling cascade is attractive and being investigated for several autoimmune and cancer disorders.

JAK-STAT signalling has been identified as having a potential role in sustaining vascular inflammation. In particular, STAT-1 signalling appears to regulate the activity of vasDCs as well as controlling T cell trafficking and retention of inflammatory T cells in the vascular lesions [95]. Hartmann and colleagues evaluated the presence of STAT-1 transcripts in an experimentally induced vasculitis of human temporal arteries grafted in immunodeficient mice and found STAT-1 abundantly expressed in arteritic tissue lesions. Interferon-gamma, the major inducer of STAT-1, was, 10-fold higher in patients affected by GCA compared to controls. In the experimental model, while high-dose GCs effectively suppressed the activity of vasDCs and reduced IL-6 in the lesional tissue, the Th1 cellular infiltrate was not affected. Conversely, administration of the JAK/STAT inhibitor, tofacitinib, effectively prevented Th1 cell accumulation in the vessel wall and reduced interferon-gamma production [95]. Compared to TCZ, which mediates its effect primarily through the IL-6/gp130/STAT3 signalling axis [96]; JAK inhibitors can exert control over multiple pathogenic cellular lineages by impeding the proinflammatory signal of more than one cytokine signalling pathway (Fig. 2). The benefit of JAK inhibition in patients with GCA is currently unknown but a phase 2 trial evaluating baricitinib (oral selective JAK1, JAK2 inhibitor) in patients with relapsing GCA is currently ongoing (ClinicalTrials.gov Identifier NCT03026504).

Future treatment options

The Notch signalling pathway is critical for regulating cellular proliferation, differentiation, apoptosis, and homeostasis. Dysregulation of this highly preserved pathway has been associated with several malignancies and autoimmune conditions [97, 98]. Interaction between lymphocytes and vascular smooth muscles cells and endothelial cells involves the activity of the Notch pathway. Immunohistochemical and gene expression analysis of inflamed temporal arteries have identified overexpression of Notch receptors and their associated ligands (Jagged1, Delta1). Blockade of Notch signalling in a humanized vasculitis mouse model effectively depleted both Th1 and Th17 cells from vascular infiltrates [99]. In addition, it has been shown that systemic vascular endothelial growth factor (VEGF) can trigger aberrant Notch signalling through upregulation of the Notch ligand Jagged1 and induces pathogenic effector cell function via adventitial microvascular endothelial cells [100].

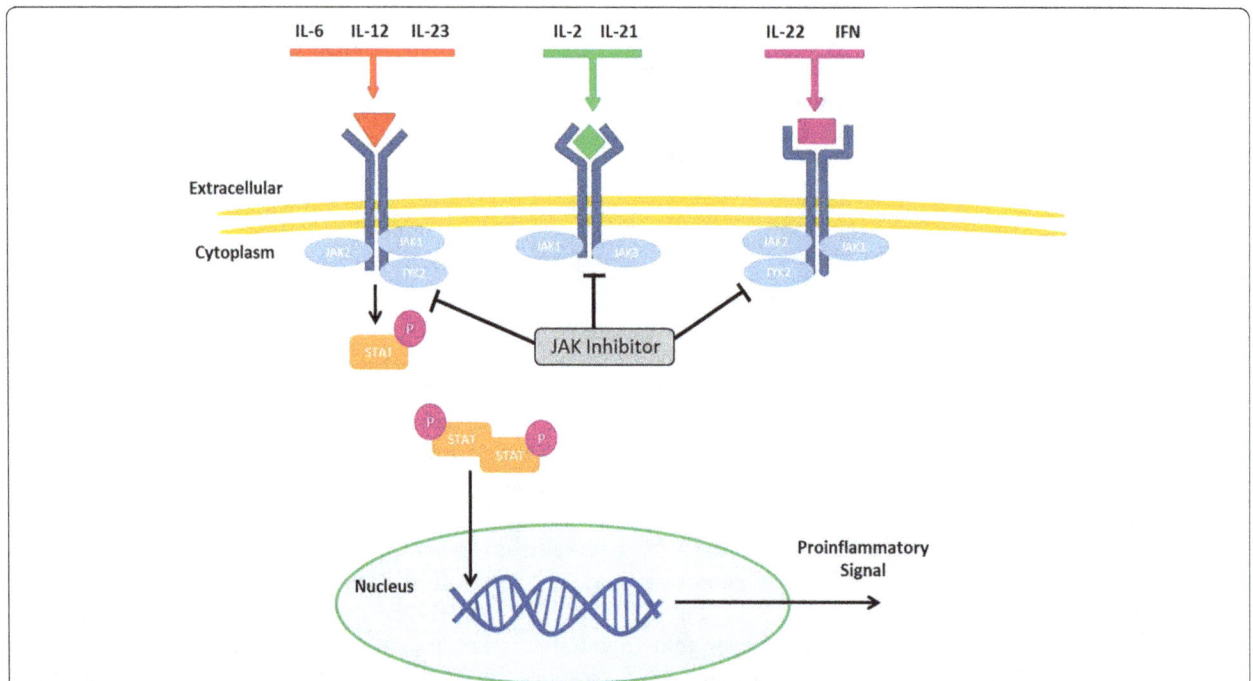

Fig. 2 Effector cytokines can stimulate transcription of proinflammatory signals through the Janus kinase–signal transducers and activators of transcription (JAK-STAT) signalling pathway. Intracellular JAK and tyrosine kinase (TYK) proteins are activated when a ligand binds to its receptor which induces phosphorylation and activation, which in turn activate STAT proteins. The STAT proteins dimerize and translocate to the nucleus where they bind STAT-specific response elements in target gene promotors and regulate gene transcription; including proinflammatory signals. JAK inhibitors (e.g. baricitinib and tofacitinib) are able to abrogate signalling cascades from more than one effector cytokine pathway

The arterial microvascular network appears to be essential in the recruitment of activated T cells and may therefore provide additional therapeutic targets. Multiple phase 1 and phase 2 trials evaluating different classes of Notch inhibition are underway in treatment of various forms of cancer, but Notch inhibition as of yet has not been attempted in patients with GCA.

The role of the pro-inflammatory cytokine IL-1-beta in GCA is uncertain; however, expression of IL-1-beta has been found in 60–80% of circulating monocytes in patients with untreated GCA and 20% of macrophages in temporal artery lesions produce this cytokine [33]. Limited information is available to determine the clinical efficacy of IL-1 blockade in patients with GCA but a small case series utilizing the IL-1 inhibitor, anakinra, showed benefit in three refractory cases [101]. A randomized, double-blind, placebo-controlled study evaluating gevokizumab (monoclonal antibody targeting IL-1 beta) for the treatment of patients with relapsing GCA is ongoing and has recruited 13 patients to date (EudraCT number 2013–002778-38).

Conclusion

Recent advances have provided a greater understanding of the pathomechanisms involved in GCA; however, further studies are required to fully elucidate the aetiology and pathogenesis of this inflammatory vasculopathy. The complex interaction of genetics, vascular factors and immunologic pathways in this disease is responsible for the variability in both the clinical presentation and response to immunosuppressive therapy. After decades of treating GCA almost exclusively with glucocorticoids, clinicians are finally able to reach for novel and targeted biologic agents. IL-6 is a key mediator in GCA and tocilizumab is the first agent to show a profound effect on disease control and GC reduction. This agent is quickly being incorporated into the treatment algorithm of both newly diagnosed and relapsing patients with GCA. More information is needed to understand tocilizumab's effect on long-term outcomes and the optimal length of therapy required for maintenance in this disease. Abatacept and ustekinumab have shown preliminary evidence of potential efficacy in the treatment of GCA but confirmation in larger trials is needed before either is utilized in clinical care. The proposed benefit of JAK-STAT inhibition seen in preclinical studies of vasculitis is encouraging and the evaluation of baricitinib in patient trials is underway. The era of glucocorticoid monotherapy for GCA may be coming to a close, a most welcome prospect for patients with this condition.

Abbreviations

APC: antigen presenting cell; CTLA-4: cytotoxic T-lymphocyte associated protein-4; GC: glucocorticoids; GCA: giant cell arteritis; HLA: human leukocyte antigen; IL: interleukin; JAK-STAT: Janus kinase–signal transducers and activators of transcription; LVV: large vessel vasculitis; PD-1: programmed cell death-1; TAB: temporal artery biopsy; TCZ: tocilizumab; Th1: type 1 helper T cell; Th17: type 17 helper T cell; vasDC: vascular dendritic cell; VZV: varicella zoster virus

Acknowledgements
We wish to thank those who reviewed the manuscript for their constructive comments (Additional file 1).

Funding
None.

Author's contributions
Manuscript design/conception: MJK, KJW. Drafting of manuscript: MJK, KJW. Critical revision: MJK, KJW.
Approval of manuscript: MJK, KJW. Both authors read and approved the final manuscript.

Competing interests
The authors declare that they have no competing interests.

References
1. Weyand CM, Goronzy JJ. Clinical practice. Giant-cell arteritis and polymyalgia rheumatica. N Engl J Med. 2014;371(1):50–7.
2. Combe B, Sany J, Le Quellec A, Clot J, Eliaou JF: Distribution of HLA-DRB1 alleles of patients with polymyalgia rheumatica and giant cell arteritis in a Mediterranean population. J Rheumatol. 1998;25(1):94-98.
3. Dababneh A, Gonzalez-Gay MA, Garcia-Porrua C, Hajeer A, Thomson W, Ollier W. Giant cell arteritis and polymyalgia rheumatica can be differentiated by distinct patterns of HLA class II association. J Rheumatol. 1998;25(11):2140–5.
4. Jacobsen S, Baslund B, Madsen HO, Tvede N, Svejgaard A, Garred P. Mannose-binding lectin variant alleles and HLA-DR4 alleles are associated with giant cell arteritis. J Rheumatol. 2002;29(10):2148–53.
5. Martinez-Taboda VM, Bartolome MJ, Lopez-Hoyos M, Blanco R, Mata C, Calvo J, Corrales A, Rodriguez-Valverde V. HLA-DRB1 allele distribution in polymyalgia rheumatica and giant cell arteritis: influence on clinical subgroups and prognosis. Semin Arthritis Rheum. 2004;34(1):454–64.
6. Salvarani C, Boiardi L, Mantovani V, Ranzi A, Cantini F, Olivieri I, Viggiani M, Bragliani M, Macchioni P. HLA-DRB1, DQA1, and DQB1 alleles associated with giant cell arteritis in northern Italy. J Rheumatol. 1999;26(11):2395–9.
7. Weyand CM, Hicok KC, Hunder GG, Goronzy JJ. The HLA-DRB1 locus as a genetic component in giant cell arteritis. Mapping of a disease-linked sequence motif in the antigen binding site of the HLA-DR molecule. J Clin Invest. 1992;90(6):2355–61.
8. Carmona FD, Vaglio A, Mackie SL, Hernandez-Rodriguez J, Monach PA, Castaneda S, Solans R, Morado IC, Narvaez J, Ramentol-Sintas M, et al. A genome-wide association study identifies risk alleles in Plasminogen and P4HA2 associated with Giant cell Arteritis. Am J Hum Genet. 2017;100(1):64–74.
9. Weyand CM, Schonberger J, Oppitz U, Hunder NN, Hicok KC, Goronzy JJ. Distinct vascular lesions in giant cell arteritis share identical T cell clonotypes. J Exp Med. 1994;179(3):951–60.
10. Duhaut P, Bosshard S, Ducroix JP. Is giant cell arteritis an infectious disease? Biological and epidemiological evidence. Presse Med. 2004;33(19 Pt 2):1403–8.
11. Ljungstrom L, Franzen C, Schlaug M, Elowson S, Viidas U. Reinfection with Chlamydia pneumoniae may induce isolated and systemic vasculitis in small and large vessels. Scand J Infect Dis Suppl. 1997;104:37–40.
12. Wagner AD, Gerard HC, Fresemann T, Schmidt WA, Gromnica-Ihle E, Hudson AP, Zeidler H. Detection of Chlamydia pneumoniae in giant cell vasculitis and correlation with the topographic arrangement of tissue-infiltrating dendritic cells. Arthritis Rheum. 2000;43(7):1543–51.
13. Elling P, Olsson AT, Elling H. Synchronous variations of the incidence of temporal arteritis and polymyalgia rheumatica in different regions of Denmark; association with epidemics of Mycoplasma pneumoniae infection. J Rheumatol. 1996;23(1):112–9.
14. Koening CL, Katz BJ, Hernandez-Rodriguez J. Identification of a Burkholderia-like strain from temporal arteries of subjects with giant cell arteritis. Arthritis Rheum. 2012;64:S373.

15. Alvarez-Lafuente R, Fernandez-Gutierrez B, Jover JA, Judez E, Loza E, Clemente D, Garcia-Asenjo JA, Lamas JR. Human parvovirus B19, varicella zoster virus, and human herpes virus 6 in temporal artery biopsy specimens of patients with giant cell arteritis: analysis with quantitative real time polymerase chain reaction. Ann Rheum Dis. 2005;64(5):780–2.

16. Gabriel SE, Espy M, Erdman DD, Bjornsson J, Smith TF, Hunder GG. The role of parvovirus B19 in the pathogenesis of giant cell arteritis: a preliminary evaluation. Arthritis Rheum. 1999;42(6):1255–8.

17. Powers JF, Bedri S, Hussein S, Salomon RN, Tischler AS. High prevalence of herpes simplex virus DNA in temporal arteritis biopsy specimens. Am J Clin Pathol. 2005;123(2):261–4.

18. Giardina A, Rizzo A, Ferrante A, Capra G, Triolo G, Ciccia F. Giant cell arteritis associated with chronic active Epstein-Barr virus infection. Reumatismo. 2013;65(1):36–9.

19. Cooper RJ, D'Arcy S, Kirby M, Al-Buhtori M, Rahman MJ, Proctor L, Bonshek RE. Infection and temporal arteritis: a PCR-based study to detect pathogens in temporal artery biopsy specimens. J Med Virol. 2008;80(3):501–5.

20. Helweg-Larsen J, Tarp B, Obel N, Baslund B. No evidence of parvovirus B19, Chlamydia pneumoniae or human herpes virus infection in temporal artery biopsies in patients with giant cell arteritis. Rheumatology (Oxford). 2002; 41(4):445–9.

21. Rodriguez-Pla A, Bosch-Gil JA, Echevarria-Mayo JE, Rossello-Urgell J, Solans-Laque R, Huguet-Redecilla P, Stone JH, Vilardell-Tarres M. No detection of parvovirus B19 or herpesvirus DNA in giant cell arteritis. J Clin Virol. 2004;31(1):11–5.

22. Nagel MA, White T, Khmeleva N, Rempel A, Boyer PJ, Bennett JL, Haller A, Lear-Kaul K, Kandasmy B, Amato M, et al. Analysis of Varicella-zoster virus in temporal arteries biopsy positive and negative for Giant cell Arteritis. JAMA Neurol. 2015;72(11):1281–7.

23. Gilden D, White T, Khmeleva N, Katz BJ, Nagel MA. Blinded search for varicella zoster virus in giant cell arteritis (GCA)-positive and GCA-negative temporal arteries. J Neurol Sci. 2016;364:141–3.

24. Gilden D, Nagel MA. Varicella zoster virus and giant cell arteritis. Curr Opin Infect Dis. 2016;29(3):275–9.

25. Muratore F, Croci S, Tamagnini I, Zerbini A, Bellafiore S, Belloni L, Boiardi L, Bisagni A, Pipitone N, Parmeggiani M, et al. No detection of varicella-zoster virus in temporal arteries of patients with giant cell arteritis. Semin Arthritis Rheum. 2017.

26. Procop GW, Eng C, Clifford A, Villa-Forte A, Calabrese LH, Roselli E, Svensson L, Johnston D, Pettersson G, Soltesz E, et al. Varicella zoster virus and large vessel Vasculitis, the absence of an association. Pathog Immun. 2017;2(2):228–38.

27. Schafer VS, Kermani TA, Crowson CS, Hunder GG, Gabriel SE, Ytterberg SR, Matteson EL, Warrington KJ. Incidence of herpes zoster in patients with giant cell arteritis: a population-based cohort study. Rheumatology (Oxford). 2010;49(11):2104–8.

28. Rhee RL, Grayson PC, Merkel PA, Tomasson G. Infections and the risk of incident giant cell arteritis: a population-based, case-control study. Ann Rheum Dis. 2017;76(6):1031–5.

29. Weyand CM, Goronzy JJ. Medium- and large-vessel vasculitis. N Engl J Med. 2003;349(2):160–9.

30. Weyand CM, Goronzy JJ. Immune mechanisms in medium and large-vessel vasculitis. Nat Rev Rheumatol. 2013;9(12):731–40.

31. Ma-Krupa W, Jeon MS, Spoerl S, Tedder TF, Goronzy JJ, Weyand CM. Activation of arterial wall dendritic cells and breakdown of self-tolerance in giant cell arteritis. J Exp Med. 2004;199(2):173–83.

32. Krupa WM, Dewan M, Jeon MS, Kurtin PJ, Younge BR, Goronzy JJ, Weyand CM. Trapping of misdirected dendritic cells in the granulomatous lesions of giant cell arteritis. Am J Pathol. 2002;161(5):1815–23.

33. Wagner AD, Goronzy JJ, Weyand CM. Functional profile of tissue-infiltrating and circulating CD68+ cells in giant cell arteritis. Evidence for two components of the disease. J Clin Invest. 1994;94(3):1134–40.

34. Rittner HL, Kaiser M, Brack A, Szweda LI, Goronzy JJ, Weyand CM. Tissue-destructive macrophages in giant cell arteritis. Circ Res. 1999;84(9):1050–8.

35. Xie J, Lee S, Chen X. Nanoparticle-based theranostic agents. Adv Drug Deliv Rev. 2010;62(11):1064–79.

36. Patel SK, Janjic JM. Macrophage targeted theranostics as personalized nanomedicine strategies for inflammatory diseases. Theranostics. 2015;5(2): 150–72.

37. Weyand CM, Liao YJ, Goronzy JJ. The immunopathology of giant cell arteritis: diagnostic and therapeutic implications. J Neuroophthalmol. 2012; 32(3):259–65.

38. Deng J, Younge BR, Olshen RA, Goronzy JJ, Weyand CM. Th17 and Th1 T-cell responses in giant cell arteritis. Circulation. 2010;121(7):906–15.

39. Samson M, Audia S, Fraszczak J, Trad M, Ornetti P, Lakomy D, Ciudad M, Leguy V, Berthier S, Vinit J, et al. Th1 and Th17 lymphocytes expressing CD161 are implicated in giant cell arteritis and polymyalgia rheumatica pathogenesis. Arthritis Rheum. 2012;64(11):3788–98.

40. Miyabe C, Miyabe Y, Strle K, Kim ND, Stone JH, Luster AD, Unizony S. An expanded population of pathogenic regulatory T cells in giant cell arteritis is abrogated by IL-6 blockade therapy. Ann Rheum Dis. 2017;76(5):898–905.

41. Hodi FS, O'Day SJ, McDermott DF, Weber RW, Sosman JA, Haanen JB, Gonzalez R, Robert C, Schadendorf D, Hassel JC, et al. Improved survival with ipilimumab in patients with metastatic melanoma. N Engl J Med. 2010;363(8):711–23.

42. Robert C, Schachter J, Long GV, Arance A, Grob JJ, Mortier L, Daud A, Carlino MS, McNeil C, Lotem M, et al. Pembrolizumab versus Ipilimumab in Advanced Melanoma. N Engl J Med. 2015;372(26):2521–32.

43. Tarhini A, Lo E, Minor DR. Releasing the brake on the immune system: ipilimumab in melanoma and other tumors. Cancer Biother Radiopharm. 2010;25(6):601–13.

44. Goldstein BL, Gedmintas L, Todd DJ. Drug-associated polymyalgia rheumatica/giant cell arteritis occurring in two patients after treatment with ipilimumab, an antagonist of ctla-4. Arthritis Rheumatol. 2014;66(3):768–9.

45. Rosenblatt J, Glotzbecker B, Mills H, Vasir B, Tzachanis D, Levine JD, Joyce RM, Wellenstein K, Keefe W, Schickler M, et al. PD-1 blockade by CT-011, anti-PD-1 antibody, enhances ex vivo T-cell responses to autologous dendritic cell/myeloma fusion vaccine. J Immunother. 2011;34(5):409–18.

46. Zhang H, Watanabe R, Berry GJ, Vaglio A, Liao YJ, Warrington KJ, Goronzy JJ, Weyand CM. Immunoinhibitory checkpoint deficiency in medium and large vessel vasculitis. Proc Natl Acad Sci U S A. 2017;114(6):E970–9.

47. Abdel-Wahab N, Shah M, Suarez-Almazor ME. Adverse events associated with immune checkpoint blockade in patients with cancer: a systematic review of case reports. PLoS One. 2016;11(7):e0160221.

48. Micaily I, Chernoff M. An unknown reaction to Pembrolizumab: Giant cell Arteritis. Ann Oncol. 2017.

49. Maleszewski JJ, Younge BR, Fritzlen JT, Hunder GG, Goronzy JJ, Warrington KJ, Weyand CM. Clinical and pathological evolution of giant cell arteritis: a prospective study of follow-up temporal artery biopsies in 40 treated patients. Mod Pathol. 2017;30(6):788–96.

50. Espinoza LR, Jara LJ, Silveira LH, Martinez-Osuna P, Zwolinska JB, Kneer C, Aguilar JL. Anticardiolipin antibodies in polymyalgia rheumatica-giant cell arteritis: association with severe vascular complications. Am J Med. 1991; 90(4):474–8.

51. Baerlecken NT, Linnemann A, Gross WL, Moosig F, Vazquez-Rodriguez TR, Gonzalez-Gay MA, Martin J, Kotter I, Henes JC, Melchers I, et al. Association of ferritin autoantibodies with giant cell arteritis/polymyalgia rheumatica. Ann Rheum Dis. 2012;71(6):943–7.

52. Grosse K, Schmidt RE, Witte T, Baerlecken NT. Epitope mapping of antibodies against ferritin heavy chain in giant cell arteritis and polymyalgia rheumatica. Scand J Rheumatol. 2013;42(3):215–9.

53. Navarro M, Cervera R, Font J, Reverter JC, Monteagudo J, Escolar G, Lopez-Soto A, Ordinas A, Ingelmo M. Anti-endothelial cell antibodies in systemic autoimmune diseases: prevalence and clinical significance. Lupus. 1997;6(6):521–6.

54. Kistner A, Bigler MB, Glatz K, Egli SB, Baldin FS, Marquardsen FA, Mehling M, Rentsch KM, Staub D, Aschwanden M, et al. Characteristics of autoantibodies targeting 14-3-3 proteins and their association with clinical features in newly diagnosed giant cell arteritis. Rheumatology (Oxford). 2017;56(5):829–34.

55. van der Geest KS, Abdulahad WH, Chalan P, Rutgers A, Horst G, Huitema MG, Roffel MP, Roozendaal C, Kluin PM, Bos NA, et al. Disturbed B cell homeostasis in newly diagnosed giant cell arteritis and polymyalgia rheumatica. Arthritis Rheumatol. 2014;66(7):1927–38.

56. Ciccia F, Rizzo A, Maugeri R, Alessandro R, Croci S, Guggino G, Cavazza A, Raimondo S, Cannizzaro A, Iacopino DG, et al. Ectopic expression of CXCL13, BAFF, APRIL and LT-beta is associated with artery tertiary lymphoid organs in giant cell arteritis. Ann Rheum Dis. 2017;76(1):235–43.

57. Bhatia A, Ell PJ, Edwards JC. Anti-CD20 monoclonal antibody (rituximab) as an adjunct in the treatment of giant cell arteritis. Ann Rheum Dis. 2005; 64(7):1099–100.

58. Mayrbaeurl B, Hinterreiter M, Burgstaller S, Windpessl M, Thaler J. The first case of a patient with neutropenia and giant-cell arteritis treated with rituximab. Clin Rheumatol. 2007;26(9):1597–8.

59. Dimitrijevic I, Andersson C, Rissler P, Edvinsson L. Increased tissue endothelin-1 and endothelin-B receptor expression in temporal arteries from patients with giant cell arteritis. Ophthalmology. 2010;117(3):628–36.

60. Lozano E, Segarra M, Corbera-Bellalta M, Garcia-Martinez A, Espigol-Frigole G, Pla-Campo A, Hernandez-Rodriguez J, Cid MC. Increased expression of the endothelin system in arterial lesions from patients with giant-cell arteritis: association between elevated plasma endothelin levels and the development of ischaemic events. Ann Rheum Dis. 2010;69(2):434–42.

61. Planas-Rigol E, Terrades-Garcia N, Corbera-Bellalta M, Lozano E, Alba MA, Segarra M, Espigol-Frigole G, Prieto-Gonzalez S, Hernandez-Rodriguez J, Preciado S, et al. Endothelin-1 promotes vascular smooth muscle cell migration across the artery wall: a mechanism contributing to vascular remodelling and intimal hyperplasia in giant-cell arteritis. Ann Rheum Dis. 2017;76(9):1624–34.

62. Regent A, Ly KH, Groh M, Khifer C, Lofek S, Clary G, Chafey P, Baud V, Broussard C, Federici C, et al. Molecular analysis of vascular smooth muscle cells from patients with giant cell arteritis: targeting endothelin-1 receptor to control proliferation. Autoimmun Rev. 2017;16(4):398–406.

63. Dunstan E, Lester SL, Rischmueller M, Dodd T, Black R, Ahern M, Cleland LG, Roberts-Thomson P, Hill CL. Epidemiology of biopsy-proven giant cell arteritis in South Australia. Intern Med J. 2014;44(1):32–9.

64. Proven A, Gabriel SE, Orces C, O'Fallon WM, Hunder GG. Glucocorticoid therapy in giant cell arteritis: duration and adverse outcomes. Arthritis Rheum. 2003;49(5):703–8.

65. Labarca C, Koster MJ, Crowson CS, Makol A, Ytterberg SR, Matteson EL, Warrington KJ. Predictors of relapse and treatment outcomes in biopsy-proven giant cell arteritis: a retrospective cohort study. Rheumatology (Oxford). 2016;55(2):347–56.

66. Dasgupta B, Borg FA, Hassan N, Alexander L, Barraclough K, Bourke B, Fulcher J, Hollywood J, Hutchings A, James P, et al. BSR and BHPR guidelines for the management of giant cell arteritis. Rheumatology (Oxford). 2010;49(8):1594–7.

67. Mahr AD, Jover JA, Spiera RF, Hernandez-Garcia C, Fernandez-Gutierrez B, Lavalley MP, Merkel PA. Adjunctive methotrexate for treatment of giant cell arteritis: an individual patient data meta-analysis. Arthritis Rheum. 2007;56(8):2789–97.

68. De Silva M, Hazleman BL. Azathioprine in giant cell arteritis/polymyalgia rheumatica: a double-blind study. Ann Rheum Dis. 1986;45(2):136–8.

69. Adizie T, Christidis D, Dharmapaliah C, Borg F, Dasgupta B. Efficacy and tolerability of leflunomide in difficult-to-treat polymyalgia rheumatica and giant cell arteritis: a case series. Int J Clin Pract. 2012;66(9):906–9.

70. Diamantopoulos AP, Hetland H, Myklebust G. Leflunomide as a corticosteroid-sparing agent in giant cell arteritis and polymyalgia rheumatica: a case series. Biomed Res Int. 2013;2013:120638.

71. Sciascia S, Piras D, Baldovino S, Russo A, Naretto C, Rossi D, Alpa M, Roccatello D. Mycophenolate mofetil as steroid-sparing treatment for elderly patients with giant cell arteritis: report of three cases. Aging Clin Exp Res. 2012;24(3):273–7.

72. Hernandez-Rodriguez J, Segarra M, Vilardell C, Sanchez M, Garcia-Martinez A, Esteban MJ, Queralt C, Grau JM, Urbano-Marquez A, Palacin A, et al. Tissue production of pro-inflammatory cytokines (IL-1beta, TNFalpha and IL-6) correlates with the intensity of the systemic inflammatory response and with corticosteroid requirements in giant-cell arteritis. Rheumatology (Oxford). 2004;43(3):294–301.

73. Hoffman GS, Cid MC, Rendt-Zagar KE, Merkel PA, Weyand CM, Stone JH, Salvarani C, Xu W, Visvanathan S, Rahman MU, et al. Infliximab for maintenance of glucocorticosteroid-induced remission of giant cell arteritis: a randomized trial. Ann Intern Med. 2007;146(9):621–30.

74. Martinez-Taboada VM, Rodriguez-Valverde V, Carreno L, Lopez-Longo J, Figueroa M, Belzunegui J, Mola EM, Bonilla G. A double-blind placebo controlled trial of etanercept in patients with giant cell arteritis and corticosteroid side effects. Ann Rheum Dis. 2008;67(5):625–30.

75. Seror R, Baron G, Hachulla E, Debandt M, Larroche C, Puechal X, Maurier F, de Wazieres B, Quemeneur T, Ravaud P, et al. Adalimumab for steroid sparing in patients with giant-cell arteritis: results of a multicentre randomised controlled trial. Ann Rheum Dis. 2014;73(12):2074–81.

76. Dasgupta B, Panayi GS. Interleukin-6 in serum of patients with polymyalgia rheumatica and giant cell arteritis. Br J Rheumatol. 1990;29(6):456–8.

77. Weyand CM, Fulbright JW, Hunder GG, Evans JM, Goronzy JJ. Treatment of giant cell arteritis: interleukin-6 as a biologic marker of disease activity. Arthritis Rheum. 2000;43(5):1041–8.

78. Beyer C, Axmann R, Sahinbegovic E, Distler JH, Manger B, Schett G, Zwerina J. Anti-interleukin 6 receptor therapy as rescue treatment for giant cell arteritis. Ann Rheum Dis. 2011;70(10):1874–5.

79. Loricera J, Blanco R, Castaneda S, Humbria A, Ortego-Centeno N, Narvaez J, Mata C, Melchor S, Aurrecoechea E, Calvo-Alen J, et al. Tocilizumab in refractory aortitis: study on 16 patients and literature review. Clin Exp Rheumatol. 2014;32(3 Suppl 82):S79–89.

80. Lurati A, Bertani L, Re KA, Marrazza M, Bompane D, Scarpellini M. Successful treatment of a patient with giant cell vasculitis (horton arteritis) with tocilizumab a humanized anti-interleukin-6 receptor antibody. Case Rep Rheumatol. 2012;2012:639612.

81. Pazzola G, Padovano I, Boiardi L, Versari A, Pipitone N, Catanoso M, Pulsatelli L, Meliconi R, Salvarani C. Tocilizumab in glucocorticoid-naive large-vessel vasculitis. Clin Exp Rheumatol. 2013;31(1 Suppl 75):S59–61.

82. Salvarani C, Magnani L, Catanoso M, Pipitone N, Versari A, Dardani L, Pulsatelli L, Meliconi R, Boiardi L. Tocilizumab: a novel therapy for patients with large-vessel vasculitis. Rheumatology (Oxford). 2012;51(1):151–6.

83. Sciascia S, Rossi D, Roccatello D. Interleukin 6 blockade as steroid-sparing treatment for 2 patients with giant cell arteritis. J Rheumatol. 2011;38(9):2080–1.

84. Seitz M, Reichenbach S, Bonel HM, Adler S, Wermelinger F, Villiger PM. Rapid induction of remission in large vessel vasculitis by IL-6 blockade. A case series. Swiss Med Wkly. 2011;w131(56):141.

85. Unizony S, Arias-Urdaneta L, Miloslavsky E, Arvikar S, Khosroshahi A, Keroack B, Stone JR, Stone JH. Tocilizumab for the treatment of large-vessel vasculitis (giant cell arteritis, Takayasu arteritis) and polymyalgia rheumatica. Arthritis Care Res (Hoboken). 2012;64(11):1720–9.

86. Stone JH, Tuckwell K, Dimonaco S, Klearman M, Aringer M, Blockmans D, Brouwer E, Cid MC, Dasgupta B, Rech J, et al. Trial of Tocilizumab in Giant-cell Arteritis. N Engl J Med. 2017;377(4):317–28.

87. Villiger PM, Adler S, Kuchen S, Wermelinger F, Dan D, Fiege V, Butikofer L, Seitz M, Reichenbach S. Tocilizumab for induction and maintenance of remission in giant cell arteritis: a phase 2, randomised, double-blind, placebo-controlled trial. Lancet. 2016;387(10031):1921–7.

88. Hunder GG, Bloch DA, Michel BA, Stevens MB, Arend WP, Calabrese LH, Edworthy SM, Fauci AS, Leavitt RY, Lie JT, et al. The American College of Rheumatology 1990 criteria for the classification of giant cell arteritis. Arthritis Rheum. 1990;33(8):1122–8.

89. Langford CA, Cuthbertson D, Ytterberg SR, Khalidi N, Monach PA, Carette S, Seo P, Moreland LW, Weisman M, Koening CL, et al. A randomized, double-blind trial of Abatacept (CTLA-4Ig) for the treatment of Giant cell Arteritis. Arthritis Rheumatol. 2017;69(4):837–45.

90. Samson M, Ghesquiere T, Berthier S, Bonnotte B. Ustekinumab inhibits Th1 and Th17 polarisation in a patient with giant cell arteritis. Ann Rheum Dis. 2017.

91. Conway R, O'Neill L, O'Flynn E, Gallagher P, McCarthy GM, Murphy CC, Veale DJ, Fearon U, Molloy ES. Ustekinumab for the treatment of refractory giant cell arteritis. Ann Rheum Dis. 2016;75(8):1578–9.

92. Banerjee S, Biehl A, Gadina M, Hasni S, Schwartz DM. JAK-STAT signaling as a target for inflammatory and autoimmune diseases: current and future prospects. Drugs. 2017;77(5):521–46.

93. Clark JD, Flanagan ME, Telliez JB. Discovery and development of Janus kinase (JAK) inhibitors for inflammatory diseases. J Med Chem. 2014;57(12):5023–38.

94. Gadina M. Janus kinases: an ideal target for the treatment of autoimmune diseases. J Investig Dermatol Symp Proc. 2013;16(1):S70–2.

95. Hartmann B, Mohan SV, Goronzy JJ, Weyand CM: JAK/STAT-signaling in giant cell arteritis. Circulation Conference: American Heart Association. 2013, 128(22 SUPPL. 1).

96. Garbers C, Aparicio-Siegmund S, Rose-John S. The IL-6/gp130/STAT3 signaling axis: recent advances towards specific inhibition. Curr Opin Immunol. 2015;34:75–82.

97. Shang Y, Smith S, Hu X. Role of Notch signaling in regulating innate immunity and inflammation in health and disease. Protein Cell. 2016;7(3):159–74.

98. Yuan X, Wu H, Xu H, Xiong H, Chu Q, Yu S, GS W, Wu K. Notch signaling: an emerging therapeutic target for cancer treatment. Cancer Lett. 2015;369(1):20–7.

99. Piggott K, Deng J, Warrington K, Younge B, Kubo JT, Desai M, Goronzy JJ, Weyand CM. Blocking the NOTCH pathway inhibits vascular inflammation in large-vessel vasculitis. Circulation. 2011;123(3):309–18.

100. Wen Z, Shen Y, Berry G, Shahram F, Li Y, Watanabe R, Liao YJ, Goronzy JJ, Weyand CM. The microvascular niche instructs T cells in large vessel vasculitis via the VEGF-Jagged1-Notch pathway. Sci Transl Med. 2017;9(399)

101. Ly KH, Stirnemann J, Liozon E, Michel M, Fain O, Fauchais AL. Interleukin-1 blockade in refractory giant cell arteritis. Joint Bone Spine. 2014;81(1):76–8.

102. Carmona FD, Mackie SL, Martin JE, Taylor JC, Vaglio A, Eyre S, Bossini-Castillo L, Castaneda S, Cid MC, Hernandez-Rodriguez J, et al. A large-scale genetic analysis reveals a strong contribution of the HLA class II region to giant cell arteritis susceptibility. Am J Hum Genet. 2015;96(4):565–80.

103. Espigol-Frigole G, Corbera-Bellalta M, Planas-Rigol E, Lozano E, Segarra M, Garcia-Martinez A, Prieto-Gonzalez S, Hernandez-Rodriguez J, Grau JM, Rahman MU, et al. Increased IL-17A expression in temporal artery lesions is a predictor of sustained response to glucocorticoid treatment in patients with giant-cell arteritis. Ann Rheum Dis. 2013;72(9):1481–7.

104. Marquez A, Hernandez-Rodriguez J, Cid MC, Solans R, Castaneda S, Fernandez-Contreras ME, Ramentol M, Morado IC, Narvaez J, Gomez-Vaquero C, et al. Influence of the IL17A locus in giant cell arteritis susceptibility. Ann Rheum Dis. 2014;73(9):1742–5.

105. Marquez A, Solans R, Hernandez-Rodriguez J, Cid MC, Castaneda S, Ramentol M, Rodriguez-Rodriguez L, Narvaez J, Blanco R, Ortego-Centeno N, et al. A candidate gene approach identifies an IL33 genetic variant as a novel genetic risk factor for GCA. PLoS One. 2014;9(11):e113476.

106. Serrano A, Carmona FD, Castaneda S, Solans R, Hernandez-Rodriguez J, Cid MC, Prieto-Gonzalez S, Miranda-Filloy JA, Rodriguez-Rodriguez L, Morado IC, et al. Evidence of association of the NLRP1 gene with giant cell arteritis. Ann Rheum Dis. 2013;72(4):628–30.

107. Carmona FD, Rodriguez-Rodriguez L, Castaneda S, Miranda-Filloy JA, Morado IC, Narvaez J, Mari-Alfonso B, Unzurrunzaga A, Rios-Fernandez R, Blanco R, et al. Role of the CCR5/Delta32CCR5 polymorphism in biopsy-proven giant cell arteritis. Hum Immunol. 2011;72(5):458–61.

108. Boiardi L, Casali B, Nicoli D, Farnetti E, Chen Q, Macchioni P, Catanoso MG, Pulsatelli L, Meliconi R, Salvarani C. Vascular endothelial growth factor gene polymorphisms in giant cell arteritis. J Rheumatol. 2003;30(10):2160–4.

109. Rueda B, Lopez-Nevot MA, Lopez-Diaz MJ, Garcia-Porrua C, Martin J, Gonzalez-Gay MA. A functional variant of vascular endothelial growth factor is associated with severe ischemic complications in giant cell arteritis. J Rheumatol. 2005;32(9):1737–41.

110. Enjuanes A, Benavente Y, Hernandez-Rodriguez J, Queralt C, Yague J, Jares P, de Sanjose S, Campo E, Cid MC. Association of NOS2 and potential effect of VEGF, IL6, CCL2 and IL1RN polymorphisms and haplotypes on susceptibility to GCA–a simultaneous study of 130 potentially functional SNPs in 14 candidate genes. Rheumatology (Oxford). 2012;51(5):841–51.

111. Salvarani C, Casali B, Farnetti E, Pipitone N, Nicoli D, Macchioni P, Cimino L, Bajocchi G, Catanoso MG, Boiardi L. Interleukin-6 promoter polymorphism at position −174 in giant cell arteritis. J Rheumatol. 2005;32(11):2173–7.

112. Gonzalez-Gay MA, Hajeer AH, Dababneh A, Garcia-Porrua C, Mattey DL, Amoli MM, Thomson W, Ollier WE. IL-6 promoter polymorphism at position −174 modulates the phenotypic expression of polymyalgia rheumatica in biopsy-proven giant cell arteritis. Clin Exp Rheumatol. 2002;20(2):179–84.

113. Amoli MM, Garcia-Porrua C, Llorca J, Ollier WE, Gonzalez-Gay MA. Endothelial nitric oxide synthase haplotype associations in biopsy-proven giant cell arteritis. J Rheumatol. 2003;30(9):2019–22.

114. Salvarani C, Casali B, Nicoli D, Farnetti E, Macchioni P, Catanoso MG, Chen Q, Bajocchi G, Boiardi L. Endothelial nitric oxide synthase gene polymorphisms in giant cell arteritis. Arthritis Rheum. 2003;48(11):3219–23.

115. Mattey DL, Hajeer AH, Dababneh A, Thomson W, Gonzalez-Gay MA, Garcia-Porrua C, Ollier WE. Association of giant cell arteritis and polymyalgia rheumatica with different tumor necrosis factor microsatellite polymorphisms. Arthritis Rheum. 2000;43(8):1749–55.

116. Boiardi L, Casali B, Farnetti E, Pipitone N, Nicoli D, Macchioni P, Cimino L, Bajocchi G, Catanoso MG, Pattacini L, et al. Interleukin-10 promoter polymorphisms in giant cell arteritis. Arthritis Rheum. 2006;54(12):4011–7.

117. Palomino-Morales RJ, Vazquez-Rodriguez TR, Torres O, Morado IC, Castaneda S, Miranda-Filloy JA, Callejas-Rubio JL, Fernandez-Gutierrez B, Gonzalez-Gay MA, Martin J. Association between IL-18 gene polymorphisms and biopsy-proven giant cell arteritis. Arthritis Res Ther. 2010;12(2):R51.

15

Prevalence of chronic widespread pain in a population-based cohort of patients with spondyloarthritis

Elisabeth Mogard[1]* (ID), Ann Bremander[2,3,4], Elisabet Lindqvist[1] and Stefan Bergman[2,4,5]

Abstract

Background: Chronic pain, regional or widespread, is a frequent and multidimensional symptom in arthritis. There is still limited information on chronic pain in spondyloarthritis, which is important to recognize for adequate diagnosis and treatment. Our objective was to study differences in prevalence of chronic widespread pain in two spondyloarthritis subgroups: ankylosing spondylitis (AS) and undifferentiated spondyloarthritis (USpA).

Methods: A population-based postal survey involving questions on the duration, distribution, and intensity of pain was answered by 940 patients with AS (ICD-10 M45.9) or USpA (ICD-10 M46.1-0, M46.8-9). The patients were categorized as having chronic widespread pain, chronic regional pain, or no chronic pain, and prevalence estimates for the pain groups were calculated, including age- and sex-adjusted prevalence.

Results: The prevalence of chronic widespread pain was 45.3% in AS vs. 49.3% in USpA, and that of chronic regional pain was 17.7% vs. 21.9% ($p = 0.033$). More women than men reported having chronic widespread pain (54.1% vs. 41.2%, $p \leq 0.001$), while the sex distribution for chronic regional pain was equal. Reports of pain intensity were equal in AS and USpA, with no significant difference in pain intensity between women and men who had chronic regional pain or chronic widespread pain. In the multiple logistic regression analysis, chronic widespread pain was associated to female sex, being an ever-smoker, and having a higher body mass index, controlled for SpA subgroup and disease duration.

Conclusions: The prevalence of chronic widespread pain in patients with AS and USpA is high, and with a female predominance, but with no difference in pain intensity between women and men. Chronic pain can complicate the clinical evaluation in patients with SpA, and highlights the need for a thorough clinical examination, including evaluation of inflammation and an accurate pain analysis, to individualize non-pharmacological and pharmacological treatment decisions.

Keywords: Spondyloarthritis, Ankylosing spondylitis, Undifferentiated spondyloarthritis, Chronic widespread pain, Sex

Background

Pain is a frequent and multidimensional symptom in patients with arthritis [1, 2]. Apart from the common inflammatory nociceptive pain, inflammation and nociceptive stimuli in peripheral and axial joints may also cause a heightened pain perception due to both peripheral sensitization, with nociceptors responding to light pressure and normal movement, and central sensitization with hyperexcitability of the neurons in the spinal cord [1, 3, 4]. This heightened pain perception could lead to a persistence of the pain and development of a chronic pain condition [5]. Chronic pain can be divided into chronic regional pain (CRP) and chronic widespread pain (CWP). CWP is usually defined as pain present in both sides of the body, above and below the waist and in axial body regions [6], and has a prevalence of about 11% in the adult population [7, 8]. In patients with rheumatoid arthritis (RA), CWP has been reported in one-third of the patients [9], but in other chronic rheumatic diseases such as spondyloarthritis (SpA), information regarding prevalence rates for CWP are limited.

* Correspondence: elisabeth.mogard@med.lu.se
[1]Department of Clinical Sciences Lund, Rheumatology, Lund University, Skane University Hospital, Lund, Sweden
Full list of author information is available at the end of the article

SpA is a group of chronic rheumatic diseases with similar clinical features such as back pain, asymmetrical peripheral arthritis, enthesitis, and extra-articular manifestations, and includes—among others—AS and undifferentiated spondyloarthritis (USpA) [10]. In Sweden, all diagnoses in clinical practice are set in accordance with the International Classification of Diseases and Related Health Problems, Tenth Revision (ICD-10). The AS diagnosis confirms with both the 1984 modified New York criteria [11] and the more recent criteria for axial spondyloarthritis (axSpA) [12]. The USpA diagnosis refers to a less well studied and variable group of patients [10, 13], including patients with non-radiographic axial SpA and peripheral SpA, or a combination [12, 14, 15]. It has been argued that USpA, in some cases, can represent an early form of AS [16–19], and in a recent review, a relatively large group of patients with USpA (39.9%) developed into AS after 10 years [20]. Functional impairment, reduced quality of life, fatigue, reduced ability to work, anxiety, and depression, are well-known findings for patients with SpA in general [21–25].

There is an increased attention regarding difficulties of managing chronic pain in SpA in the clinic. But as to date, the few studies exploring chronic pain in SpA have mainly concentrated on patients with AS and pain corresponding to the more complex fibromyalgia (FM) syndrome [6], with prevalence estimates of FM varying between 4% and 15%, and with higher frequencies in women [26–29]. CWP can include pain from different origins, and be seen as a continuum, with FM representing the more severe form. Therefore, studies that aim to identify patients with early and less severe CWP could be important. Not only, for an accurate diagnosis, but most importantly, for optimal and early treatment of both the inflammatory disease, and a possible co-existing sensitization of the nervous system, requiring other treatment strategies.

The aim of the study was to assess differences in prevalence of self-reported CWP in a population-based cohort of patients diagnosed with AS or USpA, including differences between women and men.

Methods

The Skåne Health Care Register (SHCR)

The county of Skåne is the most southerly region of Sweden. All healthcare visits, for both inpatients, and outpatients, are registered in the Skåne Health Care Register (SHCR) using unique personal identification numbers. About one-eighth of the Swedish population is covered in the SHCR. Information on the healthcare provider, on the date of visit, and on ICD-10 diagnoses is included in the SHCR. More details of this register are given elsewhere [30, 31].

Study population

This cross-sectional study made use of the population-based SpAScania cohort ($n = 3711$), which was identified through the SHCR during the period 2003–2007. For inclusion in the cohort, a diagnosis of SpA (with ICD-10 codes), was required to be registered, either by a rheumatologist or an internist on one occasion, or twice by any other physician in primary or secondary care on two separate occasions. A validation of the accuracy of the SpA diagnosis in the SHCR has previously been performed, with a valid diagnosis in 98% of the cases [30].

In 2009, a postal questionnaire was sent out to all patients in the cohort who were 18 years of age and over. Out of the 2162 patients who answered the survey (58%), 940 with a diagnosis of AS (ICD-10 code; M45.9) or USpA (ICD-10 codes; M46.0, M46.1, M46.8, M46.9) were included in the study. All patients with a diagnosis corresponding to psoriatic arthritis, IBD-related arthritis, or reactive arthritis were excluded. An analysis of non-responders within the large SpAScania cohort has previously been published [32]. This showed that patients with AS were more likely to respond, and that higher age predicted a higher response in men. There was an increased response with age also in women, except for women with AS, who tended to respond less with age.

The questionnaire

The questionnaire consisted of several validated patient-reported outcome measures as described elsewhere [32]. Data on socio-demographics (age, sex), disease duration, pain (duration, distribution and intensity), fatigue, smoking habits (smoker/ever, smoker/never), body mass index (BMI), synthetic and biologic disease-modifying antirheumatic drugs (sDMARDs and bDMARDs), corticosteroids, and disease activity (according to the Bath Ankylosing Spondylitis Disease Activity Index, BASDAI) [33], were used in this study.

Details of pain

For assessing pain intensity, a numerical rating scale (NRS) was used, ranging from 0 (meaning no pain) to 10 (meaning worst possible pain). For pain to be considered chronic, it had to be persistent or recurrent for more than 3 months during the previous 12 months [6]. The overall question for musculoskeletal chronic pain was: "have you during the last twelve months experienced any aches or pains lasting more than three months?" To distinguish between chronic regional pain (CRP) and chronic widespread pain (CWP), a pain mannequin, with 18 predefined body regions, and explanatory names for each region, was used [7]. For CWP to be considered present, according to the 1990 American College of Rheumatology (ACR) criteria [6], pain was required to be marked (I) on both the left side and the right side of the body, (II) above and below the waist, and (III) in the axial regions (the cervical spine, anterior chest, thoracic spine, and lower back) of the mannequin. When the criteria for chronic pain were met, but not those for the widespread condition, patients were considered to have CRP. Patients, who answered "no" to the question defining chronic pain were regarded as having no chronic pain (NCP).

Statistical analyses

Prevalence estimates for self-reported pain in AS and USpA, including age- and sex-adjusted prevalence, were calculated and differences in mean values were analysed with Student's t-test. Differences in proportions were analysed with chi-square test. Multivariate logistic regression analysis was used to study the associations with (i) chronic pain (CRP and CWP) vs. NCP, (ii) and CWP vs. NCP/CRP, as dependent variables. Age, sex, SpA subgroup, smoking status, and BMI were all included in the analyses as independent variables, and thereby controlled for each other in the analyses. The multivariate logistic regression analyses were done with simple contrast to a reference group for each of the variables. Age- and sex- adjusted prevalence rates were adjusted by the direct method using the Swedish census population of 2009 as a standard population, to adjust for the differences in age and sex distribution in the AS and USpA groups. Analyses were performed using SPSS software version 20 for Windows (IBM Corp., NY, USA).

The study is reported according to the STROBE (STrengthening the Reporting of OBservational studies in Epidemiology) guidelines [34].

Results

Patients with AS ($n = 570$) were older, with a mean age of 54.2 (SD 13.9) years vs. 49.1 (13.6) years, were more

often men (65.6% vs. 41.6%), and had a mean disease duration that was twice as long (20.3 (SD 13.5) years vs. 10.3 (9.5) years) as that of patients with USpA ($n = 370$). There was no significant difference in pain intensity between AS and USpA, but patients with USpA reported having a higher number of pain regions than patients with AS (mean 5.3 (SD 4.9) vs. 4.5 (4.5), $p = 0.019$) (Table 1). In general, women reported having higher pain intensity (mean 4.2 (SD 2.5) vs. 3.5 (2.4), $p \leq 0.001$) and a higher number of pain regions than men (mean 5. 7 (SD 4.8) vs. 4.1 (4.6), $p \leq 0.001$). Differences between women and men in the AS and USpA subgroups are presented in Table 2. The use of DMARDs and corticosteroids (solely or in combination) were reported by 50. 4% of the patients. The frequency of sDMARDs and corticosteroids were similar between patients with AS and USpA, but more patients with AS reported using bDMARDs (AS: 19.3% vs. USpA: 14.6%, $p = 0.005$). In addition, self-reported use of sDMARDs and bDMARDs were similar between patients in the three pain groups (NCP, CRP, CWP), but more patients with CWP reported using corticosteroids compared to patients belonging to NCP or CRP (CWP: 16.8%, CRP: 5.2%, NCP: 7.7%, $p < 0.001$).

Five per cent (53/940) of the patients could not be categorized into any of the pain groups (NCP, CRP, or CWP) due to missing responses on the chronic pain question and the pain mannequin, leaving 536 patients with AS and 351 patients with USpA. The patients not responding to the chronic pain questions had a mean age of 55.5 (SD 12.9) years (AS 57.5 (SD 12.8) vs. USpA 52.0 (SD 12.7), $p = 0.137$), and were more often men (62.3%). In addition, 64.2% of the non-responders had AS.

The prevalence of CRP and CWP

The one-year period prevalence of CRP was 19.4% (17.7% with AS vs. 21.9% with USpA), and that of

Table 1 Clinical characteristics of the patients with AS and USpA ($n = 940$)

Variables	AS	USpA	p-value
	$n = 570$	$n = 370$	
Age, years	54.2 (13.9)	49.1 (13.6)	≤ 0.001
Women/Men, n (%)	196/374 (34.4/65.6)	216/154 (58.4/41.6)	≤ 0.001
Disease duration, years	20.3 (13.5)	10.3 (9.5)	≤ 0.001
Pain intensity (0–10)	3.7 (2.7)	4.0 (2.5)	0.081
Fatigue (0–10)	4.4 (2.7)	4.7 (2.8)	0.222
Pain regions	4.5 (4.6)	5.3 (4.9)	0.019
Smoking ever %	53.7	38.6	≤ 0.001
BMI	25.9 (4.0)	25.6 (4.3)	0.256
BASDAI (0–10)	3.9 (2.2)	4.2 (2.2)	0.031

Values are given in mean (SD) unless otherwise indicated

AS ankylosing spondylitis, *USpA* undifferentiated spondyloarthritis, *BMI* body mass index, *BASDAI* the Bath Ankylosing Spondylitis Disease Activity Index

Table 2 Clinical characteristics of women and men with AS (*n* = 570) and USpA (n = 370)

Variables	AS			USpA		
	Women	Men	*p-value*	Women	Men	*p-value*
	n = 196	*n* = 374		*n* = 216	*n* = 154	
Age, years	52.2 (14.2)	55.2 (13.6)	*0.016*	49.1 (13.8)	49.0 (13.4)	*0.924*
Disease duration, years	16.7 (12.4)	22.0 (13.7)	*≤0.001*	9.7 (8.9)	11.1 (10.3)	*0.207*
Pain intensity (0–10)	4.2 (2.6)	3.4 (2.4)	*0.001*	4.2 (2.5)	3.6 (2.4)	*0.022*
Fatigue (0–10)	5.0 (2.9)	4.1 (2.6)	*≤0.001*	5.0 (2.9)	4.2 (2.6)	*0.010*
Pain regions	5.2 (4.7)	4.2 (4.6)	*0.022*	6.2 (4.9)	4.0 (4.5)	*≤0.001*
Smoking ever, %	48.0	56.7	*0.054*	38.4	39.0	*0.878*
BMI	25.0 (4.4)	26.4 (3.7)	*≤0.001*	25.4 (4.7)	25.9 (3.7)	*0.272*
BASDAI (0–10)	4.2 (2.3)	3.7 (2.2)	*0.033*	4.6 (2.1)	3.8 (2.2)	*0.001*

Values are given in mean (SD) unless otherwise indicated
AS ankylosing spondylitis, *USpA* undifferentiated spondyloarthritis, *BMI* body mass index, *BASDAI* the Bath Ankylosing Spondylitis Disease Activity Index

CWP 46.9%. CWP was significantly more common in USpA than in AS (49.3% vs. 45.3%, *p* = 0.033). CWP was also more common in women than in men, with a prevalence for the total SpA group of 54.1% vs. 41.2% (*p* ≤ 0.001), while there was an equal sex distribution regarding CRP (Table 3).

Pain intensity was not significantly different between women and men in patients reporting CRP (mean (SD) 4.0 (2.3) vs. 3.5 (2.0), *p* = 0.095) or in those reporting CWP (5.1 (2.3) vs. 5.0 (2.2), *p* = 0.622).

Age- and sex-adjusted prevalence rates for CWP

Assuming that those who did not answer the pain duration and distribution questions had NCP, this would give a minimum age- and sex-adjusted prevalence of CWP for the total group (*n* = 940) of 44.9% (95% Cl 39.1–50.7), being higher for women (53.5%, 95% Cl 43.8–63.1) than for men (36.2%, 95% Cl 29.9–42.6). For patients with AS, the minimum age- and sex-adjusted prevalence of CWP was 42.7% (95% Cl 34.4–51.0) as compared to 47.8% (95% Cl 37.4–58.2) in patients with USpA, and this was mainly explained by the higher prevalence of CWP in women with USpA (57%, 95% Cl 42.4–71.6) than in women with AS (50.4%, 95% Cl 35.4–65.3).

Variables associated with chronic pain

In the multivariate logistic regression analyses, female sex was associated with chronic pain vs. NCP (odds ratio (OR) 1.78), and with CWP vs. NCP/CRP (OR 1.70), controlled for age, SpA subgroup (AS or USpA), smoking status, BMI, and disease duration. A higher BMI was associated with chronic pain (OR 1.05), and CWP (OR 1.05), while being an ever-smoker was associated with CWP only (OR 1.44). Belonging to a specific subgroup (AS vs. USpA), or experiencing a longer disease duration was not associated with either chronic pain, or CWP, when controlling for all other variables (Table 4).

Discussion

In this study, we found a high prevalence of self-reported chronic pain in both AS and USpA. CWP was present in half of the patients with USpA, and just slightly less in patients with AS, and was overall more common in women. About one-fifth of the patients with either AS or USpA reported having CRP, with no differences between women and men. Female sex, a higher BMI, and being an ever-smoker were associated with CWP in contrast to NCP/CRP, while diagnosis (AS or USpA) and disease duration were not. These findings can complicate the evaluation of disease activity and response to treatment in patients with AS and USpA, and

Table 3 Prevalence of pain (%) in men and women, for AS and USpA respectively, based on the pain groups: no chronic pain (NCP), chronic regional pain (CRP), and chronic widespread pain (CWP)

	AS				USpA			
	Women	Men	Total		Women	Men	Total	
	n = 184	*n* = 352	*n* = 536	*p-value*	*n* = 208	*n* = 143	*n* = 351	*p-value*
NCP	30.4	40.3	36.9		22.1	38.5	28.8	
CRP	17.9	17.6	17.7		21.6	22.4	21.9	
CWP	51.6	42.0	45.3	*0.059[a]*	56.2	39.2	49.3	*0.002[a]*

Statistical comparison by chi square test
AS ankylosing spondylitis, *USpA* undifferentiated spondyloarthritis
[a]for whole table with NCP, CRP and CWP

Table 4 Results from the logistic regression analysis with odds ratios (OR) and 95% confidence interval for having (i) chronic pain vs. NCP, and (ii) CWP vs. NCP or CRP. The independent variables were all included, and thereby controlled for each other in the analyses

	Chronic pain (n = 773)		CWP (n = 767)	
	OR (95% CI)	p-value	OR (95% CI)	p-value
Sex				
Men	1		1	
Women	1.91 (1.37–2.67)	≤0.001	1.70 (1.25–2.32)	0.001
Age	1.01 (1.00–1.03)	0.080	1.01 (1.0–1.03)	0.088
Diagnosis				
AS	1		1	
USpA	1.41 (0.99–2.00)	0.055	1.11 (0.80–1.53)	0.546
Smoking				
Never	1		1	
Ever	1.33 (0.97–1.83)	0.081	1.44 (1.07–1.95)	0.016
BMI	1.05 (1.10–1.10)	0.022	1.05 (1.01–1.09)	0.010
Disease duration	0.99 (0.97–1.01)	0.184	1.00 (0.98–1.01)	0.656

AS ankylosing spondylitis, *USpA* undifferentiated spondyloarthritis, *NCP* no chronic pain, *CRP* chronic regional pain, *CWP* chronic widespread pain, *BMI* body mass index

emphasise the need of an early and thorough clinical examination, including not only evaluation of inflammation, but also an accurate and careful pain analysis.

The results from the present study are difficult to compare in relation to previous research on SpA, since to our knowledge, there have been no studies on the prevalence of CWP in AS and USpA without limiting it to FM. However, the prevalence of CWP in AS and USpA was clearly higher than in the general population [7, 8], and also, higher than in a previous report on the prevalence of CWP in RA (34%) [9]. We used the same pain mannequin and definition of chronic pain as the two previous Swedish studies [7, 9].

Previous research has found that it is important to consider that the evaluation and diagnosis of SpA, particularly in women, can be delayed [35] and complicated by the presence of CWP. Symptoms such as chronic back pain, stiffness, and fatigue are common in patients with both SpA and FM, and can be interpreted, as indicating an increase in disease activity [26, 27, 36, 37]. Also difficulties in distinguishing fibromyalgia tender points and enthesitis sites in SpA have been reported [38], with an overlap of about 30% between the inflammatory back pain (IBP) criteria and the FM criteria. Even though we could not examine for tender points or enthesitis and the study population was different, it is important to acknowledge that CWP can include pain from different causes. CWP is a prerequisite for FM, and patients with CWP could already have FM, or be at risk of developing FM at a later date [39]. Interestingly, the opposite scenario has also

been found, where almost half of the patients, particularly women, were incorrectly diagnosed with FM instead of an inflammatory rheumatic condition [40]. With the above in mind, it is important to stress the fact that a thorough evaluation, including a pain assessment to identify signs of a widespread nature, is important in all patients who report prolonged and increased pain, and other symptoms such as fatigue and poor quality of life. In addition, the origin of pain is important when it comes to treatment, but the presence of enthesitis does not exclude a co-existing sensitivity in the pain system—which is why individualized pain management, including both non-pharmacological and pharmacological treatment, is emphasized.

The women in our study had a higher prevalence of CWP, and CWP was associated with female sex in the logistic regression analysis. These findings are in accordance with the results of previous studies that have investigated FM in SpA [26–29, 36], and with a recent review [41], reporting evidence of a higher risk of developing chronic pain in women than in men. In the same review, some evidence—although inconclusive—was found that women experience more severe clinical pain than men, and this was contributed to multiple bio-psychosocial mechanisms including hormones, neurochemistry, social roles, and coping mechanisms [41]. In the present study, no sex-related difference in the prevalence rates of CRP were found, and although the prevalence of CWP was lower in men than in women, men with AS and USpA reported a high prevalence of CWP, compared to men in the general population [7]. Interestingly, we also found that pain intensity was not significantly different in women and men, when studied separately in those with CRP or CWP, and that an overall higher pain intensity in women was due to the higher prevalence of CWP in women. These findings are new, and highlight the fact that it is important to be aware of and recognize a concomitant CWP also in men with SpA.

In agreement with earlier studies in the general population [42, 43], CWP was also associated with being an ever-smoker and having a higher BMI. People with obesity can have a low-grade systemic inflammation, due to the production of pro-inflammatory cytokines and adipokines in the white adipose tissue [44]. The association between obesity and chronic pain has accordingly, been reported to partly be mediated by pro-inflammatory cytokines, but biomechanical and structural changes, mood, poor sleep, lifestyle factors and personal factors have also been found to be important mediators [45].

We found no association between SpA disease duration and chronic pain in this study. One reason for this may be that personal or other factors are more important than disease duration when it comes to developing chronic pain, and especially CWP.

Strengths of the present study were that patients from both primary and specialist health care were included, and the relatively large sample size. Another strength was that the instruments represent different dimensions of pain (duration, distribution, and intensity), and are commonly used and validated [7, 46, 47]. There were also some important limitations of the study. One was the low response rate, even though this was comparable to that in other population-based surveys [7, 42, 43]. Another limitation was that the patients were identified by their clinical ICD-10 diagnosis so we cannot be certain how many patients with USpA that would be categorized as having axial or peripheral SpA. However, in this study patients with psoriatic arthritis, IBD-related arthritis, or reactive arthritis were excluded, and 65% of the patients with USpA (M46.0-1 and M46.8-9) reported current chronic axial involvement, possibly representing an early form of AS. Moreover, the questionnaire lacked information on other comorbid diseases that could have impact on chronic pain. Also, information regarding socio-demographic variables would have been interesting with regard to CWP. The self-reported data regarding medication should due to the large proportion of missing data, be interpreted with care. Finally, the cross-sectional design makes us unable to draw conclusions as to the causality of the associations detected. In future research, longitudinal studies will be important to help us gain a better understanding of predictive factors for development of CWP in patients with SpA.

Conclusion

We found a high prevalence of concomitant CWP in patients with AS or USpA, with an even higher prevalence in women, but with no difference in the intensity of pain in women and men who experienced CWP. The results highlight the importance of a thorough pain analysis included in the clinical examination, to identify patients with high and/or increasing pain levels and multiple pain regions. It may also guide appropriate and individualized treatment decisions, including non-pharmacological and pharmacological treatment options.

Abbreviations

ACR: American College of Rheumatology; AS: Ankylosing spondylitis; ASAS: The Assessment of Spondyloarthritis Society; BASDAI: The Bath Ankylosing Spondylitis Disease Activity Index; bDMARDs: Biologic disease-modifying antirheumatic drugs; BMI: Body mass index; CRP: Chronic regional pain; CWP: Chronic widespread pain; FM: Fibromyalgia syndrome; ICD-10: The International Classification of Diseases and Related Health Problems, Tenth Revision; NCP: No chronic pain; NRS: Numerical rating scale; OR: Odds ratio; RA: Rheumatoid arthritis; sDMARDs: Synthetic disease-modifying antirheumatic drugs; SHCR: The Skåne Health Care Register; SpA: Spondyloarthritis; USpA: Undifferentiated spondyloarthritis

Acknowledgements
We thank the staff of RC-Syd for assistance in data extraction.

Funding
The study received financial support by the Region Skåne, Sweden, the Swedish Rheumatism Association and the Stig Thunes Foundation. All fundings were unrestricted grants.

Authors' contributions
EM, AB, EL and SB substantially contributed to the study conception and design. AB contributed to the acquisition of the data. EM and SB analysed the data, and all authors critically interpreted the data. EM and SB drafted the first manuscript. All authors critically revised the manuscript versions for important intellectual content, and read and approved the final manuscript.

Competing interests
The authors declare that they have no competing interests.

Author details
[1]Department of Clinical Sciences Lund, Rheumatology, Lund University, Skane University Hospital, Lund, Sweden. [2]Department of Clinical Sciences Lund,Rheumatology, Lund University, Faculty of Medicine, Lund, Sweden. [3]School of Business, Engineering and Science, Rydberg Laboratory for Applied Science, Halmstad University, Halmstad, Sweden. [4]Spenshult Research and Development Center, Halmstad, Sweden. [5]Primary Health Care Unit, Department of Public Health and Community Medicine, Institute of Medicine, Sahlgrenska Academy, University of Gothenburg, Gothenburg, Sweden.

References
1. Schaible HG, Ebersberger A, Von Banchet GS. Mechanisms of pain in arthritis. Ann N Y Acad Sci. 2002;966:343–54.
2. Goldenberg DL, Clauw DJ, Fitzcharles MA. New concepts in pain research and pain management of the rheumatic diseases. Semin Arthritis Rheum. 2011;41:319–34.
3. Meeus M, Vervisch S, De Clerck LS, Moorkens G, Hans G, Nijs J. Central sensitization in patients with rheumatoid arthritis: a systematic literature review. Semin Arthritis Rheum. 2012;41:556–67.
4. Woolf CJ. Central sensitization: implications for the diagnosis and treatment of pain. Pain. 2011;152(Suppl 3):S2–15.
5. Bergman S, Herrstrom P, Jacobsson LT, Petersson IF. Chronic widespread pain: a three year followup of pain distribution and risk factors. J Rheumatol. 2002;29:818–25.
6. Wolfe F, Smythe HA, Yunus MB, Bennett RM, Bombardier C, Goldenberg DL, et al. The American College of Rheumatology 1990 criteria for the classification of fibromyalgia. Report of the multicenter criteria committee. Arthritis Rheum. 1990;33:160–72.
7. Bergman S, Herrstrom P, Hogstrom K, Petersson IF, Svensson B, Jacobsson LT. Chronic musculoskeletal pain, prevalence rates, and sociodemographic associations in a Swedish population study. J Rheumatol. 2001;28:1369–77.
8. Croft P, Rigby AS, Boswell R, Schollum J, Silman A. The prevalence of chronic widespread pain in the general population. J Rheumatol. 1993;20:710–3.
9. Andersson ML, Svensson B, Bergman S. Chronic widespread pain in patients with rheumatoid arthritis and the relation between pain and disease activity measures over the first 5 years. J Rheumatol. 2013;40:1977–85.
10. Dougados M, van der Linden S, Juhlin R, Huitfeldt B, Amor B, Calin A. Cats et al. the European Spondylarthropathy study group preliminary criteria for the classification of spondylarthropathy. Arthritis Rheum. 1991;34:1218–27.
11. van der Linden S, Valkenburg HA, Cats A. Evaluation of diagnostic criteria for ankylosing spondylitis. A proposal for modification of the New York criteria. Arthritis Rheum. 1984;27:361–8.
12. Rudwaleit M, van der Heijde D, Landewe R, Listing J, Akkoc N, Brandt J, et al. The development of assessment of SpondyloArthritis international society classification criteria for axial spondyloarthritis (part II): validation and final selection. Ann Rheum Dis. 2009;68:777–83.
13. Baraliakos X, Braun J. Spondyloarthritides. Best Pract Res Clin Rheumatol. 2011;25:825–42.

Prevalence of chronic widespread pain in a population-based cohort of patients...

135

14. Rudwaleit M, van der Heijde D, Landewe R, Akkoc N, Brandt J, Chou CT, et al. The assessment of SpondyloArthritis international society classification criteria for peripheral spondyloarthritis and for spondyloarthritis in general. Ann Rheum Dis. 2011;70:25–31.

15. Paramarta JE, De Rycke L, Ambarus CA, Tak PP, Baeten D. Undifferentiated spondyloarthritis vs ankylosing spondylitis and psoriatic arthritis: a real-life prospective cohort study of clinical presentation and response to treatment. Rheumatology (Oxford). 2013;52:1873–8.

16. Burgos-Vargas R. Undifferentiated spondyloarthritis: a global perspective. Curr Rheumatol Rep. 2007;9:361–6.

17. Zochling J, Brandt J, Braun J. The current concept of spondyloarthritis with special emphasis on undifferentiated spondyloarthritis. Rheumatology (Oxford). 2005;44:1483–91.

18. Burgos-Vargas R, Casasola-Vargas JC. From retrospective analysis of patients with undifferentiated spondyloarthritis (SpA) to analysis of prospective cohorts and detection of axial and peripheral SpA. J Rheumatol. 2010;37: 1091–5.

19. Burgos-Vargas R. Spondyloarthritis: from undifferentiated SpA to ankylosing spondylitis. Nat Rev Rheumatol. 2013;9:639–41.

20. Xia Q, Fan D, Yang X, Li X, Zhang X, Wang M, et al. Progression rate of ankylosing spondylitis in patients with undifferentiated spondyloarthritis: a systematic review and meta-analysis. Medicine (Baltimore). 2017;96:e5960. 10.1097/MD.0000000000005960

21. Heikkila S, Viitanen JV, Kautiainen H, Kauppi M. Functional long-term changes in patients with spondylarthropathy. Clin Rheumatol. 2002;21:119–22.

22. Da Costa D, Zummer M, Fitzcharles MA. Biopsychosocial determinants of physical and mental fatigue in patients with spondyloarthropathy. Rheumatol Int. 2011;31:473–80.

23. Singh JA, Strand V. Spondyloarthritis is associated with poor function and physical health-related quality of life. J Rheumatol. 2009;36:1012–20.

24. Haglund E, Bremander A, Bergman S, Jacobsson LT, Petersson IF. Work productivity in a population-based cohort of patients with spondyloarthritis. Rheumatology (Oxford). 2013;52:1708–14.

25. Meesters JJ, Petersson IF, Bergman S, Haglund E, Jacobsson LT, Bremander A. Sociodemographic and disease-related factors are associated with patient-reported anxiety and depression in spondyloarthritis patients in the Swedish SpAScania cohort. Clin Rheumatol. 2014;33:1649–56.

26. Almodovar R, Carmona L, Zarco P, Collantes E, Gonzalez C, Mulero J, et al. Fibromyalgia in patients with ankylosing spondylitis: prevalence and utility of the measures of activity, function and radiological damage. Clin Exp Rheumatol. 2010;28(6 Suppl 63):S33–9.

27. Azevedo VF, Paiva Edos S, Felippe LR, Moreira RA. Occurrence of fibromyalgia in patients with ankylosing spondylitis. Rev Bras Reumatol. 2010;50:646–50.

28. Haliloglu S, Carlioglu A, Akdeniz D, Karaaslan Y, Kosar A. Fibromyalgia in patients with other rheumatic diseases: prevalence and relationship with disease activity. Rheumatol Int. 2014;34:1275–80.

29. Salaffi F, De Angelis R, Carotti M, Gutierrez M, Sarzi-Puttini P, Atzeni F. Fibromyalgia in patients with axial spondyloarthritis: epidemiological profile and effect on measures of disease activity. Rheumatol Int. 2014;34:1103–10.

30. Haglund E, Bremander AB, Petersson IF, Strombeck B, Bergman S, Jacobsson LT, et al. Prevalence of spondyloarthritis and its subtypes in southern Sweden. Ann Rheum Dis. 2011;70:943–8.

31. Englund M, Joud A, Geborek P, Felson DT, Jacobsson LT, Petersson IF. Prevalence and incidence of rheumatoid arthritis in southern Sweden 2008 and their relation to prescribed biologics. Rheumatology (Oxford). 2010;49:1563–9.

32. Haglund E, Bergman S, Petersson IF, Jacobsson LT, Strombeck B, Bremander A. Differences in physical activity patterns in patients with spondylarthritis. Arthritis Care Res. 2012;64:1886–94.

33. Garrett S, Jenkinson T, Kennedy LG, Whitelock H, Gaisford P, Calin A. A new approach to defining disease status in ankylosing spondylitis: the bath ankylosing spondylitis disease activity index. J Rheumatol. 1994;21:2286–91.

34. von Elm E, Altman DG, Egger M, Pocock SJ, Gotzsche PC, Vandenbroucke JP. Strengthening the reporting of observational studies in epidemiology (STROBE) statement: guidelines for reporting observational studies. BMJ. 2007;335:806–8.

35. Slobodin G, Reyhan I, Avshovich N, Balbir-Gurman A, Boulman N, Elias M, et al. Recently diagnosed axial spondyloarthritis: gender differences and factors related to delay in diagnosis. Clin Rheumatol. 2011;30:1075–80.

36. Aloush V, Ablin JN, Reitblat T, Caspi D, Elkayam O. Fibromyalgia in women with ankylosing spondylitis. Rheumatol Int. 2007;27:865–8.

37. Heikkila S, Ronni S, Kautiainen HJ, Kauppi MJ. Functional impairment in spondyloarthropathy and fibromyalgia. J Rheumatol. 2002;29:1415–9.

38. Roussou E, Ciurtin C. Clinical overlap between fibromyalgia tender points and enthesitis sites in patients with spondyloarthritis who present with inflammatory back pain. Clin Exp Rheumatol. 2012;30(6 Suppl 74):24–30.

39. Yunus MB. Fibromyalgia and overlapping disorders: the unifying concept of central sensitivity syndromes. Semin Arthritis Rheum. 2007;36:339–56.

40. Fitzcharles MA, Boulos P. Inaccuracy in the diagnosis of fibromyalgia syndrome: analysis of referrals. Rheumatology (Oxford). 2003;42:263–7.

41. Bartley EJ, Fillingim RB. Sex differences in pain: a brief review of clinical and experimental findings. Br J Anaesth. 2013;111:52–8.

42. Mundal I, Grawe RW, Bjorngaard JH, Linaker OM, Fors EA. Prevalence and long-term predictors of persistent chronic widespread pain in the general population in an 11-year prospective study: the HUNT study. BMC Musculoskelet Disord. 2014;15:213.

43. Schaefer C, Mann R, Masters ET, Cappelleri JC, Daniel SR, Zlateva G, et al. The comparative burden of chronic widespread pain and fibromyalgia in the United States. Pain Pract. 2016;16:565–79.

44. Trayhurn P. The biology of obesity. Proc Nutr Soc. 2005;64:31–8.

45. Okifuji A, Hare BD. The association between chronic pain and obesity. J Pain Res. 2015;8:399–408.

46. Hunt IM, Silman AJ, Benjamin S, McBeth J, Macfarlane GJ. The prevalence and associated features of chronic widespread pain in the community using the 'Manchester' definition of chronic widespread pain. Rheumatology (Oxford). 1999;38:275–9.

47. Sendlbeck M, Araujo EG, Schett G, Englbrecht M. Psychometric properties of three single-item pain scales in patients with rheumatoid arthritis seen during routine clinical care: a comparative perspective on construct validity, reproducibility and internal responsiveness. RMD open. 2015;1(1):e000140. https://doi.org/10.1136/rmdopen-2015-000140.

16

Possible giant cell arteritis symptoms are common in newly diagnosed patients with Polymyalgia Rheumatica: results from an incident primary care PMR cohort

William Masson[1], Sara Muller[1], Rebecca Whittle[1], James Prior[1], Toby Helliwell[1], Christian Mallen[1] and Samantha L. Hider[1,2*]

Abstract

Background: To examine the frequency of possible giant cell arteritis (GCA) symptoms (including headache, temporal/scalp tenderness, jaw claudication and visual symptoms) in newly diagnosed polymyalgia rheumatica (PMR) patients in UK primary care.

Methods: The PMR Cohort Study is a primary care inception cohort of 652 adults with newly diagnosed polymyalgia rheumatica (PMR). At baseline, participants were asked to report (yes/no) on the presence of seven potential GCA symptoms: sudden headache, tender scalp, disturbed/double vision, jaw claudication, fever, appetite loss and unintentional weight loss.

Results: Of the 652 patients, 405 (62%) were female, with a mean (SD) age of 72.5 (8.9) years. Sudden headache was the commonest symptom in 161 patients (24.7%). The least commonly reported symptom was jaw claudication in 66 (10.1%) patients. Females had a higher prevalence of headache, tender scalp and jaw pain. Sudden onset headache and fever were commoner in younger patients, (OR (95% CI) per 10 year age band increase: headache 0.76 (0.62–0.92), fever 0.63 (0.49, 0.79)). In those reporting sudden headache ($n = 161$), 19.9% ($n = 32$) also reported double/disturbed vision and a tender scalp, whilst 11.8% ($n = 19$) reported double/disturbed vision and jaw pain.

Conclusion: The data suggests possible GCA symptoms are common in PMR patients, particularly sudden headache, appetite loss and weight loss. These symptomatic PMR patients warrant careful monitoring and consideration for early referral to specialist services.

Keywords: Polymyalgia rheumatica, Giant cell arteritis, Headache

Background

Giant cell arteritis (GCA, or temporal arteritis) is a systemic large vessel vasculitis with a tendency to affect the aortic and extracranial branches, such as superficial temporal arteries [1]. GCA affects older adults (typically those >50 years) with an estimated annual incidence of 1 per 10,000 per year in those over 40 years [2]. Its aetiology is currently unknown, other than it is an immune mediated disease which has a clear association with polymyalgia rheumatica (PMR) and females are affected up to three times more frequently than males [3].

Prompt diagnosis and treatment of GCA is essential to prevent complications such as irreversible blindness [4]. Common symptoms of GCA include headache, temporal/scalp tenderness, jaw claudication and diplopia. However, studies suggest that there may be an over-reliance on headache as a presenting feature of GCA with one study suggesting a prevalence of headache of 72%, [5], but with audit data suggesting those without headache are at increased risk of visual loss, perhaps as a consequence of delayed recognition [6]. It is especially important for those

* Correspondence: s.hider@keele.ac.uk
[1]Arthritis Research UK Primary Care Centre, Primary Care Sciences, Keele University, Keele, Staffordshire ST5 5BG, UK
[2]Rheumatology Department, Haywood Rheumatology Centre, Staffordshire ST6 7AG, UK

with PMR to be monitored for signs and symptoms of GCA, as it has been reported in secondary care populations that between 16 and 21% [3, 7, 8] of those with PMR will develop GCA at some point in their disease course. However, this may be different in community populations with PMR, and it is not clear to what extent this overlap is present in the community setting. This study aims to describe the prevalence of common symptoms that are potentially indicative of GCA in a cohort of English adults with incident PMR diagnosed in primary care.

Methods

Study design

The PMR Cohort Study is a cohort of 652 adults with newly diagnosed PMR recruited in primary care. The study has been described in detail elsewhere [9, 10]. Briefly, GP's entering a first Read Code for PMR were invited to refer patients into the study and encouraged to request the recommended blood tests. All participating general practices were provided with copies of the British Society for Rheumatology guidelines for the management of PMR [11]. Between June 2012 and June 2014, patients with a new primary care diagnosis of PMR were referred into the study by their GP and mailed a baseline questionnaire. This included information regarding PMR symptoms (current pain and stiffness using a numeric rating scale (NRS)), lifestyle factors and socio-demographics. Participants were also asked to report (yes/no) on the presence of seven potential symptoms of GCA including sudden onset headache, tender scalp, disturbed/double vision, jaw pain on chewing, temperature/fever, appetite loss and unintentional weight loss. Following completion of the baseline questionnaire, participants were followed-up by postal questionnaire at regular intervals for two years, with medical record review at the end of the study in those consenting, for recorded symptoms, treatment and diagnoses. The current study uses data from the baseline questionnaire only.

Statistical analysis

Descriptive statistics were used to describe the sample. The prevalence of GCA symptoms was calculated as a percentage. Comparisons of prevalence were made across genders and age (in 10-year age bands) using cross tabulation and odds ratios with 95% confidence intervals. The prevalence of pairs of GCA symptoms was also investigated using simple descriptive statistics. As headache is an important symptom of GCA, but is relatively common in the general non-PMR population, the prevalence of combinations of symptoms with headache were also investigated.

Results

Of the 652 incident PMR cases the mean (SD) age was 72.5 (8.9) years and 405 (62%) were female. Table 1

Table 1 Baseline Characteristics of the sample

	$N = 652$
Age (Mean, SD)	72.5 (8.9)
Gender (N %)	
Female	405 (62.1)
Male	247 (37.9)
Median (IQR) pain score (NRS) at presentation	8 (7, 9)
Median (IQR) stiffness score (NRS) at presentation	8 (7, 9)
Morning stiffness >45 min duration (n, %)	524 (80.3)
Current steroid dose for PMR treatment (mg/day)[a] N (%)	
<10 mg	64 (12.3)
10 < 15 mg	87 (16.7)
15 < 20 mg	218 (41.9)
20 < 25 mg	111 (21.4)
25-30 mg	6 (1.2)
≥30 mg	34 (6.5)
Smoking (n, %)	
Never	317 (49.3%)
Previously	286 (44.5%)
Currently	40 (6.2%)

[a] Data on current steroid dose not available for 132 patients. NRS- numerical rating scale, where 0 = none and 10 is very severe.

shows the baseline demographics and clinical features of the cohort. The median (IQR) time from referral into the cohort to the baseline postal questionnaire being received was 16 (11, 23) days. Sudden onset headache (161, 24.7% patients), appetite loss (140, 21.5%) and unintended weight loss (137, 21%) were the most common symptoms (Table 2). Females were significantly more likely to report all symptoms than men, with the exception of unintentional weight loss, where there was no gender difference. (Table 2). Sudden onset headache and fever were the only symptoms significantly associated with age, with younger patients more likely to experience these symptoms (OR (95% CI) for headache per 10-year increase 0.76; 0.62–0.92) and fever (OR (95% CI) per 10-year increase 0.63 (0.49, 0.79)).

Pairs of GCA symptoms

In terms of symptom pairs, headache and tender scalp were the most common combination pair of symptoms with a prevalence of 10.1%, followed by headache and double vision (9.5%) (Table 3). In those reporting sudden headache (n = 161) (Table 2), 19.9% (n = 32) also reported double/disturbed vision and a tender scalp, whilst 11.8% (n = 19) reported double/disturbed vision and jaw pain. Double/disturbed vision, tender scalp and jaw pain was reported by 13 individuals (8.1%) reporting sudden headache.

Table 2 Possible GCA Symptoms

	All (n = 652)	Female (n = 405)	Male (n = 247)	Odds Ratio (95% CI): females vs. males (ref. category)	Mean (sd) age with symptoms	Mean (sd) age no symptoms	Odds Ratio (95% CI): per 10 year age increase
Sudden headache	161 (24.7)	123 (30.4)	38 (15.4)	2.40 (1.60, 3.60)	70.8 (9.5)	73.1 (8.7)	0.76 (0.62, 0.92)
Appetite loss	140 (21.5)	102 (25.2)	38 (15.4)	1.85 (1.23, 2.80)	73.1 (9.2)	72.4 (8.9)	1.09 (0.88, 1.35)
Unintended weight loss	137 (21.0)	83 (20.5)	54 (21.9)	0.92 (0.63, 1.36)	73.3 (8.8)	72.3 (9.0)	1.14 (0.92, 1.42)
Tender scalp	123 (18.9)	87 (21.5)	36 (14.6)	1.60 (1.04, 2.45)	72.8 (8.9)	72.4 (9.0)	1.05 (0.84, 1.31)
Disturbed / double vision	110 (16.9)	84 (20.7)	26 (10.5)	2.22 (1.39, 3.57)	71.6 (9.5)	72.7 (8.8)	0.87 (0.70, 1.09)
Temperature/ fever	99 (15.2)	72 (17.8)	27 (10.9)	1.76 (1.10, 2.83)	69.2 (9.4)	73.1 (8.7)	0.63 (0.49, 0.79)
Jaw pain on chewing	66 (10.1)	50 (12.4)	16 (6.5)	2.03 (1.13, 3.66)	72.3 (8.0)	72.5 (9.0)	0.98 (0.74, 1.30)

All are N (%) unless otherwise stated

Discussion

This study of incident PMR cases suggests that classical GCA symptoms are common in newly diagnosed PMR patients, with 1 in 4 patients reporting sudden headache, appetite loss or unintentional weight loss. Jaw pain on chewing was the least common reported symptom. Except for unintentional weight loss, a higher proportion of females reported all symptoms, whilst sudden headache, double vision and fever were reported by fewer people at older ages. Given that older patients seem to be at greater risk of both developing GCA and of visual loss (7) it may be that reporting of these symptoms is more specific in older individuals, who may report fewer symptoms but be at greater risk of complications. The most common combination of symptoms was headache with tender scalp and headache with double vision, each affecting approximately 10% of the cohort at diagnosis. Further follow up of the cohort will determine the proportion of patients who were formally diagnosed as having GCA.

The PMR Cohort study is the first inception cohort study of PMR patients in primary care and is of a substantial size. Although primary care recruitment can be seen as a weakness, because no specialist opinion as to the diagnosis was sought, this is also a major strength of the study because the majority of patients with PMR

are diagnosed and managed exclusively in primary care [12]. This sample is therefore free of the potential spectrum bias that is likely to be present in studies conducted in specialist settings where disease may be more severe, atypical or difficult to manage. Reassuringly however, the demographic and clinical characteristics of this cohort are similar to other secondary care cohorts [13], providing confidence in the accuracy of the primary care PMR diagnosis. Furthermore symptoms were recorded from patients close to the time of diagnosis thus reducing the recall bias.

One of the limitations of this study is that at this stage it is unknown if the patient was formally diagnosed with GCA or not. The prevalence of possible GCA symptoms was higher in women in our cohort, in common with the reported higher prevalence of GCA in women. [7]. Furthermore, the study demonstrates that in patients with PMR, headache is a much commoner symptom than in the older adult general population. Work by Steiner et al. [14] demonstrated that in the older adult general population (aged 50–65) the prevalence of headache was 3.4% for males and 13.5% for females The prevalence of headache was considerably higher in our cohort (males 15.4%, females 30.4%), suggesting that PMR is associated with an increase in reported headaches, which may reflect the overlap with giant cell arteritis, or that some cases of GCA are not being recognised or misdiagnosed. Although females have a higher prevalence of headaches overall, males saw a much bigger increase in the prevalence of headaches compared with a similar age general population group. However, a Danish population survey suggested the prevalence of headache to be 36.5%, although only 17% had consulted primary care because of headache symptoms [15]. Previous studies comparing patients with isolated PMR and those who went onto develop GCA

Table 3 Symptom combinations in those with PMR

Symptom Combinations	n (%)
Headache & Tender Scalp	66 (10.1%)
Headache & Double/Disturbed Vision	62 (9.5%)
Headache & Jaw Pain	39 (6.0%)
Headache & Tender Scalp & Jaw Pain	22 (3.4%)
Double/Disturbed Vision & Tender Scalp	41 (6.3%)
Double/Disturbed Vision & Jaw Pain	23 (3.5%)

have suggested that new onset headache is a key predictor [16, 17], with others suggesting that the headache is over-relied on in making a GCA diagnosis [5, 6].

Given that single symptoms such as headache are common both in the general population and in those with PMR it may be that combinations of symptoms are more useful in identifying patients at risk of GCA. Headache and tender scalp are two of the most common symptoms reported in those diagnosed with GCA and were reported by around 10% of this PMR Cohort. Further follow-up will assess whether these patients were initially misdiagnosed as PMR instead of GCA, together with further assessment of the utility of combinations of symptoms in predicting those patients at higher risk of GCA.

Conclusions

In summary, within a cohort of primary care patients newly diagnosed with PMR, symptoms suggestive of possible GCA, such as headache, tender scalp and visual disturbance are common. These occur in more than 1 in 4 patients and at higher rates than in the older age UK general population. Given the risk of irreversible visual loss in those with untreated GCA it may be that PMR patients who have these symptoms warrant closer monitoring and follow up to ensure that GCA does not develop and that symptoms do not progress. Future follow-up of this cohort will enable greater understanding of the proportions of primary care PMR patients who develop GCA and the risk factors for GCA development. Enabling risk stratification of PMR patients could facilitate GP education (regarding patients at higher risk) and more effective referral or treatment interventions to reduce the impact of this potentially serious complication.

Abbreviations
GCA: giant cell arteritis; GP: general practitioner; PMR: polymyalgia rheumatica

Acknowledgements
The authors would like to thank the staff at Keele University's Arthritis Research UK Primary Care Centre, the Keele Clinical Trials Unit, and the staff and patients of the participating practices and NIHR Clinical Research Networks.
We wish to thank those who reviewed the manuscript for their constructive comments (Additional file 1).

Funding
This work was funded by an Arthritis Research UK Clinician Scientist Award. CDM is funded by the National Institute for Health Research (NIHR) Collaborations for Leadership in Applied Health Research and Care West Midlands, the NIHR School for Primary Care Research and a NIHR Research Professorship in General Practice (NIHR-RP-2014-04-026). TH is funded by a NIHR Clinical Lectureship in General Practice. SM and JP are funded by the NIHR SPCR. The views expressed are those of the author(s) and not necessarily those of the NHS, the NIHR or the Department of Health.

Authors' contributions
All authors made substantial contributions to conception and design (WM, SM, RW, JP, TH, CM, SH) or acquisition of data or analysis and interpretation of data (SM, SH, TH, CM). All authors been involved in drafting the manuscript or revising it critically for important intellectual content and have given final approval of the version to be published.

Authors' information
N/A

Competing interests
Dr. J Prior is a member of the editorial board of BMC Rheumatology. The other authors declare no competing interests.

References
1. Nordborg E, Nordborg C. Giant cell arteritis: epidemiological clues to its pathogenesis and an update on its treatment. Rheumatology. 2003 March; 42:413–21.
2. Petri H, Nevitt A, Sarsour K, Napalkov P, Collinson N, Incidence of giant cell arteritis, characteristics of patients: data-driven analysis of comorbidities. Arthritis Care Res (Hoboken). 2015;67(3):390–5.
3. Smeeth L, Cook C, Hall AJ. Incidence of diagnosed polymyalgia rheumatica and temporal arteritis in the United Kingdom, 1990–2001. Ann Rheum Dis. 2006 August;65(8):1093–8.
4. Salvarani C, Cantini F, Hunder GG. Polymyalgia rheumatica and giant-cell arteritis. Lancet. 2008 July 19;327:234–45.
5. Smith JH, Swanson JW. Giant cell arteritis. Headache. 2014 Sep;54(8):1273–89.
6. Ezeonyeji AN, Borg FA, Dasgupta B. Delays in recognition and management of giant cell arteritis: results from a retrospective audit. Clin Rheumatol. 2011 Feb;30(2):259–62.2.
7. Gonzalez-Gay MA, Vazquez-Rodriguez TR, Lopez-Diaz MJ, Miranda-Filloy JA, Gonzalez-Juanatey C, Martin J, Llorca J. Epidemiology of giant cell arteritis and polymyalgia rheumatica. Arthritis Rheum. 2009 Oct 15;61(10):1454–61.
8. Narváez J, Estrada P, López-Vives L, Ricse M, Zacarías A, Heredia S, Gómez-Vaquero C, Nolla JM. Prevalence of ischemic complications in patients with giant cell arteritis presenting with apparently isolated polymyalgia rheumatica. Semin Arthritis Rheum. 2015 Dec;45(3):328–33.
9. Muller S, Hider S, Helliwell T, Bailey J, Barraclough K, Cope L, Dasgupta B, Foskett R, Hughes R, Mayson Z, Purcell C, Roddy E, Wathall S, Zwierska I, Mallen CD. The epidemiology of polymyalgia rheumatica in primary care: a research protocol. BMC Musculoskelet Disord. 2012 Jun 15;13:102. https://doi.org/10.1186/1471-2474-13-102.
10. Muller S, Hider SL, Helliwell T, Lawton S, Barraclough K, Dasgupta B, Zwierska I, Mallen CD. Characterising those with incident polymyalgia rheumatica in primary care: results from the PMR cohort study. Arthritis Res Ther. 2016 Sep 7;18:200. https://doi.org/10.1186/s13075-016-1097-8.
11. Dasgupta B, Borg FA, Hassan N, Barraclough K, Bourke B, Fulcher J, et al. BSR and BHPR guidelines for the management of polymyalgia rheumatica. Rheumatology (Oxford). 2010 Jan;49(1):186–90.
12. Helliwell T, Hider SL, Barraclough K, Dasgupta B, Mallen CD. Diagnosis and management of polymyalgia rheumatica. Br J Gen Pract. 2012 May; 62(598):275–6.
13. Mackie SL, Hensor EM, Haugeberg G, Bhakta B, Pease CT. Can the prognosis of polymyalgia rheumatica be predicted at disease onset? Results from a 5-year prospective study. Rheumatology (Oxford). 2010 Apr;49(4):716–22.
14. Steiner TJ, Scher AI, Stewart WF, Kolodner K, Liberman J, Lipton RB. The prevalence and disability burden of adult migraine in England. Cephalalgia. 2003;23:519–27.
15. Elnegaard S, Andersen RS, Pedersen AF, Larsen PV, Søndergaard J, Rasmussen S, Balasubramaniam K, Svendsen RP, Vedsted P, Jarbøl DE. Self-reported symptoms and healthcare seeking in the general population–exploring "he symptom iceberg" BMC Public Health 2015 Jul 21;15:685. https://doi.org/10.1186/s12889-015-2034-5.
16. Rodriguez-Valverde V, Sarabia JM, González-Gay MA, Figueroa M, Armona J, Blanco R, et al. Risk factors and predictive models of giant cell arteritis in polymyalgia rheumatica. Am J Med. 1997 April;102(4):331–6.
17. González-Gay M, Blanco R, Rodríguez-Valverde V, Martínez-Taboada V, Delgado-Rodriguez M, Figueroa M, et al. Permanent visual loss and cerebrovascular accidents in giant cell arteritis: predictors and response to

17

Asymptomatic hyperuricemia and coronary flow reserve in patients with metabolic syndrome

Seoyoung C. Kim[1,2]*[iD], Marcelo F. Di Carli[3,4], Rajesh K. Garg[5], Kathleen Vanni[2], Penny Wang[2], Alyssa Wohlfahrt[2], Zhi Yu[2], Fengxin Lu[2], Anarosa Campos[2], Courtney F. Bibbo[3], Stacy Smith[6] and Daniel H. Solomon[1,2]

Abstract

Background: Patients with metabolic syndrome (MetS) are at increased risk of asymptomatic hyperuricemia (i.e., elevated serum uric acid (SUA) level without gout) and cardiovascular disease. We conducted a cross-sectional study to examine associations between SUA levels and coronary flow reserve and urate deposits in carotid arteries in patients with asymptomatic hyperuricemia and MetS.

Methods: Adults aged ≥40 years with MetS and SUA levels ≥6.5 mg/dl, but no gout, were eligible. Using a stress myocardial perfusion positron emission tomography (PET), we assessed myocardial blood flow (MBF) at rest and stress and calculated coronary flow reserve (CFR). CFR < 2.0 is considered abnormal and associated with increased cardiovascular risk. We also measured insulin resistance by homeostatic model assessment (HOMA-IR) method and urate deposits using dual-energy CT (DECT) of the neck for the carotid arteries.

Results: Forty-four patients with the median age of 63.5 years underwent a blood test, cardiac PET and neck DECT scans. Median (IQR) SUA was 7.8 (7.1–8.4) mg/dL. The median (IQR) CFR was abnormally low at 1.9 (1.7–2.4) and the median (IQR) stress MBF was 1.7 (1.3–2.2) ml/min/g. None had urate deposits in the carotid arteries detected by DECT. In multivariable linear regression analyses, SUA had no association with CFR ($\beta = -0.12$, $p = 0.78$) or stress MBF ($\beta = -0.52$, $p = 0.28$). Among non-diabetic patients ($n = 25$), SUA was not associated with HOMA-IR ($\beta = 2.08$, $p = 0.10$).

Conclusions: Among MetS patients with asymptomatic hyperuricemia, we found no relationship between SUA and CFR, stress MBF, and insulin resistance. No patients had any DECT detectable subclinical urate deposition in the carotid arteries.

Keywords: Uric acid, Metabolic syndrome, PET/CT, DECT, Coronary blood flow

Background

The association between hyperuricemia, with and without gout, and risk of coronary artery disease (CAD), metabolic syndrome and kidney disease has been well-reported [1–9]. However, debate persists as to whether serum uric acid (SUA) has a causal role in the development of these conditions. Metabolic syndrome or diabetes is a known risk factor for CAD as results of macro- and micro-angiopathy related to diabetes [10, 11]. Patients with both metabolic syndrome and hyperuricemia may be at increased cardiovascular risk.

Positron emission tomography (PET)-measured coronary flow reserve (CFR) - the ratio of peak hyperemic myocardial blood flow (MBF) over that at rest as– is shown to be a reliable imaging marker of clinical cardiovascular risk [12, 13]. A reduced CFR can be a sign of flow-limiting CAD [14] and presence of coronary vascular dysfunction involving smaller vessels, which increases the severity of inducible myocardial ischemia and sub-clinical myocardial injury beyond the effects of

* Correspondence: sykim@bwh.harvard.edu
The interim analysis of this study was presented at the 2016 American College of Rheumatology Meeting in Washington DC, USA.
[1]Division of Pharmacoepidemiology and Pharmacoeconomics, Department of Medicine, Brigham and Women's Hospital, Harvard Medical School, 1620 Tremont St, Suite 3030, Boston, MA 02120, USA
[2]Division of Rheumatology, Immunology, and Allergy, Department of Medicine, Brigham and Women's Hospital, Harvard Medical School, Boston, MA, USA
Full list of author information is available at the end of the article

upstream coronary obstruction [15]. CFR less than 2.0 has been shown to be independently associated with risk for CAD, heart failure as well as cardiovascular death [12, 13, 16, 17]. While the association between gout, hyperuricemia and cardiovascular disease has been extensively studied, it has not been studied whether asymptomatic hyperuricemia (i.e., hyperuricemia without known diagnosis of gout) is associated with coronary vascular function measured with PET-CFR.

Dual-energy computed tomography (DECT) is a highly specific imaging modality that allows specific detection and volume measurement of urate crystals in the joints or tendons among patients with tophaceous gout [18, 19]. In a recent meta-analysis of 8 studies on DECT diagnostic performance, the pooled sensitivity was 84.7% and the pooled specificity 93.7% for gout [20]. DECT also had the positive predictive value of 87% for diagnosing gout in patients with a history of gout during their intercritical period [21]. While in some studies up to 24% had DECT-positive urate deposits in the joints of asymptomatic hyperuricemic patients [22, 23], no data is available whether urate crystals exist and/or can be detected in the vasculature using DECT scans.

We, therefore, conducted a cross-sectional study to determine the association between SUA levels and CFR, insulin resistance, renal function, and systemic inflammation. In addition, we used DECT scans to examine whether we could find/visualize subclinical urate deposits in carotid arteries among patients with asymptomatic hyperuricemia and metabolic syndrome.

Methods

Study population

For this cross-sectional study, eligible patients were men and women aged 40 years or older who had asymptomatic hyperuricemia defined as SUA ≥6.5 mg/dL and metabolic syndrome defined by the presence of at least 3 out of 5 traits in the National Cholesterol Education Program – Adult Treatment Panel III (NCEP-ATP III) criteria [i.e., obesity with body mass index (BMI) > 29.4 kg/m^2, high triglyceride level, low high-density lipoprotein level, hypertension, or hyperglycemia] [24]. We excluded pregnant or nursing women, patients with diagnosis of gout, symptomatic coronary artery disease or pulmonary disease, moderate-to-severe valvular heart disease requiring surgery, end-stage renal disease, renal replacement therapy, active malignancy requiring treatment, or those who used xanthine oxidase inhibitors, colchicine or probenecid. Details of this study cohort is described elsewhere [25].

The study protocol was approved by the Institutional Review Board of the Brigham and Women's Hospital. Written informed consent was obtained in all included patients before participating the study.

Patient recruitment

We recruited patients from the Partners Healthcare Biobank (https://biobank.partners.org) or several clinical sites of the Brigham and Women's Hospital (BWH). After we identified potential patients who met the study criteria through medical record review, we contacted those patients via letter. All patients went through a structured pre-screen phone call or a visit. We measured the SUA level by enzymatic colorimetric assay at the screening visit, unless a SUA value ≥6.5 mg/dL from within the last year was available in their medical record.

Positron emission tomographic imaging

Patients underwent a whole-body PET/computed tomography scanner (Discovery RX or STE LightSpeed 64, GE Healthcare, Milwaukee, WI) after at least 4 h of fasting. The study protocol for PET is similar to our previous work described elsewhere [26]. Briefly, ^{13}N-ammonia was used as a flow tracer at rest and stress for PET, [27] and an intravenous infusion of regadenoson was given as a stressor. We quantified MBF in ml/min/g during rest and peak stress using ^{13}N-ammonia and calculated CFR as the ratio of stress MBF over rest MBF [28–31]. Clinically relevant cardiologic variables including heart rate, blood pressure, and 12-lead ECG were assessed at baseline and throughout the test. With commercially available software, we calculated left ventricular ejection fraction (LVEF) at rest and stress from gated myocardial perfusion images. In addition, summed rest, stress, and difference scores were computed. Higher summed stress scores reflect larger areas of myocardial scar and ischemia. In general, normal scans have the summed stress score ≤ 3 [32–34].

Dual-energy CT (DECT) imaging

We obtained DECT scans of the neck using a dual-source CT scanner operated at DECT mode (SOMATOM Definition Flash, Siemens Medical Systems, Forchheim, Germany) at the tube potentials of 80 kV and 140 kV with an additional tin filter. We then used a commercial software post-processing program ('Gout', Syngo CT Workplace, Siemens Medical Systems) to produce digital color-coded images, where MSU deposits were marked as green. As a part of the main study, the study patients also underwent a DECT scan of the foot described elsewhere [25].

Markers of systemic inflammation and metabolic risks

We measured markers of systemic inflammation including interleukin (IL)-6 and high-sensitivity C-reactive protein (hs-CRP), and markers of metabolic risks including lipid, insulin and glucose levels at fasting. IL-6 level was assessed by enzyme-linked immunosorbent assay (ELISA). Insulin level was measured using a 2-site electro-chemiluminescent immunoassay on the Roche automated platform. We then quantified insulin resistance using the Homeostatic Model Assessment-Insulin Resistance (HOMA-IR, normal < 3) method [35]. We also collected information on a number of predefined variables potentially related to hyperuricemia or cardiometabolic risk, including demographics, body mass index (BMI), smoking status, comorbidities, and medication use. In addition, we measured serum creatinine and urine microalbumin and estimated glomerular filtration rate (eGFR) for the kidney function.

Statistical analysis

We used descriptive statistics to characterize the study cohort. Because data were not normally distributed, we used natural log transformation of SUA levels, CFR, MBF, and other laboratory results as dependent variables in regression models. For the primary analysis, we used unadjusted and multivariable linear regression models to examine the association between SUA levels and coronary vascular function (i.e., CFR and stress MBF) in the main cohort. Our final models were adjusted for age, sex, BMI, summed stress score (i.e., a strong indicator of myocardial scar and ischemia), serum creatinine, IL-6, hs-CRP, and presence of diabetes. Because prior myocardial scar or ischemia is a major determinant of CFR, we conducted a sensitivity analysis in which we performed multivariable linear regression models only in patients with summed stress scores which measure the extent of myocardial scar and ischemia ≤3 [32–34]. For the association between SUA and HOMA-IR, we ran unadjusted and multivariable linear regression in a subgroup of patients without diabetes.

Because no patients had subclinical urate deposits in the neck DECT scan, no further analysis was done for that variable. We used SAS 9.4 Statistical Software (SAS Institute Inc., Cary, NC) for all analyses.

Results

A total of 131 patients were consented into the study. Of these, 78 (59.5%) were excluded because of absence of hyperuricemia. One patient did not complete the screening blood draw. Eight patients who had hyperuricemia did not complete the full study; three declined to participate further, three patients completed only a portion of the study, and two were withdrawn by the study investigator. Forty-four completed the full study (see Fig. 1). Median age (IQR) was 65 (64–67) years, median (IQR) SUA was 5.5 (5.0–6.1) mg/dL and 66.7% were male in 86 patients who were consented but did not complete the study visit. Among those who completed the study, median [Interquartile range (IQR)] age was 63.5 (58.0–68.5) years, median (IQR) SUA was 7.8 (7.1–8.4) mg/dL and 40.9% were male (Table 1). The median (IQR) BMI was 34.7 (32.0–41.8) kg/m^2 and 43.2%

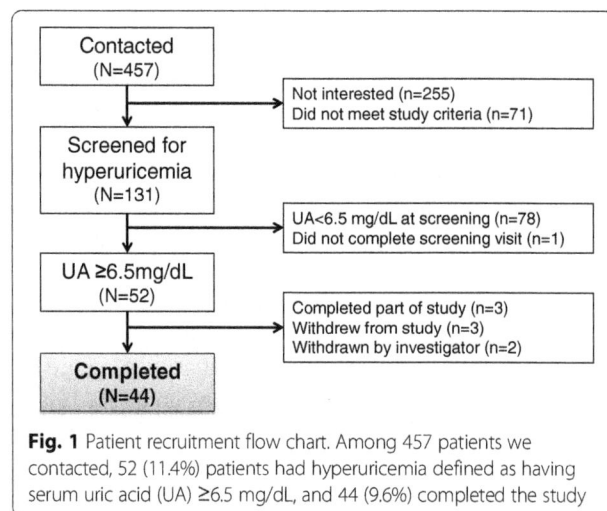

Fig. 1 Patient recruitment flow chart. Among 457 patients we contacted, 52 (11.4%) patients had hyperuricemia defined as having serum uric acid (UA) ≥6.5 mg/dL, and 44 (9.6%) completed the study

had type 2 diabetes. Half of patients had a family history of MI and 11.4% had a history of MI.

The median (IQR) CFR was 1.9 (1.7–2.4) and median (IQR) stress MBF was 1.7 (1.3–2.2) ml/min/g. Twenty-six (57.8%) patients had CFR less than 2.0 known to be associated with worse cardiovascular outcomes in a general referral population [16]. Twenty-eight (62.2%) had a normal summed stress score (≤3) which is a marker of prior myocardial scar or ischemia [32–34]. The median (IQR) HOMA-IR was 4.8 (3.4–6.5). In the unadjusted linear regression analyses (Table 2), SUA was not associated with coronary vascular function (CFR and stress MBF), systemic inflammation (IL-6 and hs-CRP), and insulin resistance (HOMA-IR). However, SUA had a positive association with serum creatinine ($\beta = 0.87$, $p = 0.01$) and an inverse association with eGFR ($\beta = -1.23$, $p = 0.002$). In the final multivariable linear regression model adjusting for age, sex, diabetes, BMI, summed stress score, serum creatinine, IL-6 and hs-CRP (Table 3), SUA was not associated with CFR ($\beta = -0.12$, $p = 0.78$) or stress MBF ($\beta = -0.52$, $p = 0.28$).

No association between SUA, CFR and stress MBF was noted in a sensitivity analysis limiting to 28 patients with a normal summed stress score (≤3). Among patients with no diabetes ($n = 25$), the median (IQR) HOMA-IR was 4.6 (3.8–5.7) and there was no significant association between SUA and HOMA-IR ($\beta = 2.08$, $p = 0.1$). None had DECT-detectable subclinical urate deposits in the neck, while 15% of these patients had subclinical urate deposits in the foot DECT scan (results published elsewhere) [25].

Discussion

Over the past few decades, growing evidence from a number of large epidemiologic studies suggests that a higher SUA is independently associated with an increased risk of cardiovascular disease including CAD [2–9, 36, 37].

Table 1 Study patient characteristics

Total number of patients	44
Demographic	
Age, year, median (IQR)	63.5 (58.0–68.5)
Male, n (%)	18 (40.9)
Comorbidities	
Body mass index, kg/m², median (IQR)	34.7 (32.0–41.8)
Current smoking, n (%)	3 (6.8%)
Type 2 diabetes, n (%)	19 (43.2%)
Insulin use, n (%)	6 (13.6%)
MI, n (%)	5 (11.4%)
Statin use, n (%)	33 (75.0%)
Family history of MI, n (%)	22 (50.0%)
10-year Reynolds risk score, %, median (IQR)	11.2 (4.2–19.4)
Laboratory data, median (IQR)	
Uric acid, mg/dL	7.8 (7.1–8.4)
Total cholesterol, mg/dL	167.5 (153.0–198.0)
Triglycerides, mg/dL	172.5 (115.0–201.5)
HDL, mg/dL	44.0 (38.0–54.0)
LDL, mg/dL	87.0 (76.5–116.5)
Fasting blood glucose, mg/dL	100.5 (92.5–135.0)
Serum creatinine, mg/dL	0.9 (0.8–1.2)
eGFR, mL/min/1.73m²	48.5 (34.5–57.5)
Fasting insulin, mIU/L	18.2 (14.4–21.9)
HOMA-IR	4.8 (3.4–6.5)
hs-CRP, mg/L	2.9 (1.1–7.4)
Interleukin-6, pg/mL	4.5 (2.4–6.8)
Urine microalbumin, mg/L	15.0 (7.5–43.4)
Cardiovascular function, median (IQR)	
Systolic blood pressure, mmHg	131 (123–146)
Diastolic blood pressure, mmHg	65 (61–76)
Rest heart rate, per minute	72 (64–78)
Stress heart rate, per minute	94 (84–103)
Rest myocardial blood flow, mL/min/g	0.8 (0.7–0.9)
Stress myocardial blood flow, mL/min/g	1.7 (1.3–2.2)
Coronary flow reserve	1.9 (1.7–2.4)
Rest left ventricular ejection fraction, %	60.0 (52.0–67.0)
Stress left ventricular ejection fraction, %	63.0 (54.5–70.0)
Summed stress score	0 (0–6)
Summed rest score	0 (0–0)
Summed difference score	0 (0–5)

IQR = interquartile range, MI = myocardial infarction, eGFR = estimated glomerular filtration rate, HDL = high-density lipoprotein, LDL = low-density lipoprotein, HOMA-IR = Homeostatic Model Assessment of Insulin Resistance (normal < 3), hs-CRP = high sensitivity C-reactive protein

Table 2 Unadjusted linear regression analysis for the association between serum uric acid and cardiometabolic function ($n = 44$)

Variables[a]	Standardized coefficient (SE)	P-value
Coronary flow reserve	0.04 (0.35)	0.90
Stress myocardial blood flow	−0.20 (0.43)	0.64
Interleukin-6	−0.46 (1.00)	0.65
Serum creatinine	0.87 (0.33)	0.01
HOMA-IR	0.76 (1.04)	0.47
hs-CRP	−1.47 (1.56)	0.35
eGFR	−1.23 (0.38)	0.002

[a]All the variables were log-transformed. SE = standard error, eGFR = estimated glomerular filtration rate, HOMA-IR = Homeostatic Model Assessment of Insulin Resistance, hs-CRP = high sensitivity C-reactive protein

Elevated serum uric acid levels are thought to cause endothelial dysfunction via oxidative stress, micro-inflammation, lipid oxidation, and inhibition of nitric oxide production [38, 39]. However, the causality of such associations has not been proven [40, 41]. In this cross-sectional study of 44 patients with metabolic syndrome and asymptomatic hyperuricemia, 58% had abnormally low CFR (i.e., CFR < 2.0) known to be an independent predictor for worse cardiovascular risk [12, 13, 16, 17]. However, we found that SUA level was not associated with CFR, stress MBF, or HOMA-IR. Both unadjusted and adjusted analyses consistently yielded the null results. Due to the nature of the cross-sectional design, we were unable to determine an association between the duration of hyperuricemia and CFR.

There are several explanations for our null findings. First, it is possible that our study did not find any association between SUA and coronary vascular function or insulin resistance because our study was limited to those with hyperuricemia. Second, it is possible that hyperuricemia is not causally associated with coronary vascular function or insulin resistance in the absence of gout. Third, moderate hyperuricemia might not have a strong relationship with CFR even if SUA itself is causally related to cardiovascular risk. However, our results are consistent with another study of 382 patients with and without gout which showed no association between SUA level and CFR [26]. Fourth, since most patients in our study are older and have many other known strong cardiovascular risk factors such as obesity, hypertension, renal dysfunction, and diabetes, SUA may not have any additional effect on patients' coronary vascular function even if it has a modest causal association with cardiometabolic risk. Third, this pilot study may be underpowered particularly at the level of moderately, not severely, high SUA. Fourth, since we did not have a normouricemic group to compare with, the difference in patients' SUA levels might have been relatively too small.

Table 3 Multivariable linear regression analysis for the association between serum uric acid and cardiometabolic function

	Adjusted for	Standardized coefficient (SE)	P-value
All patients (n = 44)			
CFR	Age, sex	0.04 (0.35)	0.92
	Age, sex, diabetes, BMI, SSS, Cr	0.07 (0.39)	0.86
	Age, sex, diabetes, BMI, SSS, Cr, IL-6, and hs-CRP	−0.12 (0.42)	0.78
Stress MBF	Age, sex	−0.19 (0.40)	0.63
	Age, sex, diabetes, BMI, SSS, Cr	−0.35 (0.44)	0.43
	Age, sex, diabetes, BMI, SSS, Cr, IL-6, and hs-CRP	−0.52 (0.47)	0.28
Patients with summed stress score ≤ 3 (n = 28)			
CFR	Age, sex	0.17 (0.43)	0.69
	Age, sex, diabetes, BMI, SSS, Cr	0.21 (0.38)	0.60
	Age, sex, diabetes, BMI, SSS, Cr, IL-6, and hs-CRP	0.09 (0.43)	0.83
Stress MBF	Age, sex	−0.13 (0.42)	0.76
	Age, sex, diabetes, BMI, SSS, Cr	−0.13 (0.43)	0.76
	Age, sex, diabetes, BMI, SSS, Cr, IL-6, and hs-CRP	−0.23 (0.47)	0.63
Patients without diabetes (n = 25)			
HOMA-IR	Age, sex	1.87 (1.30)	0.17
	Age, sex, BMI	1.36 (1.26)	0.29
	Age, sex, BMI, IL-6 and hs-CRP	2.08 (1.21)	0.10

SE = standard error, CFR = coronary flow reserve, MBF = myocardial blood flow, BMI = body mass index, SSS = summed stress score, Cr = serum creatinine, IL = interleukin, hs-CRP = high sensitivity C-reactive protein, HOMA-IR = Homeostatic Model Assessment of Insulin Resistance

A few prior studies examined the presence of subclinical urate deposits in patients with asymptomatic hyperuricemia using musculoskeletal ultrasound [42, 43]. DECT is a newer imaging modality that allows specific detection and volume measurement of urate crystals in the joints or tendons among patients with gout [18]. A validation study of DECT for gout showed a high specificity over 93% but a moderate sensitivity below 80% [19]. However, the sensitivity of DECT is noted to be low in non-tophaceous gout [44]. A few studies used DECT to assess subclinical urate deposits in patients with asymptomatic hyperuricemia. In a previous study of 25 patients with asymptomatic hyperuricemia (SUA ≥9.0 mg/dL), 24% were noted to have subclinical urate deposits in the joints and tendons based on the DECT scans of the feet [23]. In a cohort of renal transplant patients with asymptomatic hyperuricemia (n = 27, median SUA = 7.9 mg/dL), only 1 patient had quadriceps tendon deposition. However, none had articular or renal urate deposits [22]. In the present study, we also did not find any DECT-detectable urate deposits in the carotid arteries among hyperuricemic patients. It may be partially explained by the fact that most patients were hyperuricemic but their SUA were not too high with the upper quartile SUA level of 8.4 mg/dL. Furthermore, the sensitivity of DECT for the vasculature in asymptomatic hyperuricemia patient may be too low as 15% of the study cohort had DECT-positive urate deposits in their feet [25].

While it has been reported that urate deposits were present in the mitral valve, aortic and tricuspid valves and the endocardium in patients with gout, [45–47]. it remains unknown whether patients with asymptomatic hyperuricemia have urate deposits in the vasculature including the carotid arteries.

There are limitations in this study. First, this is a cross-sectional study without longitudinal followup. While we found no association between SUA and coronary vascular function and insulin resistance at one point in time, there could be an association between changes in SUA and changes in cardiometabolic risks. Second, since we included only asymptomatic hyperuricemic patients, the association between SUA and cardiometabolic risks may be different for patients with gout. Third, this study was performed at a single academic center and relied on active patient participation. Thus, the generalizability of our results may be limited. Patients who were enrolled but did not complete the study visit were older and more likely to be male and had lower SUA levels. Fourth, while this is one of the largest studies on asymptomatic hyperuricemia, the study size may not be adequate. In particular, only 25 patients (56.8%) had no diabetes. Thus, the subgroup analysis that included only non-diabetic patients on the association between SUA and HOMA-IR may be underpowered. Fifth, the final models were adjusted for several important predictors of cardiometabolic risk including age, sex, renal function, a summed stress score (i.e., a marker of myocardial scar and ischemia), and markers of systemic inflammation (i.e., IL-6 and hs-CRP), there may be residual confounding.

Conclusions

In this cross-sectional study of patients with metabolic syndrome and asymptomatic hyperuricemia, we found no relationship between SUA, coronary vascular function, and other cardiometabolic markers. Further studies are needed to confirm our findings. None of the patients had DECT-detectable subclinical urate deposits in the neck.

Abbreviations

BMI: body mass index; CAD: coronary artery disease; CFR: coronary flow reserve; CRP: c-reactive protein; DECT: dual-energy computed tomography; HOMA-IR: Homeostatic Model Assessment of Insulin Resistance; IL: interleukin; IQR: interquartile range; MBF: myocardial blood flow; MetS: metabolic syndrome; PET: positron emission tomography; SUA: serum uric acid

Funding

This study was funded by an investigator-initiated research grant from AstraZeneca. However, the study was conducted by the authors independent of the sponsor. The sponsor was given the opportunity to make non-binding comments on a draft of the manuscript, but the authors retained the right of publication and to determine the final wording.

Disclosures

This study was supported by an investigator-initiated grant from AstraZeneca/Ironwood Pharmaceuticals. The study was conducted by the authors independent of the sponsor. The sponsor was given the opportunity to make non-binding comments on a draft of the manuscript, but the authors retained the right of publication and to determine the final wording.

Authors' contributions

SCK had full access to all of the data in the study and takes responsibility for the integrity of the data and the accuracy of the data analysis. She is the guarantor for the study. SCK, MFD, RKG, KV, PW, AW, ZY, FL, AC, CFB, SS, and DHS conceived and designed the study. SCK, MFD, RKG, KV, PW, AW, ZY, FL, AC, CFB, SS, and DHS collected and analyzed the data. SCK, MFD, RKG, KV, PW, AW, ZY, FL, AC, CFB, SS, and DHS interpreted the data together and critically revised the manuscript for important intellectual content. SCK drafted the paper. All authors have given final approval of the version to be published.

Competing interests

Kim has received research support from Lilly, Pfizer, Genentech, Bristol-Myers Squibb, and Merck for unrelated studies.
Solomon has received research/funding support from Amgen, AstraZeneca, Genentech, Lilly and CORRONA, received royalties from UpToDate and served in unpaid roles in studies funded by Pfizer.
Di Carli, Garg, Vanni, Wang, Wohlfahrt, Yu, Lu, Campos, Bibbo, and Smith have nothing to disclose.

Author details

[1]Division of Pharmacoepidemiology and Pharmacoeconomics, Department of Medicine, Brigham and Women's Hospital, Harvard Medical School, 1620 Tremont St, Suite 3030, Boston, MA 02120, USA. [2]Division of Rheumatology, Immunology, and Allergy, Department of Medicine, Brigham and Women's Hospital, Harvard Medical School, Boston, MA, USA. [3]Division of Nuclear Medicine, Department of Radiology, Brigham and Women's Hospital, Harvard Medical School, Boston, MA, USA. [4]Division of Cardiovascular Medicine, Department of Medicine, Brigham and Women's Hospital, Harvard Medical School, Boston, MA, USA. [5]Division of Endocrinology, Diabetes & Hypertension, Department of Medicine, Brigham and Women's Hospital, Harvard Medical School, Boston, MA, USA. [6]Department of Radiology, Brigham and Women's Hospital, Harvard Medical School, Boston, MA, USA.

References

1. Kim S, Garg R, Smith S, Wohlfahrt A, Campos A, Vanni K, Lee L, Wang P, Yu Z, Di Carli M, et al. Cardiometabolic Risk and Subclinical Urate Deposits in Patients with Symptomatic Hyperuricemia and Metabolic Syndrome [abstract]. Arthritis Rheumatol (Hoboken, NJ). 2016;68(suppl 10).
2. Choi HK, Ford ES, Li C, Curhan G. Prevalence of the metabolic syndrome in patients with gout: the third National Health and nutrition examination survey. Arthritis Rheum. 2007;57(1):109–15.
3. Kim SY, Guevara JP, Kim KM, Choi HK, Heitjan DF, Albert DA. Hyperuricemia and risk of stroke: a systematic review and meta-analysis. Arthritis Rheum. 2009;61(7):885–92.
4. Kim SY, Guevara JP, Kim KM, Choi HK, Heitjan DF, Albert DA. Hyperuricemia and coronary heart disease: a systematic review and meta-analysis. Arthritis Care Res (Hoboken). 2010;62(2):170–80.
5. Kok VC, Horng JT, Lin HL, Chen YC, Chen YJ, Cheng KF. Gout and subsequent increased risk of cardiovascular mortality in non-diabetics aged 50 and above: a population-based cohort study in Taiwan. BMC Cardiovasc Disord. 2012;12:108.
6. Kuo CF, See LC, Yu KH, Chou IJ, Chiou MJ, Luo SF. Significance of serum uric acid levels on the risk of all-cause and cardiovascular mortality. Rheumatology (Oxford). 2013;52(1):127–34.
7. Lottmann K, Chen X, Schadlich PK. Association between gout and all-cause as well as cardiovascular mortality: a systematic review. Curr Rheumatol Rep. 2012;14(2):195–203.
8. Krishnan E, Akhras KS, Sharma H, Marynchenko M, Wu EQ, Tawk R, Liu J, Shi L. Relative and attributable diabetes risk associated with hyperuricemia in US veterans with gout. QJM : monthly journal of the Association of Physicians. 2013;106(8):721–9.
9. Krishnan E, Pandya BJ, Chung L, Hariri A, Dabbous O. Hyperuricemia in young adults and risk of insulin resistance, prediabetes, and diabetes: a 15-year follow-up study. Am J Epidemiol. 2012;176(2):108–16.
10. Alexanderson E, Garcia-Rojas L, Jimenez M, Jacome R, Calleja R, Martinez A, Ochoa JM, Meave A, Alexanderson G. Effect of ezetimibe-simvastatine over endothelial dysfunction in dyslipidemic patients: assessment by 13N-ammonia positron emission tomography. J Nucl Cardiol : official publication of the American Society of Nuclear Cardiology. 2010;17(6):1015–22.
11. Di Carli MF, Janisse J, Grunberger G, Ager J. Role of chronic hyperglycemia in the pathogenesis of coronary microvascular dysfunction in diabetes. J Am Coll Cardiol. 2003;41(8):1387–93.
12. Fukushima K, Javadi MS, Higuchi T, Lautamaki R, Merrill J, Nekolla SG, Bengel FM. Prediction of short-term cardiovascular events using quantification of global myocardial flow reserve in patients referred for clinical 82Rb PET perfusion imaging. J Nucl Medi : official publication, Society of Nuclear Medicine. 2011;52(5):726–32.
13. Herzog BA, Husmann L, Valenta I, Gaemperli O, Siegrist PT, Tay FM, Burkhard N, Wyss CA, Kaufmann PA. Long-term prognostic value of 13N-ammonia myocardial perfusion positron emission tomography added value of coronary flow reserve. J Am Coll Cardiol. 2009;54(2):150–6.
14. Taqueti VR, Everett BM, Murthy VL, Gaber M, Foster CR, Hainer J, Blankstein R, Dorbala S, Di Carli MF. Interaction of impaired coronary flow reserve and cardiomyocyte injury on adverse cardiovascular outcomes in patients without overt coronary artery disease. Circulation. 2015;131(6):528–35.
15. Gould KL, Ornish D, Scherwitz L, Brown S, Edens RP, Hess MJ, Mullani N, Bolomey L, Dobbs F, Armstrong WT, et al. Changes in myocardial perfusion abnormalities by positron emission tomography after long-term, intense risk factor modification. Jama. 1995;274(11):894–901.

16. Murthy VL, Naya M, Foster CR, Hainer J, Gaber M, Di Carli G, Blankstein R, Dorbala S, Sitek A, Pencina MJ, et al. Improved cardiac risk assessment with noninvasive measures of coronary flow reserve. Circulation. 2011;124(20):2215–24.

17. Ziadi MC, Dekemp RA, Williams KA, Guo A, Chow BJ, Renaud JM, Ruddy TD, Sarveswaran N, Tee RE, Beanlands RS. Impaired myocardial flow reserve on rubidium-82 positron emission tomography imaging predicts adverse outcomes in patients assessed for myocardial ischemia. J Am Coll Cardiol. 2011;58(7):740–8.

18. Choi HK, Al-Arfaj AM, Eftekhari A, Munk PL, Shojania K, Reid G, Nicolaou S. Dual energy computed tomography in tophaceous gout. Ann Rheum Dis. 2009;68(10):1609–12.

19. Choi HK, Burns LC, Shojania K, Koenig N, Reid G, Abufayyah M, Law G, Kydd AS, Ouellette H, Nicolaou S. Dual energy CT in gout: a prospective validation study. Ann Rheum Dis. 2012;71(9):1466–71.

20. Lee YH, Song GG. Diagnostic accuracy of dual-energy computed tomography in patients with gout: a meta-analysis. Semin Arthritis Rheum. 2017;47(1):95–101. https://doi.org/10.1016/j.semarthrit.2017.03.002. Epub 2017 Mar 8

21. Breuer GS, Bogot N, Nesher G. Dual-energy computed tomography as a diagnostic tool for gout during intercritical periods. Int J Rheum Dis. 2016; 19(12):1337–41.

22. Kimura-Hayama E, Criales-Vera S, Nicolaou S, Betanzos JL, Rivera Y, Alberu J, Rull-Gabayet M, Hernandez-Molina G. A pilot study on dual-energy computed tomography for detection of urate deposits in renal transplant patients with asymptomatic hyperuricemia. J Clin Rheumatol : practical reports on rheumatic & musculoskeletal diseases. 2014;20(6):306–9.

23. Dalbeth N, House ME, Aati O, Tan P, Franklin C, Horne A, Gamble GD, Stamp LK, Doyle AJ, McQueen FM. Urate crystal deposition in asymptomatic hyperuricaemia and symptomatic gout: a dual energy CT study. Ann Rheum Dis. 2015;74(5):908–11.

24. Third Report of the National Cholesterol Education Program. NCEP expert panel on detection, evaluation, and treatment of high blood cholesterol in adults adult treatment panel III final report. Circulation. 2002;106(25):3143–421.

25. Wang P, Smith SE, Garg R, Lu F, Wohlfahrt A, Campos A, Vanni K, Yu Z, Solomon DH, Kim SC. Identification of monosodium urate crystal deposits in patients with asymptomatic hyperuricemia using dual-energy CT. RMD open. 2018;4(1):e000593.

26. Kim SC, Shah NR, Rogers JR, Bibbo CF, Di Carli MF, Solomon DH. Assessment of coronary vascular function with cardiac PET in relation to serum uric acid. PLoS One. 2018;13(2):e0192788.

27. Di Carli MF, Dorbala S, Meserve J, El Fakhri G, Sitek A, Moore SC. Clinical myocardial perfusion PET/CT. J Nucl Med : official publication, Society of Nuclear Medicine. 2007;48(5):783–93.

28. Beanlands RS, Muzik O, Melon P, Sutor R, Sawada S, Muller D, Bondie D, Hutchins GD, Schwaiger M. Noninvasive quantification of regional myocardial flow reserve in patients with coronary atherosclerosis using nitrogen-13 ammonia positron emission tomography. Determination of extent of altered vascular reactivity. J Am Coll Cardiol. 1995;26(6):1465–75.

29. Di Carli M, Czernin J, Hoh CK, Gerbaudo VH, Brunken RC, Huang SC, Phelps ME, Schelbert HR. Relation among stenosis severity, myocardial blood flow, and flow reserve in patients with coronary artery disease. Circulation. 1995;91(7):1944–51.

30. El Fakhri G, Kardan A, Sitek A, Dorbala S, Abi-Hatem N, Lahoud Y, Fischman A, Coughlan M, Yasuda T, Di Carli MF. Reproducibility and accuracy of quantitative myocardial blood flow assessment with (82) Rb PET: comparison with (13) N-ammonia PET. J Nucl Med : official publication, Society of Nuclear Medicine. 2009;50(7):1062–71.

31. El Fakhri G, Sitek A, Guerin B, Kijewski MF, Di Carli MF, Moore SC. Quantitative dynamic cardiac 82Rb PET using generalized factor and compartment analyses. J Nucl Med : official publication, Society of Nuclear Medicine. 2005;46(8):1264–71.

32. Cerqueira MD, Weissman NJ, Dilsizian V, Jacobs AK, Kaul S, Laskey WK, Pennell DJ, Rumberger JA, Ryan T, Verani MS. Standardized myocardial segmentation and nomenclature for tomographic imaging of the heart. A statement for healthcare professionals from the cardiac imaging Committee of the Council on clinical cardiology of the American Heart Association. Int J Cardiovasc Imaging. 2002;18(1):539–42.

33. Machac J, Bacharach SL, Bateman TM, Bax JJ, Beanlands R, Bengel F, Bergmann SR, Brunken RC, Case J, Delbeke D, et al. Positron emission tomography myocardial perfusion and glucose metabolism imaging. J Nucl Cardiol : official publication of the American Society of Nuclear Cardiology. 2006;13(6):e121–51.

34. Yoshinaga K, Chow BJ, Williams K, Chen L, deKemp RA, Garrard L, Lok-Tin Szeto A, Aung M, Davies RA, Ruddy TD, et al. What is the prognostic value of myocardial perfusion imaging using rubidium-82 positron emission tomography? J Am Coll Cardiol. 2006;48(5):1029–39.

35. Matthews DR, Hosker JP, Rudenski AS, Naylor BA, Treacher DF, Turner RC. Homeostasis model assessment: insulin resistance and beta-cell function from fasting plasma glucose and insulin concentrations in man. Diabetologia. 1985;28(7):412–9.

36. Grayson PC, Kim SY, LaValley M, Choi HK. Hyperuricemia and incident hypertension: a systematic review and meta-analysis. Arthritis Care Res (Hoboken). 2011;63(1):102–10.

37. Perez-Ruiz F, Martínez-Indart L, Carmona L, Herrero-Beites AM, Pijoan JI, Krishnan E. Tophaceous gout and high level of hyperuricaemia are both associated with increased risk of mortality in patients with gout. Ann Rheum Dis. 2013;73(1):177–82. https://doi.org/10.1136/annrheumdis-2012-202421. Epub 2013 Jan 12

38. Wang Y, Bao X. Effects of uric acid on endothelial dysfunction in early chronic kidney disease and its mechanisms. Eur J Med Res. 2013;18(1):26.

39. Khosla UM, Zharikov S, Finch JL, Nakagawa T, Roncal C, Mu W, Krotova K, Block ER, Prabhakar S, Johnson RJ. Hyperuricemia induces endothelial dysfunction. Kidney Int. 2005;67(5):1739–42.

40. Keenan T, Zhao W, Rasheed A, Ho WK, Malik R, Felix JF, Young R, Shah N, Samuel M, Sheikh N, et al. Causal assessment of serum urate levels in Cardiometabolic diseases through a Mendelian randomization study. J Am Coll Cardiol. 2016;67(4):407–16.

41. White J, Sofat R, Hemani G, Shah T, Engmann J, Dale C, Shah S, Kruger FA, Giambartolomei C, Swerdlow DI, et al. Plasma urate concentration and risk of coronary heart disease: a Mendelian randomisation analysis. Lancet Diabetes Endocrinol. 2016;4(4):327–36.

42. De Miguel E, Puig JG, Castillo C, Peiteado D, Torres RJ, Martin-Mola E. Diagnosis of gout in patients with asymptomatic hyperuricaemia: a pilot ultrasound study. Ann Rheum Dis. 2012;71(1):157–8.

43. Puig JG, Beltran LM, Mejia-Chew C, Tevar D, Torres RJ. Ultrasonography in the diagnosis of asymptomatic hyperuricemia and gout. Nucleosides Nucleotides Nucleic Acids. 2016;35(10–12):517–23.

44. Baer AN, Kurano T, Thakur UJ, Thawait GK, Fuld MK, Maynard JW, McAdams-DeMarco M, Fishman EK, Carrino JA. Dual-energy computed tomography has limited sensitivity for non-tophaceous gout: a comparison study with tophaceous gout. BMC Musculoskelet Disord. 2016;17:91.

45. Emmerson BT. Atherosclerosis and urate metabolism. Aust NZ J Med. 1979; 9(4):451–4.

46. Jr.MH: Pathology of the cardiovascular system in chronic Ren Fail In: Management of Cardiovascular Disease in Ren Fail Volume 1, EDN Edited by DT L, RL P, W L. Phiadelphia: FA Davis; 1981.

47. McAllister H Jr, Buja L, Ferrans V. Valvular heart disease: anatomic abnormalities. In: Willerson J, Cohn J, Wellens H, Holmes Jr D, editors. Cardiovascular Medicine, vol. 20007. 3rd ed: Springer Science & Business Media. p. 372.

18

Perceptions of first-degree relatives of patients with rheumatoid arthritis about lifestyle modifications and pharmacological interventions to reduce the risk of rheumatoid arthritis development

Gwenda Simons[1*†] , Rebecca J Stack[1,2†], Michaela Stoffer-Marx[3,4], Matthias Englbrecht[5], Erika Mosor[3,6], Christopher D Buckley[1,7,8], Kanta Kumar[9,10], Mats Hansson[11], Axel Hueber[5], Tanja Stamm[3,6], Marie Falahee[1] and Karim Raza[1,7,8]

Abstract

Background: There is increasing interest in the identification of people at risk of rheumatoid arthritis (RA) to monitor the emergence of early symptoms (and thus allow early therapy), offer lifestyle advice to reduce the impact of environmental risk factors and potentially offer preventive pharmacological treatment for those at high risk. Close biological relatives of people with RA are at an increased risk of developing RA and are therefore potential candidates for research studies, screening initiatives and preventive interventions. To ensure the success of approaches of this kind, a greater understanding of the perceptions of this group relating to preventive measures is needed.

Methods: Twenty-four first-degree relatives of patients with an existing diagnosis of RA from the UK, three from Germany and seven from Austria (age: 21–67 years) took part in semi-structured interviews exploring their perceptions of RA risk, preventive medicine and lifestyle changes to reduce RA risk. Interviews were audio-recorded, transcribed verbatim and analysed using thematic analysis.

Results: Many first-degree relatives indicated that they anticipated being happy to make lifestyle changes such as losing weight or changing their diet to modify their risk of developing RA. Participants further indicated that in order to make any lifestyle changes it would be useful to know their personal risk of developing RA. Others implied they would not contemplate making lifestyle changes, including stopping smoking, unless this would significantly reduce or eliminate their risk of developing RA. Many first-degree relatives had more negative perceptions about taking preventive medication to reduce their risk of RA, and listed concerns about potential side effects as one of the reasons for not wanting to take preventive medicines. Others would be more willing to consider drug interventions although some indicated that they would wish to wait until symptoms developed.

(Continued on next page)

* Correspondence: g.simons@bham.ac.uk
†Gwenda Simons and Rebecca J Stack contributed equally to this work.
[1]Institute for Inflammation and Aging, Rheumatology Research Group, College of Medical and Dental Sciences, University of Birmingham, Birmingham B15 2TT, UK
Full list of author information is available at the end of the article

(Continued from previous page)

Conclusions: Information targeted at those considered to be at risk of RA should contain information about RA, the extent to which risk can be quantified at an individual level and how risk levels may differ depending on whether early symptoms are present. The benefits (and risks) of lifestyle changes and pharmacological interventions as potential preventive measures should be clearly described.

Keywords: Rheumatoid arthritis, Risk, Qualitative, Relatives, Preventive medicine, Lifestyle changes,

Background

Rheumatoid arthritis (RA) is a common chronic inflammatory disease with a prevalence of 1% [1]. The disease has a significant negative impact at both individual and societal levels [2]. Early diagnosis and treatment reduce the risk of future joint damage and disability [3–8] and increase the chance of drug-free remission [9]. As a result, there is now a drive to identify and treat people as early in the disease process as possible, potentially before the onset of joint swelling [10].

Genetic factors contribute significantly to a person's risk of developing RA [11]. Having a family history, especially having one or more first-degree relatives with RA, increases the risk of developing RA by approximately 3–5 fold [12–14]. Modifiable environmental factors such as smoking [15], alcohol intake [16, 17], and diet [18–20] also influence the risk of developing RA [21]. Interactions between these risk factors are likely [22]. Gathering information about an individual's genotype, environmental exposures, systemic and joint related immune abnormalities may thus allow clinicians to predict future RA development in those who are currently asymptomatic [22]. Among those people with a close relative with RA, current risk models using both environmental and genetic factors have been shown to be highly discriminative for both seropositive and seronegative RA [23].

Relatives of RA patients are a prime target population for both risk stratification and preventive interventions [24, 25]. First-degree relatives of RA patients are currently in the focus of prospective observational cohort studies [26–28] and interventional trials [21, 25]. However, difficulties recruiting first-degree relatives to such studies have been reported [29]. As recruitment of first-degree relatives is usually dependent on the cooperation of RA patients themselves, it is also important to understand patients' perceptions of RA risk, risk modification and the communication about these issues with their relatives. Qualitative studies have already started to explore the views of RA patients in this context [30].

In order to develop effective recruitment strategies and potential future preventive strategies for first-degree relatives we also need to have a good understanding of the perceptions this group, and their willingness to engage with preventive approaches. We have recently reported data from interviews with first-degree relatives in three European countries looking at their perceptions of being at risk of RA and of predictive testing. Relatives reported having a range of concerns about both predictive testing and risk information related to RA, including the possibility that knowing ones risk might increase anxiety and reported concerns about the level of uncertainty associated with predictive testing. Those relatives who expressed positive views about predictive testing indicated that they would need support to understand risk information [22].

Recent qualitative research has suggested that uptake of preventive medication by first-degree relatives might be related to perceived baseline risk and experience of the disease through their relative(s) [31]. Furthermore, preliminary data from a choice experiment with first-degree relatives suggest that acceptance of such medication would depend on its effectiveness and side effect profile [24]. In relation to lifestyle changes, one recent trial looked at the effect of disclosure of first-degree relatives' RA risk personalised with genetics, biomarkers, and lifestyle factors on their health behaviour intentions and actual behaviour [21] and found that those at risk were motivated to and actually changed certain behaviours after such personalised information. However, there is currently no information available about first-degree relatives' perceptions around these lifestyle changes and pharmacological interventions aimed at reducing the risk of RA development. This paper provides an exploration of previously unreported data collected during our earlier interview study [22] with first-degree relatives examining these issues in more detail.

Methods
Participants

Eligible participants were the first-degree relatives of people with an existing diagnosis of RA. Patients with RA were approached during their routine secondary care clinic appointments in Birmingham (United Kingdom), Erlangen (Germany) and Vienna (Austria) and asked to consider contacting a first-degree relative about participation in an interview study about risk and predictive testing for RA. Full procedural details are presented elsewhere [22]. We restricted the selection of relatives to offspring and siblings and excluded parents. In order to be eligible to take part, first-degree relatives had to be

Perceptions of first-degree relatives of patients with rheumatoid arthritis about lifestyle...

149

aged 18 years or over and not diagnosed with inflammatory arthritis at the time of the study.

Data collection and analysis

The semi-structured interviews were conducted either face to face at the recruiting hospital sites or by telephone and were guided by an interview schedule (Table 1). The schedule was informed by a literature review [32, 33] and in consultation with an international team of healthcare professionals, researchers and patient research partners participating in the EuroTEAM (Towards Early diagnosis and biomarker validation in Arthritis Management) project [34]. The interviewers in the UK were conducted by RS (female research fellow with a psychology background) and KK (female researcher and nurse specialist)). Interviews in Germany were conducted by AH (male senior clinical research fellow) and interviews in Austria were conducted by EM (female occupational therapist and researcher). All interviewers had previous experience of conducting interviews and RS, KK, and EM have extensive experience of qualitative methods. Interviewees received information about EuroTEAM in the participant information sheet (i.e. that it is a multi-country research project funded by the EU) and were told the name of the person interviewing them, as well as their role in the project. All interviews were audio recorded and transcribed by a professional transcription service. Interviews conducted in Germany and Austria were translated from German into English following transcription by bilingual native speakers and the translations were checked by the respective research teams.

Table 1 Outline Interview schedule

• Tell me what you know about RA?

• Do you ever worry about the possibility of developing RA in the future?

• What would you think if you were told that you could have a test that would tell you how likely you were to develop RA?

• What would your concerns be if you knew what your risk of developing RA was?

• What kind of tests do you think people might be able to do to work out whether or not you might develop RA (tests that are available now and tests that might become available in the future)?

• Various tests can currently be done, and various tests are currently being developed to predict the development of RA. What are your thoughts about:
  ° Blood tests looking at biomarkers, molecules in the blood
  ° Blood tests looking at genes
  ° Tests involving scanning the joints with either an ultrasound or MRI
  ° Tests involving taking tissue out of a joint or elsewhere (e.g. lymph nodes)

• What are your thoughts about taking medicines to reduce the risk of RA developing in the future?

• What are your thoughts about changing your lifestyle (e.g. stop smoking, more exercise, change diet) to reduce the risk of developing RA in the future?

All transcripts were analysed centrally at the University of Birmingham, United Kingdom.

Data collection and analysis were carried out in parallel to allow for an assessment of when thematic saturation had been achieved. Transcripts were analysed thematically [35] using NVivo (software programme for qualitative data analysis; [36]). One researcher (RJS) coded all the transcripts and three patient research partners blind coded three transcripts. The coding framework was discussed with the patient research partners and coding categories that lacked concordance were absorbed into the coding framework. The initial codes were then grouped into the most noteworthy and frequently occurring categories by RJS, KK and GS.

Results

Thirty-four first-degree relatives of RA patients were interviewed; 24 from the UK, three from Germany and seven from Austria. Participants were aged between 21 and 67 years ($M = 39$, $SD = 10.8$), and 76% ($n = 26$) were female. All but two British participants were white. Table 2 gives the individual participant characteristics including age, gender, relation to relative with RA and current musculoskeletal symptoms.

Interviews lasted between 30 and 90 min. The results presented here represent a new analysis of the resulting transcribed data. Findings related to an analysis of perceptions of risk and predictive testing are presented elsewhere [22]. The core themes presented here focus on perceptions of first-degree relatives about the possibility of making lifestyle changes and taking preventive medicine to modify their risk of developing RA. An overview of the organising themes and subthemes can be found in Table 3. Quotations referred to in the text can be found in Tables 4 and 5.

Modifying risk through lifestyle intervention

Many participants expressed positive views about undertaking lifestyle changes to reduce their risk of developing RA in the future (Table 4, Quote 1 (T4Q1)) or to delay the start of the disease (T4Q2). The main lifestyle factors identified by participants included healthy eating, increasing levels of exercise and smoking cessation. Some participants indicated that they were already trying to live as healthily as possible (although not necessarily focused on preventing RA), but that they would be willing to make additional changes (T4Q3–4). Diet in particular was highlighted as a modifiable risk factor for development of RA and one which patients could take control of (T4Q5). Some participants felt that being overweight and ageing were risk factors for the development of RA (T4Q6).

Participants felt it would be useful to know their personal risk of developing RA so they could modify their lifestyle as a preventive measure (T4Q7). Many participants indicated that they would need information about if and

Table 2 Interviewee characteristics

Participant number	Gender	Age	Ethnicity	Interview Country	First degree relative with RA	Experience of (blood) testing[a]	Reported musculoskeletal problems[a]
1	Female	18–40	White	UK	Parent	None	None
2	Female	41–60	White	UK	Parent	None	Yes (Historic)
3	Male	61–80	White	UK	Sibling	None	None
4	Male	18–40	White	UK	Parent	None	None
5	Female	18–40	White	UK	Parent	None	None
6	Male	18–40	White	UK	Parent	Yes	None
7	Female	18–40	White	UK	Parent	None	Yes
8	Female	18–40	White	UK	Parent	Yes	Yes
9	Female	41–60	White	UK	Sibling	None	Yes
10	Female	18–40	White	UK	Parent	None	Yes
11	Female	41–60	White	UK	Sibling/Parent	None	Yes
12	Female	41–60	White	UK	Sibling	None	Yes
13	Female	41–60	White	UK	Sibling/Parent	Yes	Yes
14	Female	41–60	White	UK	Parent	Yes	Yes
15	Female	18–40	White	UK	Parent	None	None
16	Female	18–40	White	UK	Parent	None	None
17	Female	41–60	Asian	UK	Parent	None	None
18	Female	18–40	White	UK	Parent	None	None
19	Male	41–60	Asian	UK	Parent	None	None
20	Female	18–40	White	UK	Parent	None	None
21	Female	41–60	White	UK	Parent	None	Yes (Historic)
22	Female	18–40	White	UK	Sibling	None	None
23	Female	41–60	White	UK	Parent	None	None
24	Male	41–60	White	UK	Parent	None	None
25	Female	18–40	White	Germany	Parent	None	None
26	Female	18–40	White	Germany	Parent	None	None
27	Female	41–60	White	Germany	Parent	None	None
28	Female	18–40	White	Austria	Parent	None	None
29	Male	18–40	White	Austria	Parent	None	None
30	Female	61–80	White	Austria	Sibling	None	None
31	Female	18–40	White	Austria	Sibling	Yes	None
32	Male	18–40	White	Austria	Parent	None	None
33	Male	18–40	White	Austria	Parent	None	None
34	Female	18–40	White	Austria	Parent	None	None

[a]Data on testing and musculoskeletal problems are based on self-reports of the interviewees as interviewers had no access to health records of the interviewees

how certain factors such as exercise and diet might impact on the risk of developing RA before deciding what they would do (T4Q8–9).

Some participants expressed more negative views and indicated that they might not be prepared to make lifestyle changes as a preventive measure. Some were more concerned about the perceived negative consequences of making such changes and as a result of that might not want to engage with them (T4Q10). One person indicated

that if the only information they have, is that they are at a heightened risk of RA they would not make a change to their diet (T4Q11).

Only a small proportion of the first-degree relatives were current smokers (five, one of whom smoked very rarely) and 2 were ex-smokers. Whereas one smoker described their willingness to give up smoking if a test result identified him as being a person at risk (T4Q12–13), another smoker indicated that a 50% baseline risk would not

Table 3 Overview of themes related to the sub-analysis focused on modifying risk through lifestyle and preventive medicines

Modifying risk through lifestyle intervention

- Positive view of lifestyle changes and/or continuing to engage with healthy living to reduce risk of developing RA

- Healthy eating, diet and exercise as examples of life style changes

- Being overweight considered a risk factor

- Knowing risk is useful as it allows you to make life style changes as a preventive measure

- Need for more information about effectiveness in order to make a decision about lifestyle changes

- Perceived negative consequences of making life style changes

- Unwilling to make lifestyle changes including smoking cessation, unless it is clear that there will be a significant reduction in risk

Willingness to take preventive medicines to modify risk

- Uncertainty and worry about potential short term and long term side effects

- Perceived need to consider pros and cons carefully

- Weighing perceived uncertainty of developing RA against perceived certainty of side effects

- Level of likelihood of getting RA affects consideration of preventive medicine

- Negative opinion about taking medicines in general

- Preference for making lifestyle changes over taking preventive medication

- Recognition why medication might be used

- Preference for starting medication only when first symptoms appear

- Screening will put at risk individuals on alert for early symptoms

- Perceived effectiveness of intervention (medication or lifestyle changes) makes a significant impact on acceptability

be enough to consider stopping (T4Q14). A third smoker indicated that they were only prepared to give up smoking if it was confirmed to them that this would definitely prevent them from developing RA (T4Q15). Participants who were not current smokers either identified or accepted that smoking is a risk factor for the development of RA and contemplated how smokers may react negatively to risk information (T4Q16). Another participant pointed out that it can be difficult to avoid passive smoking (T4Q17) and hence the exposure to this risk factor.

Willingness to take preventive medicines to modify risk
When discussing the possibility of taking preventive medicines if identified as being at high risk of developing RA, many participants highlighted that they would be worried about possible side effects of these medications (T5Q1). They indicated that they would need to think very carefully about the pros and cons of taking preventive medication before making a decision (T5Q2–3). Some participants further worried about the effect of the preventive medication on their existing medical conditions and the potential interaction with current medication (T5Q4–5). Other

participants considered the long-term implications of taking medicines, and whether it would, for example, have an impact on family planning in the future (T5Q6). The immunosuppressive properties of disease modifying anti-rheumatic drugs were a particular concern for participants, especially those who had seen the side-effects of such medicines (e.g. an increased frequency of infections) experienced by their family members with RA (T5Q7).

For some participants, weighing up the side-effects of preventive treatment, which were often described as if they were highly likely or certain to occur, against the relative uncertainty of developing RA in the future, meant that they would most likely decline to have preventive medication unless it was shown to be highly effective (T5Q8). Many participants indicated that they would not be willing to take a preventive medication based on a "*probability*" provided by a predictive test and that they would need more "*definitive*" evidence (T5Q9). It was felt that this type of probability information (E.g. 'You have a 50-50 chance to develop RA') was too uncertain to inform a choice about medication. Participants reported that a preventive pharmacological therapy would be considered only if the medicine was highly effective in reducing their risk (T5Q10). There were further worries about potentially taking medication for the rest of their lives and the potential consequences of stopping medication (T5Q11). Participants suggested that if a test showed that there was a 50% risk that they would develop RA, this would not be enough for them to accept preventive medication, though they felt that this information might encourage them to monitor for the onset of potential symptoms of RA. Others suggested a relatively high predicted baseline risk might be high enough to convince them to accept preventive medication (e.g. one interviewee suggested this would be a 70–80% risk that they would develop RA; T5Q12).

In addition, several participants expressed negative opinions about taking medicines in general, in some cases as a result of past experiences with being prescribed medication that they perceived to be unnecessary,-and they anticipated that this attitude would stop them from taking medication to prevent the onset of RA (T5Q13–14). Others indicated that, based on the assumption of an equal level of risk reduction, they would rather prefer to make lifestyle changes as opposed to taking long term medication (T5Q15) in order to reduce their risk of developing RA.

There was also a group of participants who could understand why preventive medicine may be prescribed if they were found to be at risk of developing RA in the future and anticipated that they would be willing to accept such treatment (T5Q16). This was

Table 4 Modifying risk through lifestyle changes

1   "Well, I would gather information ahead of time about this disease, so, what issues are there, what characteristics, and how can you get rid of it, how can you prevent it so that it doesn't break out. Well, I would be more careful about my life or my health than I have up to now." (Participant 33; male)

2   "…...it would strike a chord with me to eat healthier and be healthier if they said I can have five years extra when I'm possibly not going to get it. I'd rather not have RA than have it and I'd do everything in my power not to have it because it doesn't seem that much fun." (Participant 5; female)

3   "Well, I don't smoke and I hope I've got a reasonably healthy diet. Yes, if there are changes necessary to be made, I'd be happy to make them." (Participant 3; male)

4   "Lifestyle changes, I'm up for any kind really, yeah. Healthy eating and exercise, although I can't do a lot but I do try and do as much as I can." (Participant 13; female)

5   "How I look at it is, it's part of… if you get it the only way that you can actually do something about it is change … what you eat, the foods you consume and stuff like that. So I'm the only one in my family that eats organic or free range food and I drink whole milk and I eat saturated fat as well so I avoid low fat stuff so I believe it's to do with your diet as well. By changing your diet you can actually change the way your body functions and what happens to it." (Participant 14; female).

6   "I think it probably half depend on what kind of person you are, I know for my sister she was much more worried than I was only because she's a lot older than me and she's overweight and she saw that as kind of, like without reading the letters I could figure she was going to get it more than me." (Participant 5; female)

7   "I would prefer to know about (my risk of developing RA) because then I can potentially try and manage my lifestyle better in general …..." (Participant 24; male)

8   "So,… lifestyle changes, yeah definitely, particularly with things like exercise, because that's something, I'm not a particularly sporty person, and I know my dad's been very, very sporty throughout his life and, you know, what are the risks I suppose, of that? Or whether (it is) osteoarthritis that puts the weight on your joints or, you know, that kind of information that I wouldn't necessarily know; that'd be the kind of thing I'd be looking to find out." (Participant 1; female)

9   "I think that I might behave more consciously in ways of diet or, yes generally, maybe I would try somehow to prevent that it actually happens. Well, of course, I would have to read up on what is possible in that regard, but I think I would do that." (Participant 31; female)

10 "Well, I wouldn't change anything about my diet and concerning sports, as I said, that's the question, I don't think so, due to the fact that I think it wouldn't stress me, I wouldn't change my habits in sports as in doing less or doing more, whatever, because I just think, then I would become so careful that in the end I would just sit around and not do anything anymore or exaggerate everything. That wouldn't be a good idea, well I can't really imagine that, because basically I would change little or nothing." (Participant 28; female)

11 "If all I know that I am at a heighted risk, I don't think I would change my diet" (Participant 28; female)

12 "Yeah, I think it would have, because after seeing what my mum can go through, when it does trigger and it kicks in, yeah, without a doubt, I think, it brings reality home. So, yeah, I think if, I'd have probably walked out and chucked the fags in the bin there and then if, certainly if they'd come back and said, 'Yeah, you're in this category,' and I thought, certainly if it was in, probably, middle to upwards, I definitely would have. If it had been the other way, I'd have thought, 'Right, I need to quit,' and worked on a couple of months' timescale to do it." (Participant 6; male)

13 "I've been smoking since I was 14. I'm 31 now, so I'm thinking, 'Well, I've been smoking longer than half of my life.' I wanna be around for my son when he's older, … I know smoking is – because unfortunately I am a smoker – and my mum was, like, 'You need to pack it in, anyway, but even more so after it had …' Certain things can trigger it …Yeah. I'm trying to quit smoking anyway, at the moment, so I've reduced the fags down to four at the moment, so I'm working down to getting to nothing." (Participant 6; male)

14 "Yes, that's a very good question. Since I'm a smoker and to be honest my diet isn't really that great, I don't know if I'd really – if someone could confirm to me, 100%, that if I stopped smoking and had a healthier diet I could stop myself from developing RA, then I would consider it – I would try to stop smoking and live a healthier life." (Participant 26; female)

15 "Regarding smoking, I mean I smoke, I wouldn't know, well if I say I have a heightened risk and that chances are 50:50 I develop it or not, then I don't know whether I would consider it worth it to stop smoking." (Participant 28; female)

16 "… ..People can be very touchy, particularly about smoking. About dietary things, people are more willing to take on board the advice about leafy green vegetables and those kind of things, but not smoking. I think there's a little bit of them that makes them a bit over-defensive about their choice. They get hammered from so many different aspects; I think that it's, like, one more person, that they don't wanna be told from another person, that they shouldn't smoke, so it's quite a delicate subject. You can, sort of, give them the facts without trying to scare them, I guess." (Participant 1; female)

17 "I'd be happy to change my lifestyle, if I thought it was going to have an impact on me developing the disease. But like you say, the only real strong lifestyle – well, the only one that I'm really aware of that has a massive impact, is smoking. I don't smoke. You can't really help but come into contact with people that do smoke, as much as you try and limit it, and it's not that much now." (Participant 10; female)

especially the case for those participants who had experienced the negative impact of the illness on their relatives (T5Q17).

Participants were supportive of the idea that predictive testing could be useful to alert those who are at high risk to be vigilant for the early symptoms of RA, so that treatment could be initiated as soon as symptoms appeared (T5Q18).

Many participants suggested that they would prefer this strategy of early intervention during the symptomatic phase as opposed to taking a preventive medicine prior to the onset of symptoms (T5Q19).

Finally, for some participants the issue of engaging with a preventive intervention depended on an expectation that it would definitely be effective (T5Q20).

Perceptions of first-degree relatives of patients with rheumatoid arthritis about lifestyle...

153

Table 5 Modifying risk through preventive medicine

1   *"For me, it would depend, if I knew for sure that the danger of my developing it within the next 5 years was very high, then I would definitely try to find out what kind of side effects it has. Most medicine has side effects and in the long run that might not be so good".* (Participant 31; female)

2   *"I would definitely want to find out more about taking the medication. I do worry about the side-effects of some of the drugs. I'd have to take that into account as well. Mild side-effects would be fine. If it was something that affected my everyday life in a negative way now then I would have to weigh-up the pros and cons, even if it was worthwhile in the future. I'd want to know the side-effects, or the possible side-effects. Maybe even give it a trial run. Maybe I would just do that. Try it out and see because it affects people in different ways, doesn't it? It's not guaranteed that you would get all of the side-effects."* (Participant 20; female)

3   *"I do think sometimes prevention is better than a cure but when I say prevention's better than a cure I mean sometimes you know just by looking after yourself and things like that. Whether I could take medication for something that's not there I'm not sure about because I would presume, I'd have to know a bit about the medication, would it be some sort of steroid you know because some medications can affect you in other ways so I would have to know what it was and what my effects would be before I would consider something like that."* (Participant 21; female)

4   *"Side effects. I would be concerned about side effects. I know with a lot of medicines you get a lot of side effects. You're taking the medication for one thing and then you've got something else developing or something else coming out of it. And being a diabetic and suffer with diabetes, blood pressure as well, and the digestive system. So I'm a bit worried about side effects that the medication would have."* (Participant 13; female)

5   *"I don't know really. I'd have to try it but then I'd probably read up more about it, what the side effects are, because if they'll clash with my other medication, because if they did then the side effects I'd probably just leave it as it is then if there's going to be worse side - if I'm going to be feeling worse than I already am or with the pain. And then maybe it all depends. I might just stick to the painkillers and try to avoid the pain. I really don't want too many side effects."* (Participant 13; female)

6   *"If I had to start taking that medication would that affect me having kids."* (Participant 5; female)

7   *"They've got side effects, because I know that my mum came off the methotrexate because I think, she'd got some – I think on the x-rays of her lungs and that, there was some shadowing, so I think he took her off the methotrexate because of that."* (Participant 2; female)

8   *"So, unless you can tell me it's going to be a significant benefit at preventing onset of disease, again, I wouldn't want to take any medication unless it was going to really significantly reduce my chances of developing it. So it would depend on the sort of risk ... benefit profile of the two."* (Participant 10; female)

9   *"I would be disinclined to take any medicines purely based on a probability factor. I would want more definitive evidence before I'd start taking medicines."* (Participant 4; male)

10 *"I've got to take a medication for how long, the rest of my life? ... It's a big commitment when the odds of developing the disease is still fairly high if I've got a 50% risk of still developing it, whereas if you tell me, 'Well, actually, if you take it and based on what we can tell you about your predictability factors, your odds of developing the disease are gonna be down to 5%,' then I might consider it.."* (Participant 10; female).

11 *"But it's the weighing up, do I want to take a medication for the rest of my life, potentially, if it's preventative? What happens if you stop it? Again, you need trials to go on a long, long time to tell us that, and you're just not gonna have that data ... you know, even once you've got your predictive things, you're not gonna know how long somebody has to stay on that medication to prevent it. So it's a bit commitment for the rest of your life, to stay on a medication."* (Participant 10; female).

12 *"Okay, so I think if it's a number, I think it'd have to be fairly high for me to wanna take a preventative tablet. So probably that'd be something I think I'd give some thought, I guess, but I suppose 50% probably wouldn't be high enough for me to want to ...do preventative medicine, but obviously I'd be looking out for symptoms to start, you know ... medication when I developed symptoms. But, no, if it was as high as, sort of 70%, 80%, I probably be more likely to say, Okay, let's do the preventative."* (Participant 01; female)

13 *"Nothing, I don't like pills I don't want to say, but I don't think much of taking medicine, I've always been someone who didn't like taking medicine, in that case* (taking medicine to reduce the risk of developing the disease) *I would say no"* (Participant 32; male).

14 *"Just I never liked taking medication. Only if I have to I would take it. If I can get away with not taking it I will not take it. I have done it in the past. Get away with things. I've been told I've got something, not took medicine for it. They did a lot of trying to persuade me and I said no. I was adamant that I hadn't got that, which I was right. So I didn't take the medication and 12 months they said, 'Right, okay, you're clear.' They kept prescribing me the medication but I wouldn't take it."* (Participant 13; female)

15 *"I try to exercise. So, I don't know that I could modify my lifestyle, but if it was a choice – if I had options to changing my lifestyle, and it was a choice between that and the long-term medication, and the benefits were equal between the two, I'd go for lifestyle over a medication."* (Participant 10; female)

16 *"Yeah, I think (with) that kind of information, then, I'd be much more keen to, sort of, sort out what I needed to do to try and prevent that becoming a problem; if I could at that point take some medication to, sort of, reduce the antibodies or you know, head it of before it became a big problem."* (Participant 2; female, 42)

17 *"Dad's been pretty bad with it at times and fortunately, at the moment, he seems to be on a fairly even keel, which is good. So I think having seen at first- hand, I'd be much more willing to ... And then given that, if my testing came back and said I'd had a high risk, I'd be much more willing to, sort of, then consider medication - particularly if it was (going to be) affecting my arms - a mild tablet, and the side effects weren't too bad."* (Participant 1; female)

Table 5 Modifying risk through preventive medicine *(Continued)*

18   "I don't know whether, then, you'd prescribe medication type thing or whether you just leave it alone and see what happens, but be mindful that you could have symptomatic, sort of, issues going forward. And if you had those, then you'd probably want to report it, you know, to make doctors more aware, and maybe you'd be more mindful of perhaps your condition and be aware of changes in your body, perhaps." (Participant 6; male)

19   *"So there obviously are side effects to some of the drugs, so, I guess, unless you were probably showing symptoms, you probably wouldn't want to go on those sorts of things. But other things like, just, you know, for your bones or whatever, I guess there you would be more than, you know, happier to take that sort of thing in the early stages."* (Participant 2; female)

20   *"If I'm taking it I'd expect it to work for me. There's no point in taking anything that is just not going to work for you and it's not doing the job. Like I've always said, I'm not a keen person on medication but if I'm taking it then I would have expectations for it to work."* (Participant 13; female)

Discussion

Given the current impetus to identify early intervention points in the RA disease pathway, it is important to understand the perspectives of those at increased risk of developing RA about possible preventive interventions. The current study looked at one particular at risk group, first-degree relatives, and found that many anticipated being happy to make lifestyle changes such as losing weight, increasing exercise and changing diet to modify their risk of developing RA. However, there was less enthusiasm about a pharmacological approach, at either the pre-symptomatic or the symptomatic at risk stage [9, 24].

The interviewees' reactions to the possibility of making lifestyle changes might be in part due to the social desirability of giving such a response and it is unclear how many would actually adopt these behaviours. One would expect that using well trained interviewers who, with one exception were non-Rheumatologists, went some way to avoiding such responses. Further, the results from the trial conducted by Sparks and colleagues [21] indicate that first-degree relatives were both motivated to modify their behaviour and reported making actual lifestyle changes (e.g. increasing their fish intake; quitting smoking) especially after receiving personalised information about their risk status and the impact of health behaviours on their risk status. This implies that first-degree relatives might indeed follow through on making lifestyle changes after receiving relevant (and personalised) information. Indeed, some interviewees in the current study indicated that they would appreciate further information about the impact of such behavioural changes on their risk of developing RA. Others said that they would require definitive confirmation that it would lead to a significant reduction in their risk of developing RA before contemplating making such changes. Interviewees were more reluctant to contemplate making changes in their lifestyle if they considered there to be negative effects of making such changes. Stopping smoking can be a difficult lifestyle change to make due to the addictive nature of tobacco [37]. In our sample, the perceived benefits of stopping smoking in relation to RA would make some participants more likely to consider smoking cessation if they were found to be at risk of developing RA. Others would need more certainty that this lifestyle change would eliminate their risk of developing

RA altogether. These findings are in line with research in other at risk groups for chronic conditions such as diabetes or cardiovascular disease (CVD). In a study where individuals were given their actual risk score for CVD, some indicated that they had made or intended to make lifestyle changes such as diet change or stopping smoking, whereas others would not make those changes, for example, because they disbelieved the risk score or downplayed their risk, or because they actively resisted making such changes and for example 'could not be bothered' to stop smoking [38]. A person's motivation to be healthy prior to being tested for a chronic condition, will impact on how they perceive their risk and their willingness to make behavioural changes once they receive their results [32]. Further research is needed to comprehensively assess predictors of responses to information about disease risk.

The finding that first-degree relatives were more hesitant about preventive medication is in agreement with how patients with RA in previous research felt that their family members might react if given the option of preventive medicine [30]. In line with findings from previous research in RA (e.g [27, 39]), potential side effects, long-term implications of taking the medication and possible interactions with existing conditions and medications were a major concern for many of our interviewees and they indicated that they would weigh up perceived benefits and potential harms before making a decision about therapy. Personal experiences of RA in family members influenced decision making about the value of preventive medication for several interviewees. On the one hand, those who had observed the side effects of medications such as Disease Modifying Anti-Rheumatic Drugs (DMARDs) experienced by their relatives indicated that they might be more reluctant to take the medication as a preventive measure. On the other hand, some interviewees, who had witnessed the negative effects of RA on their relative's daily life, were keen to use preventive medicine to reduce the risk of developing musculoskeletal symptoms. Acceptance of preventive medication was further associated with the issue of certainty of future RA development. Many felt that uncertainty around future development of RA would discourage them from accepting medications, which they associated with negative side effects. Some interviewees indicated that they would only consider taking medication after the onset of symptoms, and the main value of predictive screening would be to identify the extent to which they should be on the alert for the start of RA symptoms – at which point they would consider therapy which is also in line with findings from a recent focus group study with first-degree relatives [39]. Interviewees in the current study were further not directly asked what they perceived their current risk of developing RA to be, but it is likely that different levels of perceived risk might have had an impact on their views on preventative measures. Future research should explore this relationship further.

Interviewees in this study were not provided with detailed information about the likely duration, frequency of method of administration of preventive treatments. Some of our interviewees appeared to assume that treatment to reduce their risk of RA would involve long-term medication and associated extended risk of side effects. This could account for negative viewpoints towards such treatment. However the trial that is currently evaluating preventive therapy (hydroxychloroquine) for this group (asymptomatic individuals) involves a 12 month course [25], which could be considered as relatively long term treatment.

A recent discrete choice experiment looking at first-degree relatives' preferences related to pharmacological interventions, suggested that method of administration may be an important determinant of preventive treatment acceptability [40]. In contrast a related best worst scaling pilot study found that the efficacy and risks of treatment were more important than method of administration in decision making about preventive treatments [24]. Further quantitative evidence is needed to clarify the relative importance of treatment related and other attributes in the choices made by at risk individuals about preventive therapy for RA.

Collectively these findings suggest that educational approaches will be needed to support preventive strategies, and should include information about the benefits and risks of lifestyle changes and pharmacological interventions as well as details about the nature of the intervention itself. This supportive information should be given in the context of personalised risk estimation with clear (and where possible quantitative) information about the potential for risk reduction associated with such interventions [41]. As predictive algorithms for RA continue to evolve and improve, the interplay between genetic and environmental factors could be highlighted and it is possible for interactive tools to give people personalised information about their risk of developing RA given their genetic make-up and current lifestyle, demonstrating how RA risk can be changed by making certain lifestyle changes. The recent trial of such a tool shows a positive impact on both intended and actual risk related behaviour change [21]. However, there remains a misalignment between public

expectations of risk assessment (e.g. being able to predict with 100% certainty whether or not an individual will develop a disease) and the realistic possibilities of predictive models – which provide probabilistic risk estimates with varying confidence intervals [30]. Levels of confidence in estimates of risk or efficacy may impact on preferences for preventive treatments [30, 40, 42], therefore informational resources accompanying preventive interventions should therefore also manage expectations around the accuracy of risk information [42].

Our results further highlight the need to communicate risk information in a way that is sensitive to the personal/family context or life situation of each individual. One could also provide information that is specifically tailored for different groups with varying experiences of RA in order to provide a richer, more personalised reflection of their own experience. First-degree relatives are a distinct at risk group and their views are likely to be influenced by their personal experiences with RA. As such, their information needs are likely to be different from those of the general population and of other at risk groups, such as patients with clinically suspect arthralgia [43] or undifferentiated arthritis. In ongoing research we are exploring the perspectives of other at risk groups and the wider public, and predictors of perceptual variability within each of these groups.

A number of limitations need to be considered when interpreting the findings of the current research. Firstly, the proportion of men in the sample was relatively small. Although this does reflect the fact that fewer men than women develop RA [1], important viewpoints may have been missed in the current study and future research should aim to include a larger sample size of men. Similarly, although we interviewed relatives in three different European countries, the current sample is not ethnically diverse and as such does not comprehensively represent the population of each of the participating countries. The sample size and qualitative approach used here do not allow for comparative analysis between the three countries and assessment of cross-cultural differences are not possible on the basis of the current data. Future research should therefore specifically address these omissions in order for screening and intervention programmes to be tailored for as wide a target population as possible and to provide related information in a way that is gender or culturally appropriate. Further quantitative evidence is needed to explore psychosocial and cultural predictors of preference heterogeneity and the degree to which at risk individuals trade off positive and negative aspects of preventive interventions for RA.

Since access to first-degree relatives is usually indirectly through patients with existing RA, future research needs to extend and quantify findings of previous research [30] related to if and how RA patients are likely to communicate with their first-degree relatives about their increased risk of developing RA and risk reduction options. This information will help to facilitate the development of efficient preventive approaches and recruitment of participants to preventive studies. The current research discussed participants' willingness to make (hypothetical) lifestyle changes. However, although there is consensus about some lifestyle factors which influence a person's personal risk of developing RA (such as smoking), more research is needed to understand the degree of risk reduction, in the context of different genetic backgrounds, associated with risk related lifestyle changes [21]. Only when such data are available can those at risk make informed decisions about preventive intervention.

Conclusion

The current research gives an indication of first-degree relatives' perceptions of lifestyle changes and preventive medication to reduce their risk of developing RA and the factors associated with acceptability of such preventive measures. It identifies factors which should be highlighted in informational materials aimed at first-degree relatives who are considering participating in related research studies or preventive approaches as well as highlighting factors which warrant further investigation.

Abbreviations
CVD: Cardiovascular Disease; DMARDs: Disease Modifying Anti-Rheumatic Drugs; RA: Rheumatoid Arthritis

Acknowledgements
The authors would like to thank the EuroTEAM Patient Research Partners Panel for their involvement in this research. In particular, we would like to thank Codruta Zabalan, Di Skingle, Mircia Dobrin who have been instrumental in the coding of the current research.

Funding
This work was supported by the European Union within the FP7 HEALTH programme under the grant agreement FP7-HEALTH-F2-2012-305549 (Euro-TEAM) and by Riksbankens Jubileumsfond (The Swedish Foundation for Humanities and Social Sciences) under Grant M13–0260:1 'Mind the Risk'. K Raza is supported by the NIHR Biomedical Research Centre, Birmingham, UK.

Authors' contributions
GS: Contributed to study conception and design; analysed and interpreted data; drafted the manuscript and revised it. RJS: Contributed to study conception and design; collected, analysed and interpreted data; was involved in the drafting and revision of the manuscript as joint first author. MS: Contributed to study conception and design; collected data; was involved in the drafting and revision of the manuscript. ME: Contributed to study conception and design; collected data; was involved in the drafting and revision of the manuscript. EM: Contributed to study conception and design; collected data; was involved in the drafting and revision of the manuscript. KK: Contributed to study conception and design; collected, analysed and interpreted data; was involved in the drafting and revision of the manuscript. MH: Contributed to study conception and design; was

involved in the drafting and revision of the manuscript. AH: Contributed to study conception and design; was involved in the drafting and revision of the manuscript. TS: Contributed to study conception and design; was involved in the drafting and revision of the manuscript. MF: Contributed to study conception and design; was involved in the drafting and revision of the manuscript. KR: Contributed to study conception and design; was involved in the drafting and revision of the manuscript. Final approval of the version of the article to be published was given by all authors.

Competing interests
Rebecca Jayne Stack is an editorial board member for this journal. All other authors declare they have no conflicts of interests.

Author details
[1]Institute for Inflammation and Aging, Rheumatology Research Group, College of Medical and Dental Sciences, University of Birmingham, Birmingham B15 2TT, UK. [2]Department of Psychology, Nottingham Trent University, 50 Shakespeare St, Nottingham NG1 4FQ, UK. [3]Section for Outcomes Research, Center for Medical Statistics, Informatics, and Intelligent Systems, Medical University of Vienna, Spitalgasse 23, BT88/E 031090 Vienna, Austria. [4]University of Applied Sciences FH Campus Wien, Vienna 1100, Austria. [5]Department of Internal Medicine 3, University of Erlangen-Nuremberg, Internistisches Zentrum (INZ), Ulmenweg 18, 91054 Erlangen, Germany. [6]Division of Rheumatology, Department of Internal Medicine III, Medical University of Vienna, Vienna, Austria. [7]Department of Rheumatology, Sandwell & West Birmingham Hospitals NHS Trust, Birmingham, UK. [8]Arthritis Research UK Rheumatoid Arthritis Pathogenesis Centre of Excellence, MRC Arthritis Research UK Centre for Musculoskeletal Ageing Research and NIHR Biomedical Research Centre, College of Medical and Dental Sciences, University of Birmingham, Birmingham, UK. [9]The Institute of Clinical Sciences, College of Medical and Dental Sciences, University of Birmingham, Birmingham B15 2TT, UK. [10]Faculty of Biology, Medicine and Health, School of Health Sciences, University of Manchester, Manchester M13 9PL, UK. [11]Centre for Research Ethics and Bioethics, Uppsala University, Box 564, SE-751 22 Uppsala, Sweden.

References
1. Gibofsky A. Overview of epidemiology, pathophysiology, and diagnosis of rheumatoid arthritis. Am J Manag Care. 2012;18(Suppl 13):295–302.
2. Filipovic I, Walker D, Forster F, Curry AS. Quantifying the economic burden of productivity loss in rheumatoid arthritis. Rheumatology (Oxford). 2011;50: 1083–90.
3. Feldman D, Bernatsky S, Beauchamp ME, Abrahamowicz M. Early consultation with a rheumatologist for RA: does it reduce subsequent use of orthopaedic surgery? Rheumatology (Oxford). 2013;52:452–9.
4. Nell V, Machold KP, Eberl G, Stamm T, Uffmann M, Smolen JS. Benefit of very early referral and very early therapy with disease-modifying anti-rheumatic drugs in patients with early rheumatoid arthritis. Rheumatology. 2004;43:906–14.
5. Raza K, Buckley CE, Salmon M, Buckley CD. Treating very early rheumatoid arthritis. Best Pract Res Clin Rheumatol. 2006;20:849–63.
6. Raza K, Filer A. The therapeutic window of opportunity in rheumatoid arthritis: does it ever close? Ann Rheum Dis. 2015;74:793–4.
7. Scott D, Hunter J, Deighton C, Scott D, Isenberg D. Treatment of rheumatoid arthritis is good medicine. BMJ. 2011;343:d6962.
8. van der Linden M, le Cessie S, Raza K, van der Woude D, Knevel R, Huizinga T, et al. Long-term impact of delay in assessment of early arthritis patients. Arthritis Rheum. 2010;62:3537–46.
9. Demoruelle MK, Deane KD. Treatment strategies in early rheumatoid arthritis and prevention of rheumatoid arthritis. Curr Rheumatol Rep. 2012;14:472–80.
10. Karlson EW, van SD, van der Helm-van Mil AH. Strategies to predict rheumatoid arthritis development in at-risk populations. Rheumatology (Oxford). 2016;55:6–15.
11. Yarwood A, Huizinga TW, Worthington J. The genetics of rheumatoid arthritis: risk and protection in different stages of the evolution of RA. Rheumatology (Oxford). 2016;55:199–209.

12. Somers EC, Antonsen S, Pedersen L, Sorensen HT. Parental history of lupus and rheumatoid arthritis and risk in offspring in a nationwide cohort study: does sex matter? Ann Rheum Dis. 2013;72:525–9.

13. Grant SF, Thorleifsson G, Frigge ML, Thorsteinsson J, Gunnlaugsdottir B, Geirsson AJ, et al. The inheritance of rheumatoid arthritis in Iceland. Arthritis Rheum. 2001;44:2247–54.

14. Frisell T, Holmqvist M, Kallberg H, Klareskog L, Alfredsson L, Askling J. Familial risks and heritability of rheumatoid arthritis: role of rheumatoid factor/anti-citrullinated protein antibody status, number and type of affected relatives, sex, and age. Arthritis Rheum. 2013;65:2773–82.

15. Sugiyama D, Nishimura K, Tamaki K, Tsuji S, Nakazawa T, Morinobu A, Kumagai S. Impact of smoking as a risk factor for developing rheumatoid arthritis: a meta-analysis of observational studies. Ann Rheum Dis. 2010;69:70–81.

16. Lu B, Solomon DH, Costenbader KH, Karlson EW. Alcohol consumption and risk of incident rheumatoid arthritis in women: a prospective study. Arthritis Rheumatol. 2014;66:1998–2005.

17. Kallberg H, Jacobsen S, Bengtsson C, Pedersen M, Padyukov L, Garred P, et al. Alcohol consumption is associated with decreased risk of rheumatoid arthritis: results from two Scandinavian case-control studies. Ann Rheum Dis. 2009;68:222–7.

18. Pattison DJ, Silman AJ, Goodson NJ, Lunt M, Bunn D, Luben R, et al. Vitamin C and the risk of developing inflammatory polyarthritis: prospective nested case-control study. Ann Rheum Dis. 2004;63:843–7.

19. Pattison DJ, Symmons DP, Lunt M, Welch A, Luben R, Bingham SA, et al. Dietary risk factors for the development of inflammatory polyarthritis: evidence for a role of high level of red meat consumption. Arthritis Rheum. 2004;50:3804–12.

20. Rosell M, Wesley AM, Rydin K, Klareskog L, Alfredsson L. Dietary fish and fish oil and the risk of rheumatoid arthritis. Epidemiology. 2009;20:896–901.

21. Sparks JA, Iversen MD, Yu Z, Triedman NA, Prado MG, Miller Kroouze R, et al. Disclosure of personalized rheumatoid arthritis risk using genetics, biomarkers, and lifestyle factors to motivate health behavior improvements: a randomized controlled trial. Arthritis Care Res. 2017. https://doi.org/10.1002/acr.23411 [Epub ahead of print].

22. Stack RJ, Stoffer M, Englbrecht M, Mosor E, Falahee M, Simons G, et al. Perceptions of risk and predictive testing held by the first-degree relatives of patients with rheumatoid arthritis in England, Austria and Germany: a qualitative study. BMJ Open. 2016;6:e010555. https://doi.org/10.1136/bmjopen-2015-010555.

23. Sparks JA, Chen CY, Jiang X, et al. Improved performance of epidemiologic and genetic risk models for rheumatoid arthritis serologic phenotypes using family history. Ann Rheum Dis. 2015;74:1522–9.

24. Finckh A, Escher M, Liang MH, Bansback N. Preventative treatments for rheumatoid arthritis: issues regarding patient preferences. Curr Rheumatol Rep. 2016;18:51.

25. Strategy to Prevent the Onset of Clinically-Apparent Rheumatoid Arthritis (StopRA). 2018. https://clinicaltrials.gov/ct2/show/record/NCT02603146?view=record. Accessed 23 March 2018.

26. Kolfenbach JR, Deane KD, Derber LA, O'Donnell C, Weisman MH, Buckner JH, et al. A prospective approach to investigating the natural history of pre-clinical rheumatoid arthritis (RA) using first-degree relatives of Probands with RA. Arthritis Rheum. 2009;61:1735–42.

27. Arthritis-Checkup: Study of an early detection of the disease. 2017 http://www.arthritis-checkup.ch/index_gb.html. Accessed 23 March 2018.

28. PREVeNT RA: a nationwide Register of First-Degree Relatives of Patients with Rheumatoid Arthritis to evaluate predictors of the development of RA. 2017.

http://research.bmh.manchester.ac.uk/Musculoskeletal/research/CfE_ARCHIVE/preventra/. Accessed on 27 July 2017.

29. Cornelis F, Finckh A. AB0225 recruitment difficulty for unaffected rheumatoid arthritis relatives due to misplaced guilt? Ann Rheum Dis. 2013;72:A855–6.

30. Falahee M, Simons G, Buckley CD, Hansson M, Stack RJ, Raza K. Patients' perceptions of their Relatives' risk of developing rheumatoid arthritis and of the potential for risk communication, prediction, and modulation. Arthritis Care Res. 2017;69:1558–65.

31. Novotny F, Haeny S, Hudelson P, Escher M, Finckh A. Primary prevention of rheumatoid arthritis: a qualitative study in a high-risk population. Joint Bone Spine. 2013;80:673–4.

32. Bayliss K, Raza K, Simons G, Falahee M, Hansson M, Starling B, Stack RJ. Perceptions of predictive testing for those at risk of developing a chronic inflammatory disease: a meta-synthesis of qualitative studies. J Risk Res. 2018;21:167–89.

33. Falahee M, Simons G, Raza K, Stack RJ. Healthcare professionals' perceptions of risk in the context of genetic testing for the prediction of chronic disease: a qualitative metasynthesis. J Risk Res. 2016;21:1–38.

34. European Commision. Final Report Summary - EURO-TEAM (Towards Early diagnosis and biomarker validation in Arthritis Management). http://cordis.europa.eu/result/rcn/194541_en.html. Accessed 2 Aug 2017.

35. Guest GS, MacQueen KM, Namey EE. Applied thematic analysis. Thousand oaks. California: Sage Publications; 2012.

36. NVivo qualitative data analysis Software; QSR International Pty Ltd. Version 10, 2012.

37. Roberts NJ, Kerr SM, Smith SMS. Behavioral interventions associated with smoking cessation in the treatment of tobacco use. Health Services Insights. 2013;6:79–85.

38. Honey S, Hill K, Murray J, Craigs C, House A. Patients' responses to the communication of vascular risk in primary care: a qualitative study. Prim Health Care Res Dev. 2015;16:61–70.

39. Munro S, Spooner L, Milbers K, Hudson M, Koehn C, Harrison M. Perspectives of patients, first-degree relatives and rheumatologists on preventive treatments for rheumatoid arthritis: a qualitative analysis. BMC Rheumatol. 2018;2:18.

40. Harrison M, Spooner L, Hudson M, Milbers K, Koehn CL, Finckh A, Bansback N. Preventing Rheumatoid Arthritis: North American Perspectives of Patients and First-Degree Relatives on the Risk of Developing the Disease and of Potential Preventative Interventions [abstract]. Arthritis Rheumatol. 2017; 69(suppl 10). https://acrabstracts.org/abstract/preventing-rheumatoid-arthritis-north-american-perspectives-of-patients-and-first-degree-relatives-on-the-risk-of-developing-the-disease-and-of-potential-preventative-interventions/. Accessed 26 Sept 2018.

41. EuroTEAM: Am I likely to develop rheumatoid arthritis: A guide for relatives of patients with rheumatoid arthritis. 2016. https://www.birmingham.ac.uk/Documents/college-mds/r2p2/Arthritis-booklet-relatives1.pdf. Accessed 23 Mar 2018.

42. Hunter DJ. Uncertainty in the era of precision medicine. N Engl J Med. 2016; 375(8):711–3.

43. van Steenbergen HW, Aletaha D, Beaart-van de Voorde LJ, Brouwer E, Codreanu C, Combe B, Fonseca JE, Hetland ML, Humby F, Kvien TK, Niedermann K, Nuño L, Oliver S, Rantapää-Dahlqvist S, Raza K, van Schaardenburg D, Schett G, De Smet L, Szücs G, Vencovský J, Wiland P, de Wit M, Landewé RL, van der Helm-van Mil AH. EULAR definition of arthralgia suspicious for progression to rheumatoid arthritis. Ann Rheum Dis. 2017;76(3):491–6.

19

Cardiovascular risk management in rheumatoid and psoriatic arthritis: online survey results from a national cohort study

Premarani Sinnathurai[1,2,3*] (iD), Alexandra Capon[2], Rachelle Buchbinder[4,5], Vibhasha Chand[6], Lyndall Henderson[3], Marissa Lassere[7,8] and Lyn March[1,2,3]

Abstract

Background: Chronic inflammatory arthritis is associated with increased cardiovascular (CV) morbidity and mortality. Pharmacological management and healthy lifestyle modification is recommended to manage these risks, but it is not known how often these are utilised and whether there is any difference in their use between patients with different types of arthritis. The aim of this study was to determine and compare the proportion of participants with rheumatoid arthritis (RA) and psoriatic arthritis (PsA) receiving pharmacological or lifestyle management strategies for CV risk factors. The secondary objective was to identify factors associated with use of management strategies.

Methods: A survey was sent to online participants in the Australian Rheumatology Association Database, a voluntary national registry for inflammatory arthritis. Participants were asked whether they took medications for hypertension, hyperlipidaemia and diabetes, and to report their height, weight, level of physical activity, and dietary changes made. The use of management strategies was compared between participants with RA and PsA. Logistic regression analyses were performed to identify factors associated with physical activity and dietary changes.

Results: There were 858 respondents with RA and 161 with PsA (response rate 64.5%). Pharmacological treatment was reported by 93% of participants with hypertension and 70% with hyperlipidaemia. All participants with diabetes reported being managed with dietary modification, pharmacological treatment, or a combination of both. Adequate physical activity was reported by 50.8%. Only 27% of overweight or obese participants reported making any dietary change for their health in the past year. There was no difference between RA and PsA in reported utilisation of management strategies. Hyperlipidaemia and being overweight were associated with making dietary change. Obesity and arthritis disease activity were negatively associated with physical activity.

Conclusions: Most participants with RA and PsA reported using pharmacological treatment for CV risk factors. Relatively few reported using lifestyle modifications. Targeted lifestyle interventions should be implemented for RA and PsA patients.

Keywords: Rheumatoid arthritis, Psoriatic arthritis, Cardiovascular diseases, Medications, Diet, Physical activity

Background

Chronic inflammatory arthritis is associated with increased cardiovascular (CV) morbidity and mortality [1]. Systemic inflammation may cause insulin resistance and endothelial dysfunction, which then leads to atherosclerosis and vascular disease [2]. An increased risk of CV

mortality is well established in rheumatoid arthritis (RA). A meta-analysis of observational studies, published in 2008, demonstrated 50% increased risk of CV death in patients with RA (meta-standardised mortality ratio (SMR) 1.50, 95% confidence interval (CI) 1.39–1.61) compared with the general population [3]. Both traditional CV risk factors and markers of severity of RA are predictors of future CV events [4]. In recent years, there seems to have been a changing trend. In two cohorts in North America, mortality from CV disease in patients with incident RA since the year 2000 appears to be

* Correspondence: Premarani.Sinnathurai@health.nsw.gov.au
[1]Institute of Bone and Joint Research, Kolling Institute, Northern Sydney Local Health District, Sydney, NSW, Australia
[2]Department of Rheumatology, Royal North Shore Hospital, Reserve Road, St Leonards, NSW 2065, Australia
Full list of author information is available at the end of the article

similar to that in general population controls [5, 6]. It is not known whether this trend may be attributed to improved management of RA or more stringent screening and treatment for CV risk factors.

Psoriatic arthritis (PsA) is associated with an increased risk of the metabolic syndrome and other CV risk factors [7–10]. Previous analysis from the Australian Rheumatology Association Database (ARAD) showed that in this cohort, diabetes mellitus and high cholesterol were more common in participants with PsA than RA [11]. In the Consortium of Rheumatology Researchers of North America (CORRONA) Registry, PsA was associated with higher rates of obesity, diabetes mellitus and hypertriglyceridaemia, compared with RA [12]. Due to this high prevalence of traditional CV risk factors in PsA, it might be expected that CV mortality in PsA might be increased at a rate similar to, or even higher than in RA. However, the evidence relating to mortality in PsA is mixed with SMRs ranging from 0.82–1.62 [13–15]. Several studies found an increase in all-cause mortality, with CV disease the most common cause of death [16, 17]. One longitudinal cohort study demonstrated an overall increase in mortality, with a trend for improvement in survival over time [18]. However, other studies have found no increase in mortality compared with the general population [19, 20].

The reasons for this discrepancy in reported mortality in PsA, and for the apparent difference in mortality between PsA and RA are not yet known. There may be inherent differences in pathophysiology contributing to the difference observed between RA and PsA, although both are associated with chronic systemic inflammation. PsA is a heterogeneous disease and variable disease phenotype may contribute to the differences in mortality. Alternatively, variability in the management of CV risk factors may account for some of the diversity in mortality trends.

A EULAR task force produced recommendations for the management of CV risk in patients with inflammatory arthritis, which were updated in 2016 [21, 22]. The evidence available from their systematic literature review was far greater for RA than for PsA or ankylosing spondylitis. They advise CV risk assessment and management should be performed in accordance with national guidelines. They advise that healthy diet, regular exercise and smoking cessation should be recommended, based on accumulating evidence that physical inactivity is common in patients with RA and exercise may have beneficial effects on CV disease and systemic inflammation. The Group for Research and Assessment of Psoriasis and Psoriatic Arthritis (GRAPPA) recommend that all PsA patients should be encouraged to achieve and maintain a healthy body weight [23]. Similarly, recommendations from Spanish expert panels emphasise the importance of screening for CV

disease and management in a multidisciplinary environment including promotion of regular exercise, healthy body weight and smoking cessation for patients with RA and PsA [24–26]. The Australian guidelines for the management of absolute CV disease risk also include a consensus-based recommendation that lifestyle advice and support be given to all adults, even those assessed to have low CV risk [27].

It is not known how often pharmacological management strategies and/or lifestyle modifications are currently being used by patients with inflammatory arthritis to manage CV risk, and whether there is any difference in the utilisation of these strategies in patients with RA or other inflammatory arthritides such as PsA. The primary objective of this study was to describe and compare the proportion of participants in ARAD with RA or PsA utilising pharmacological and/or lifestyle management strategies for CV risk factors. The secondary objective was to explore factors that are associated with reported utilisation of lifestyle modifications which can reduce CV risk.

Methods

ARAD is a voluntary national registry which collects longitudinal health information from people with inflammatory arthritis, including PsA, RA, ankylosing spondylitis and juvenile idiopathic arthritis, with diagnosis being confirmed by the treating rheumatologist [28]. The database was established in 2003 and has been previously described in detail [28]. Briefly, participants complete questionnaires every 6–12 months in online or paper format. These questionnaires include demographic data, past medical history, treatment for arthritis, adverse effects, infections and malignancies. Patient-reported pain is collected using pain visual analogue scale (VAS, 0 = no pain to 100 = pain as bad as it could be). Self-reported disease activity is also collected using global assessment VAS (0 = none to 100 = extreme). Written consent is obtained from all participants. Rigorous quality control and validation processes are undertaken to check and follow up any missing data to ensure database quality.

The Heart Health Survey was sent to all online ARAD participants with RA ($n = 1295$) and PsA ($n = 285$). This cross-sectional survey was sent in September 2015, with a reminder sent one month later to non-respondents. The survey was closed in December 2015. The survey asked participants about whether they took any medications for selected cardiovascular risk factors, and also about dietary changes and level of physical activity. Participants were asked:

- if they took any medications for hypertension, hyperlipidaemia and diabetes (yes or no);

- whether they had made any dietary changes for their health in the last year, such as seeing a dietician or participating in a weight loss program (yes or no); if they had made a dietary change, participants were asked if they had attended a weight loss program run by a dietician or a commercial program, whether they had used meal replacements, had bariatric surgery, or attended an exercise program;
- how often they performed moderate physical activity, defined as physical activity associated with a moderate, noticeable increase in the depth and rate of breathing while still being able to whistle or talk comfortably. They were given options ranging from no physical activity to 30 min of moderate physical activity every day;
- if there were any medical conditions which limited their ability to participate in physical activity, including heart conditions, breathing difficulty, problems relating to a previous stroke, their arthritis, other conditions, or if there were no medical conditions limiting their activity;
- self-reported weight and height.

For all survey recipients, demographic information, arthritis medications, comorbidities and self-reported global assessment of disease activity (reported on a 0 to 100 VAS where a higher score indicates more disease activity) and pain (0 to 100 VAS where a higher score indicates more pain) were extracted from their most recent ARAD entry.

Statistical analysis was performed using IBM SPSS Statistics 22. Descriptive analyses were used to determine the proportion of participants with CV risk factors including smoking, hypertension, hyperlipidaemia, and diabetes. Self-reported height and weight were used to calculate body mass index (BMI) for respondents. Participants were classified as overweight if they had a BMI greater than or equal to 25 kg/m^2, and obese if their BMI was greater than or equal to 30 kg/m^2 [29]. Adequate physical activity was defined as performing 30 min of moderate intensity physical activity at least three days of the week. This definition was based on a consensus recommendation developed for people with arthritis [30], and is less stringent than the World Health Organisation guideline for adults which is a minimum of 150 min of moderate intensity physical activity per week [31]. For between group comparisons, Chi-squared and student T-tests were used for categorical and continuous variables respectively. P values of 0.05 or less were considered statistically significant.

Logistic regression was used to identify factors which were associated with physical activity and dietary changes. For these regression analyses, participants with RA and PsA were combined. However, only participants

who had completed an ARAD questionnaire within 30 days of the Heart Health Survey, and therefore had recent measures of self-reported global assessment of disease activity and pain, were included in the regression analyses. Univariate analysis was first performed on potential predictors including age, gender, education level and employment status, diagnosis (RA or PsA), arthritis treatments (methotrexate, prednisone, biologic disease modifying anti-rheumatic drug (DMARD)), CV risk factors (hypertension, hyperlipidaemia, diabetes, smoking, obesity), disease duration, and disease activity as measured by patient global assessment and pain VAS. Low disease activity was defined as a patient global assessment score less than or equal to 20. Variables which were associated with the outcome of interest with $p \leq 0.25$ in the univariate logistic regression were entered into a multivariate logistic regression model and non-significant covariates removed via backwards stepwise elimination until only significant variables ($p < 0.05$) remained in the final model [32].

Results

Overall 1019 participants responded to the survey (overall response rate 64.5%), including 858 with RA (response rate 66.3%) and 161 with PsA (response rate 56.5%) (Fig. 1). Table 1 summarises demographic information for responders and non-responders. Overall, responders were older, and had longer disease duration. Responders were more likely to be taking a biologic DMARD and methotrexate, but less likely to be smoking or working or studying full time.

Characteristics of responders, stratified by diagnosis, are shown in Table 2. RA responders were slightly older than PsA responders, and had slightly longer disease duration. There were more female respondents with RA, in keeping with the known epidemiology of this disease. Participants with PsA were more likely than those with RA to be overweight or obese (131/161, 81.4% vs 564/858, 66.0%, $p < 0.001$). Approximately half of all respondents (518/1019, 50.8%) were classified as physically active and the proportion of physically active respondents was similar in both disease groups. However, 189/1019 (18.5%) reported that they had not performed any moderate intensity physical activity in the last week. The prevalence of other CV risk factors was similar between the two groups. Current cigarette smoking was reported by 6.1% of participants. Data regarding whether participants had received smoking cessation advice or management strategies were not collected in this study.

Pharmacological treatments, dietary changes and physical activity reported by participants are shown in Table 3. Most participants with hypertension or hyperlipidaemia reported taking medications for these risk factors (93% and 70% respectively). All participants who reported

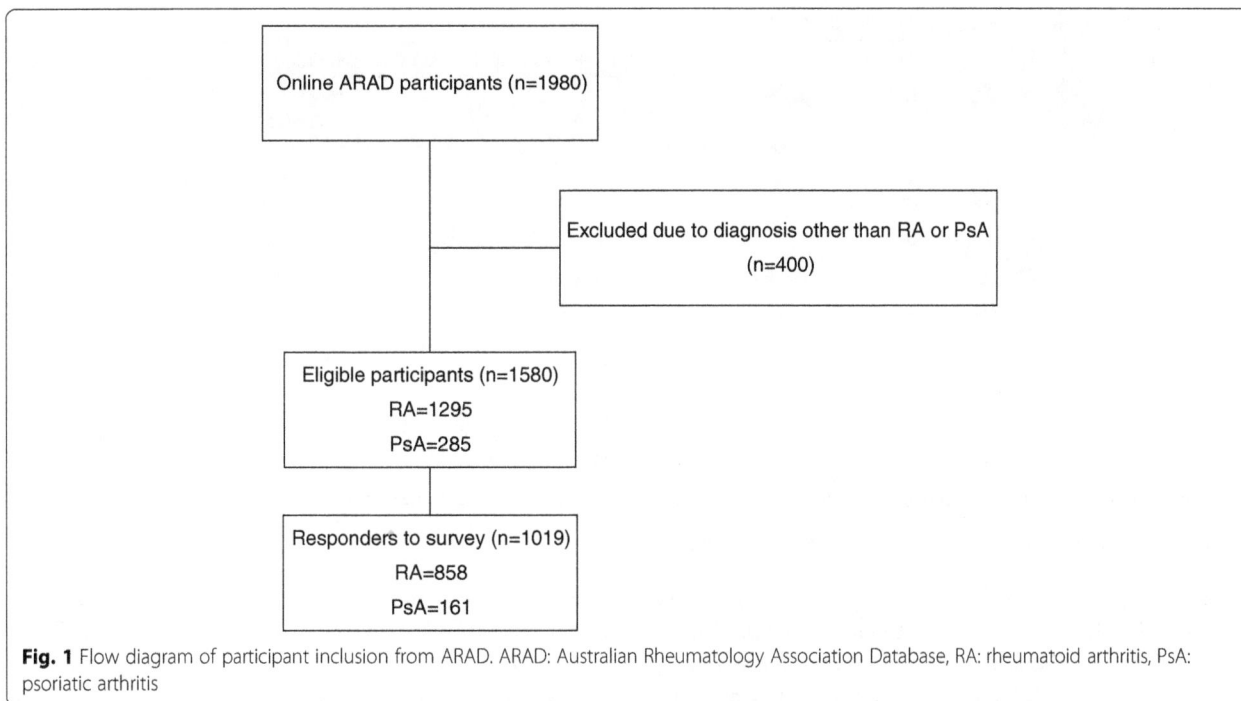

Fig. 1 Flow diagram of participant inclusion from ARAD. ARAD: Australian Rheumatology Association Database, RA: rheumatoid arthritis, PsA: psoriatic arthritis

having diabetes reported being managed with dietary modification, pharmacological treatment, or a combination of the two. Only about a quarter of RA and PsA participants who were overweight or obese reported that they had made any dietary change for their health in the past

year. For those who had made a change, use of meal replacements was the most commonly reported strategy, and 57/151 (37.8%) RA and 11/36 (30.6%) PsA reported participating in an exercise program.

In all participants, arthritis was by far the most commonly reported factor limiting physical activity (703/1019, 69.0%). In those who were classified as performing

Table 1 Characteristics of Responders and Non-Responders to Heart Health Survey

	Responders (N = 1019)	Non-Responders (N = 561)	p
	Mean (SD)	Mean (SD)	
Age, years	58 (11)	53 (13)	< 0.001
Disease duration, years	18 (11)	16 (10)	0.001
	N (%)	N (%)	
Diagnosis			0.002
RA	858 (84.2)	437 (77.9)	
PsA	161 (15.8)	124 (22.1)	
Female	752 (73.8)	407 (72.5)	0.6
University/tertiary education	605 (59.4)	313 (55.8)	0.17
Full time work or study	281 (27.6)	214 (38.1)	< 0.001
Current biologic DMARD	752 (73.8)	380 (67.7)	0.01
Current methotrexate	662 (65.0)	334 (59.5)	0.03
Current prednis(ol)one	311 (30.5)	188 (33.5)	0.22
Current smoker	62 (6.1)	49 (8.7)	0.05
Hypertension	332 (32.6)	160 (28.5)	0.10
Diabetes	87 (8.5)	42 (7.5)	0.5
Hyperlipidaemia	183 (18.0)	85 (15.2)	0.16

SD standard deviation, *RA* rheumatoid arthritis, *PsA* psoriatic arthritis, *DMARD* disease modifying antirheumatic drug

Table 2 Demographics and cardiovascular risk factors for RA and PsA Responders

	RA (N = 858)	PsA (N = 161)	p
	Mean (SD)	Mean (SD)	
Age, years	58 (12)	55 (10)	< 0.001
Disease duration, years	18 (11)	15 (9)	0.005
	N (%)	N (%)	
Female	657 (76.6)	95 (59.0)	< 0.001
University/tertiary education	504 (58.7)	101 (62.7)	0.3
Full time work or study	214 (24.9)	67 (41.6)	< 0.001
Current biologic DMARD	627 (73.1)	125 (77.6)	0.23
Current methotrexate	576 (67.1)	86 (53.4)	0.001
Current prednis(ol)one	295 (34.4)	16 (9.9)	< 0.001
Current smoker	52 (6.1)	10 (6.2)	0.9
Hypertension	279 (32.5)	53 (32.9)	0.9
Diabetes	73 (8.5)	14 (8.7)	0.9
Hyperlipidaemia	157 (18.3)	26 (16.1)	0.5
Overweight or obese	564 (66.0)	131 (81.4)	< 0.001
Physically active	418 (48.7)	83 (51.6)	0.5

RA rheumatoid arthritis, *PsA* psoriatic arthritis, *SD* standard deviation, *DMARD* disease modifying antirheumatic drug

Table 3 Reported treatment for cardiovascular risk factors

CV risk factor	Treatment	Responders with reported risk factor reporting receiving treatment		p
		RA	PsA	
		N (%)	N (%)	
Hypertension	Pharmacological	259/279 (92.8)	50/53 (94.3)	0.7
Diabetes	Diet and/or pharmacological	73/73 (100.0)	14/14 (100.0)	N/A
Hyperlipidaemia	Pharmacological	109/157 (69.4)	19/26 (73.1)	0.7
Overweight or obese	Any dietary change in the last year	151/564 (26.8)	36/131 (27.5)	0.9
	Commercial weight loss program	21/564 (3.7)	3/131 (2.3)	0.4
	Health professional weight loss program	44/564 (7.8)	7/131 (5.3)	0.3
	Meal replacements	53/564 (9.4)	10/131 (7.6)	0.5
	Exercise program	57/564 (10.1)	11/131 (8.4)	0.6
	Bariatric surgery	4/564 (0.7)	1/131 (0.8)	0.9

Treatment for hypertension, diabetes, hyperlipidaemia and being overweight or obese in RA and PsA respondents to the Heart Survey and a comparison of the two disease groups

CV cardiovascular, *RA* rheumatoid arthritis, *PsA* psoriatic arthritis, *N/A* not applicable

insufficient physical activity, 361/501 (72.1%) reported that their arthritis limited their ability to participate in physical activity. Only 26 (2.6%) reported heart conditions limited their activity, 14 (1.4%) reported stroke as a limiting factor and 95 (9.3%) reported breathing difficulties. Out of all respondents, 255 (25.0%) reported there were no medical conditions limiting their physical activity, including 100/501 (20.0%) who had insufficient physical activity. There were no significant differences in the utilisation of pharmacological or lifestyle management strategies between the RA and PsA groups.

The results for univariate and multivariate logistic regression on physical activity are shown in Table 4. There were 275 participants who had completed an ARAD questionnaire within 30 days of the Heart Health Survey and could therefore be included in the logistic regression. There were no significant demographic differences between the participants included in the logistic regression and those who were excluded (data not shown). In univariate analysis, lower self-reported disease activity was associated with higher odds of being physically active. Hypertension and being overweight or obese were associated with lower odds of physical activity. Self-reported pain and global assessment of disease activity were closely correlated (Pearson Correlation coefficient = 0.86) and therefore these variables were entered into separate multivariate regression models. However, in the multivariate analysis, pain was not significantly associated with physical activity, and therefore the results of the final model including self-reported global assessment of disease activity are presented in Table 4. In the final model, there was a statistically significant inverse association between being physically active and being overweight or obese, while low self-reported disease activity was significantly positively associated with being physically active.

Results of the logistic regression on dietary change are shown in Table 5. In univariate analysis, reporting high cholesterol or being overweight or obese were associated with a higher odds of having made a dietary change for health reasons in the last year. However, current biologic DMARD treatment and self-reported low disease activity were associated with lower odds of having made a dietary change. In multivariate analysis, the associations with biologic DMARD treatment, high cholesterol and being overweight or obese persisted, but the association with self-reported low disease activity and low pain were no longer statistically significant.

Discussion

CV risk factors were common in this cohort with RA and PsA, in keeping with other reported RA and PsA cohorts [10, 33]. Most of the participants with hypertension, hyperlipidaemia and diabetes reported receipt of pharmacological treatment, and there was no difference in utilisation rates between RA and PsA. Few studies have examined the management of CV risk factors in inflammatory arthritis. Using data from The Health Improvement Network medical record database in the United Kingdom [34], Jafri et al. reported similarly high utilisation of pharmacotherapy; approximately 85% of patients with hypertension, 65% with hyperlipidaemia and 45% with diabetes received prescriptions for pharmacotherapy. There was no difference in the frequency of prescription of therapy when comparing the PsA, RA and general population control cohorts in that study, and use of lifestyle modification was not examined as this was not readily identifiable in the coded database. In this study from ARAD, the use of lifestyle modifications known to improve CV risk was assessed by participant self-report. Only about half of the respondents reported adequate levels of physical activity, and less than one third of patients who were overweight

Table 4 Odds and adjusted odds ratios for demographic and clinical characteristics associated with being physically active

Univariate analysis			Multivariate analysis (baseline model)*		Multivariate analysis (final model)*	
Variable	OR (95% CI)	p	Adjusted OR (95% CI)	p	Adjusted OR (95% CI)	p
Sex (female vs male)	1.09 (0.70–2.05)	0.5	–	–	–	–
Diagnosis (PsA vs RA)	0.80 (0.42–1.52)	0.5	–	–	–	–
Current biologic DMARD	0.99 (0.58–1.69)	1.0	–	–	–	–
Current methotrexate	1.31 (0.81–2.12)	0.3	–	–	–	–
Current prednis(ol)one	0.90 (0.54–1.48)	0.7	–	–	–	–
Current hypertension	0.58 (0.35–0.98)	0.04	0.65 (0.38–1.11)	0.11	–	–
Current hyperlipidaemia	1.20 (0.67–2.14)	0.6	–	–	–	–
Current diabetes	1.04 (0.44–2.49)	0.9	–	–	–	–
Current smoker	1.22 (0.40–3.73)	0.7	–	–	–	–
Overweight or obese	0.51 (0.31–0.84)	0.01	0.59 (0.35–0.99)	0.04	0.56 (0.33–0.93)	0.03
University/tertiary education	1.20 (0.74–1.93)	0.5	–	–	–	–
Full time work or study	0.98 (0.57–1.66)	0.9	–	–	–	–
Age ≥ 65 years	1.17 (0.70–1.94)	0.6	–	–	–	–
Disease duration ≥5 years	0.68 (0.27–1.75)	0.4	–	–	–	–
Low self-reported disease activity (VAS ≤ 20)	1.88 (1.14–3.09)	0.01	1.69 (1.01–2.82)	0.05	1.71 (1.03–2.85)	0.04
Low pain (VAS ≤20)	1.57 (0.95–2.61)	0.08	–	–	–	–

Combined analysis including RA and PsA respondents, $N = 275$
OR odds ratio, *CI* confidence interval, *RA* rheumatoid arthritis, *PsA* psoriatic arthritis, *DMARD* disease modifying antirheumatic drug, *VAS* visual analogue scale
*Variables with $p \leq 0.25$ in the univariate logistic regression were entered into the multivariate logistic regression baseline model and non-significant covariates removed via backwards stepwise elimination until only significant covariates remained in the final model. Stepwise backwards elimination process can be seen in Additional file 1. Nagelkerke R^2 for model = 0.06

Table 5 Odds and adjusted odds ratios for demographic and clinical characteristics associated with making dietary change

Univariate analysis			Multivariate analysis (baseline model)*		Multivariate analysis (final model)*	
Variable	OR (95% CI)	p	Adjusted OR (95% CI)	p	Adjusted OR (95% CI)	p
Sex (female vs male)	1.72 (0.81–3.62)	0.16	1.90 (0.86–4.20)	0.11	–	–
Diagnosis (PsA vs RA)	0.87 (0.38–1.98)	0.7	–	–	–	–
Current biologic DMARD	0.44 (0.23–0.82)	0.01	0.42 (0.21–0.82)	0.01	0.36 (0.19–0.71)	0.003
Current methotrexate	1.12 (0.61–2.06)	0.7	–	–	–	–
Current prednis(ol)one	0.82 (0.43–1.57)	0.6	–	–	–	–
Current hypertension	1.63 (0.88–3.04)	0.12	1.26 (0.63–2.51)	0.51	–	–
Current hyperlipidaemia	2.08 (1.07–4.06)	0.03	2.06 (0.99–4.31)	0.05	2.20 (1.09–4.44)	0.03
Current diabetes	1.60 (0.60–4.31)	0.4	–	–	–	–
Current smoker	0.73 (0.16–3.42)	0.7	–	–	–	–
Overweight or obese	3.91 (1.76–8.67)	0.001	4.08 (1.76–9.47)	0.001	4.49 (1.97–10.26)	< 0.001
University/tertiary education	0.94 (0.52–1.72)	0.9	–	–	–	–
Full time work or study	0.94 (0.48–1.85)	0.9	–	–	–	–
Age ≥ 65 years	1.10 (0.59–2.08)	0.8	–	–	–	–
Disease duration ≥5 years	1.33 (0.37–4.73)	0.7	–	–	–	–
Self-reported low disease activity (VAS ≤ 20)	0.43 (0.22–0.87)	0.02	0.55 (0.26–1.16)	0.12	–	–
Low pain (VAS ≤20)	0.46 (0.22–0.94)	0.03	–	–	–	–

Combined analysis including RA and PsA respondents, $N = 275$
OR odds ratio, *CI* confidence interval, *RA* rheumatoid arthritis, *PsA* psoriatic arthritis, *DMARD* disease modifying antirheumatic drug, *VAS* visual analogue scale
*Variables with $p \leq 0.25$ in the univariate logistic regression were entered into the multivariate logistic regression baseline model and non-significant covariates removed via backwards stepwise elimination until only significant covariates remained in the final model. Stepwise backwards elimination process can be seen in Additional file 1. Nagelkerke R^2 for model = 0.15

or obese report having made a dietary change for their health in the last year.

Respondents reporting high cholesterol or obesity were more likely to have made a dietary change than those without these risk factors, and participation in a weight loss program run by a health professional was the most commonly reported method of dietary change. Use of biologic DMARDs was negatively associated with making a dietary change, but the reasons for this association are unclear. The analyses identifying factors associated with physical activity and dietary changes were exploratory, and it is possible that some significant findings may have occurred by chance.

On a global level, physical inactivity has been described as a pandemic which should be a public health priority [35]. However, arthritis has been recognised as a barrier to physical activity in patients with obesity, heart disease and diabetes [36–38]. This study from ARAD highlights the low level of physical activity in patients with inflammatory arthritis, despite the known health benefits [39, 40]. Approximately half of all respondents were classified as physically inactive, and obesity was associated with being physically inactive. Arthritis was the most commonly reported condition limiting physical activity and those with low self-reported disease activity were more likely to be physically active. However, other comorbidities and demographic factors including age and level of education were not significantly associated with physical activity. In a cross-sectional international study of patients with RA published in 2008, even higher rates of physical inactivity were reported than in this Australian cohort; only 13.8% of patients reported physical exercise three or more times weekly [41]. In the 2002 National Health Interview Survey in the United States, 63% of adults with arthritis did not meet the arthritis expert panel recommendation for physical activity, compared with 61% of those without arthritis [42]. Using data from the 2000 Behavioral Risk Factor Surveillance System survey in the general United States population, Hootman et al. reported 30.8% of people with arthritis are completely inactive, compared to 25.8% of those without arthritis [43].

There are some limitations to this study. Due to the self-reported nature of ARAD, clinical information such as blood pressure readings and blood lipid or glucose levels were not available. It is possible that some respondents in ARAD had undiagnosed CV risk factors which were not detected through self-report. Also, it was not possible to assess the severity of CV risk factors, or the adequacy of treatment. In a Dutch cross-sectional cohort study in which blood pressure and cholesterol levels were measured, 42% of patients with RA received inadequate lipid-lowering and/or antihypertensive treatment, based on Dutch CV risk management guidelines [44]. Online ARAD participants who did not respond to the survey were more likely to be working full time and less likely to be taking biologic DMARDs than survey responders. It is therefore possible that this non-responder group had less severe disease and may have different patterns of physical activity or CV risk management. The number of participants was relatively small, particularly in the PsA subgroup, and the number of participants who were included in the regression analysis, which may have affected the analysis. Furthermore, participants in ARAD are predominantly Caucasian, with English as their first language and over half of respondents had a university or other tertiary level education. Therefore, the findings from this study may not be generalisable to the wider population of people with RA and PsA.

The Heart Health survey focussed on medical conditions limiting physical activity but did not investigate social, environmental or psychological barriers to physical activity and dietary change. The R^2 values for the regression models were low (0.06 for physical activity and 0.15 for dietary change) indicating that there are factors which are not accounted for which may be associated with lifestyle modifications. In other published studies, older age, lower education, self-efficacy and pain have been associated with physical activity status in people with arthritis [42, 45]. A qualitative study among adults with arthritis identified a multitude of physical, psychological, social and environmental barriers to exercise [46]. Pain and lack of exercise programs or facilities specifically for people with arthritis emerged in almost all groups. Patients with RA have reported that fear for safety, and uncertainty regarding what type and amount of activity is recommended is a barrier to participating in physical activity or exercise [47].

There is a need for further research to identify barriers that prevent patients from taking up dietary modification and regular physical activity, so that appropriate, targeted interventions can be designed to combat these problems. The population health strategies encouraging physical activity in the general population are not always appropriate for those with arthritis who face particular challenges relating to their disease. However, even light and very light intensity exercise is associated with favourable cardiovascular markers and lower disease activity in rheumatoid arthritis [48]. Although the current goal in treat to target strategies in RA [49] and PsA [50] is to maximise long-term health-related quality of life, including physical function and participation in work and social activities, the primary method to achieve this goal is focussed on the use of DMARDs to control inflammation. Multidisciplinary models of care are needed to address not only pharmacological treatment for inflammation, but also target achievable physical activity and healthy weight goals to improve patient outcomes, both disease-specific and relating to long-term CV risk.

Conclusions

In this study, most participants with RA and PsA were managing their CV risk factors using pharmacological treatments. However, relatively few had undertaken lifestyle modifications to improve their CV risk. There was no difference in the utilisation of these management strategies between those with RA and PsA. Treating clinicians should look beyond pharmacological management and address targeted lifestyle interventions for their RA and PsA patients.

Abbreviations

ARAD: Australian Rheumatology Association Database; BMI: Body mass index; CI: Confidence interval; CORRONA: Consortium of Rheumatology Researchers of North America; CV: Cardiovascular; DMARD: Disease modifying antirheumatic drug; GRAPPA: Group for Research and Assessment of Psoriasis and Psoriatic Arthritis; OR: Odds ratio; PsA: Psoriatic arthritis; RA: Rheumatoid arthritis; SD: Standard deviation; SMR: Standardised mortality ratio; VAS: Visual analogue scale

Acknowledgements

We thank Australian rheumatologists and patients for contributing data to ARAD. We would also like to acknowledge the contributions of Joan McPhee, and the ARAD Steering Committee with special thanks to Graeme Carroll and Claire Barrett.

Funding

Premarani Sinnathurai is supported by a Commonwealth Government of Australia National Health & Medical Research Council (NHMRC) postgraduate scholarship and received the SA LSS Support Group Grant & Arthritis Australia & State and Territory Affiliate Grant funded by Arthritis South Australia 2015. Rachelle Buchbinder is funded by an NHMRC Senior Principal Research Fellowship. ARAD is currently supported by unrestricted educational grants administered through the Australian Rheumatology Association from AbbVie Pty Ltd., Pfizer Australia, Sanofi Australia, Celgene Australian & NZ, Bristol-Myers Squibb Australia Pty Ltd. Previous sponsorship for ARAD included an NHMRC Enabling Grant [384330], Amgen Australia Pty Ltd., Aventis, AstraZeneca, Roche, Monash University, Cabrini Health. Infrastructure support for ARAD received from Cabrini Health, Monash University, Royal North Shore Hospital and the Australian Rheumatology Association.

Authors' contributions

All authors (PS, AC, RB, VC, LH, ML and LM) were substantially involved in study concept and design. PS, AC and LM analysed and interpreted the data. PS drafted the manuscript. All authors, critically reviewed the manuscript and approved the final version to be published.

Competing interests

The authors declare that they have no competing interests.

Author details

¹Institute of Bone and Joint Research, Kolling Institute, Northern Sydney Local Health District, Sydney, NSW, Australia. ²Department of Rheumatology, Royal North Shore Hospital, Reserve Road, St Leonards, NSW 2065, Australia. ³Sydney Medical School, University of Sydney, Sydney, NSW, Australia. ⁴Monash Department of Clinical Epidemiology, Cabrini Institute, Malvern, VIC, Australia. ⁵Department of Epidemiology and Preventive Medicine, School of Public Health and Preventive Medicine, Monash University, Clayton, VIC, Australia. ⁶Centre of Cardiovascular Research & Education in Therapeutics, School of Public Health and Preventive Medicine, Monash University, Clayton, VIC, Australia. ⁷School of Public Health and Community Medicine, University of New South Wales, Sydney, NSW, Australia. ⁸Department of Rheumatology, St George Hospital, Kogarah, NSW, Australia.

References

1. Ogdie A, Yu Y, Haynes K, Love TJ, Maliha S, Jiang Y, et al. Risk of major cardiovascular events in patients with psoriatic arthritis, psoriasis and rheumatoid arthritis: a population-based cohort study. Ann Rheum Dis. 2015;74:326–32.
2. Boehncke W-H, Boehncke S. Cardiovascular mortality in psoriasis and psoriatic arthritis: epidemiology, pathomechanisms, therapeutic implications, and perspectives. Curr Rheumatol Rep. 2012;14:343–8.
3. Avina-Zubieta JA, Choi HK, Sadatsafavi M, Etminan M, Esdaile JM, Lacaille D. Risk of cardiovascular mortality in patients with rheumatoid arthritis: a meta-analysis of observational studies. Arthritis Rheum. 2008;59:1690–7.
4. Solomon DH, Kremer J, Curtis JR, Hochberg MC, Reed G, Tsao P, et al. Explaining the cardiovascular risk associated with rheumatoid arthritis: traditional risk factors versus markers of rheumatoid arthritis severity. Ann Rheum Dis. 2010;69:1920–5.
5. Lacaille D, Avina-Zubieta JA, Sayre EC, Abrahamowicz M. Improvement in 5-year mortality in incident rheumatoid arthritis compared with the general population—closing the mortality gap. Ann Rheum Dis. 2017;76:1057–63.
6. Myasoedova E, Gabriel SE, Matteson EL, Davis JM, Therneau TM, Crowson CS. Decreased cardiovascular mortality in patients with incident rheumatoid arthritis (RA) in recent years: Dawn of a new era in cardiovascular disease in RA? J Rheumatol. 2017;44:732–9.
7. Raychaudhuri SK, Chatterjee S, Nguyen C, Kaur M, Jialal I, Raychaudhuri SP. Increased prevalence of the metabolic syndrome in patients with psoriatic arthritis. Metab Syndr Relat Disord. 2010;8:331–4.
8. Sharma A, Gopalakrishnan D, Kumar R, Vijayvergiya R, Dogra S. Metabolic syndrome in psoriatic arthritis patients: a cross-sectional study. Int J Rheum Dis. 2013;16:667–73.
9. Pehlevan S, Yetkin DO, Bahadir C, Goktay F, Pehlevan Y, Kayatas K, et al. Increased prevalence of metabolic syndrome in patients with psoriatic arthritis. Metab Syndr Relat Disord. 2014;12:43–8.
10. Han C, Robinson DW, Hackett MV, Paramore LC, Fraeman KH, Bala MV. Cardiovascular disease and risk factors in patients with rheumatoid arthritis, psoriatic arthritis, and ankylosing spondylitis. J Rheumatol. 2006;33:2167–72.
11. Sinnathurai P, Lassere M, Buchbinder R, March L. Baseline characteristics of patients with psoriatic arthritis (PsA) from the Australian Rheumatology Association Database (ARAD) [abstract]. Intern Med J. 2015;45 Suppl 2:43.
12. Labitigan M, Bahce-Altuntas A, Kremer JM, Reed G, Greenberg JD, Jordan N, et al. Higher rates and clustering of abnormal lipids, obesity, and diabetes mellitus in psoriatic arthritis compared with rheumatoid arthritis. Arthritis Care Res (Hoboken). 2014;66:600–7.
13. Arumugam RAMA, McHugh NJ. Mortality and causes of death in psoriatic arthritis. J Rheumatol. 2012;89:32–5.
14. Jamnitski A, Symmons D, Peters MJ, Sattar N, McInnes I, Nurmohamed MT. Cardiovascular comorbidities in patients with psoriatic arthritis: a systematic review. Ann Rheum Dis. 2013;72:211–6.
15. Horreau C, Pouplard C, Brenaut E, Barnetche T, Misery L, Cribier B, et al. Cardiovascular morbidity and mortality in psoriasis and psoriatic arthritis: a systematic literature review. J Eur Acad Dermatol Venereol. 2013;27(Suppl 3):12–29.
16. Wong K, Gladman DD, Husted J, Long JA, Farewell VT. Mortality studies in psoriatic arthritis: results from a single outpatient clinic. I. Causes and risk of death. Arthritis Rheumatol. 1997;40:1868–72.
17. Mok CC, Kwok CL, Ho LY, Chan PT, Yip SF. Life expectancy, standardized mortality ratios, and causes of death in six rheumatic diseases in Hong Kong. China Arthritis Rheum. 2011;63:1182–9.
18. Ali Y, Tom BDM, Schentag CT, Farewell VT, Gladman DD. Improved survival in psoriatic arthritis with calendar time. Arthritis Rheum. 2007;56:2708–14.

19. Ogdie A, Haynes K, Troxel AB, Love TJ, Hennessy S, Choi H, et al. Risk of mortality in patients with psoriatic arthritis, rheumatoid arthritis and psoriasis: a longitudinal cohort study. Ann Rheum Dis. 2014;73:149–53.

20. Buckley C, Cavill C, Taylor G, Kay H, Waldron N, Korendowych E, et al. Mortality in psoriatic arthritis - a single-center study from the UK. J Rheumatol. 2010;37:2141–4.

21. Peters MJL, Symmons DPM, McCarey D, Dijkmans BAC, Nicola P, Kvien TK, et al. EULAR evidence-based recommendations for cardiovascular risk management in patients with rheumatoid arthritis and other forms of inflammatory arthritis. Ann Rheum Dis. 2010;69:325–31.

22. Agca R, Heslinga SC, Rollefstad S, Heslinga M, McInnes IB, Peters MJL, et al. EULAR recommendations for cardiovascular disease risk management in patients with rheumatoid arthritis and other forms of inflammatory joint disorders: 2015/2016 update. Ann Rheum Dis. 2016;76:17.

23. Coates LC, Kavanaugh A, Mease PJ, Soriano ER, Laura Acosta-Felquer M, Armstrong AW, et al. Group for Research and Assessment of psoriasis and psoriatic arthritis 2015 treatment recommendations for psoriatic arthritis. Arthritis Rheumatol. 2016;68:1060–71.

24. Loza E, Lajas C, Andreu JL, Balsa A, González-Álvaro I, Illera O, et al. Consensus statement on a framework for the management of comorbidity and extra-articular manifestations in rheumatoid arthritis. Rheumatol Int. 2015;35:445–58.

25. Torre-Alonso JC, Carmona L, Moreno M, Galíndez E, Babío J, Zarco P, et al. Identification and management of comorbidity in psoriatic arthritis: evidence- and expert-based recommendations from a multidisciplinary panel from Spain. Rheumatol Int. 2017;37:1239–48.

26. Castaneda S, Loza E, Dauden E, Carmona L. Consensus statement on the Management of Comorbidity in patients with rheumatoid arthritis and psoriasis. J Rheumatol. 2016;43:990–1.

27. National Vascular Disease Prevention Alliance. Guidelines for the management of absolute cardiovascular disease risk. 2012. https://heartfoundation.org.au/images/uploads/publications/Absolute-CVD-Risk-Full-Guidelines.pdf. Accessed 18th Oct 2016.

28. Buchbinder R, March L, Lassere M, Briggs AM, Portek I, Reid C, et al. Effect of treatment with biological agents for arthritis in Australia: the Australian rheumatology association database. Intern Med J. 2007;37:591–600.

29. World Health Organisation. Obesity: preventing and managing the global epidemic. Report of a WHO Consultation. In: WHO Technical Report Series. 2000. http://www.who.int/nutrition/publications/obesity/WHO_TRS_894/en/. Accessed 18th Oct 2016.

30. Work group recommendations: 2002 Exercise and Physical Activity Conference, St. Louis, Missouri. Session V: evidence of benefit of exercise and physical activity in arthritis. Arthritis Rheum. 2003;49:453–4.

31. World Health Organisation. Global Recommendations on Physical Activity for Health. 2010. http://www.who.int/dietphysicalactivity/publications/9789241599979/en/. Accessed 18th Oct 2016.

32. Zhang Z. Model building strategy for logistic regression: purposeful selection. Ann Transl Med. 2016;4:111.

33. Gulati AM, Semb AG, Rollefstad S, Romundstad PR, Kavanaugh A, Gulati S, et al. On the HUNT for cardiovascular risk factors and disease in patients with psoriatic arthritis: population-based data from the Nord-Trøndelag health study. Ann Rheum Dis. 2015;75:819–24.

34. Jafri K, Bartels CM, Shin D, Gelfand JM, Ogdie A. Incidence and management of cardiovascular risk factors in psoriatic arthritis and rheumatoid arthritis: A population-based study. Arthritis Care Res (Hoboken). 2017;69:51–7.

35. Kohl HW 3rd, Craig CL, Lambert EV, Inoue S, Alkandari JR, Leetongin G, et al. The pandemic of physical inactivity: global action for public health. Lancet. 2012;380:294–305.

36. Langham S, Langham J, Goertz HP, Ratcliffe M. Large-scale, prospective, observational studies in patients with psoriasis and psoriatic arthritis: a systematic and critical review. BMC Med Res Methodol. 2011;11:32.

37. Centers for Disease Control and Prevention (CDC). Arthritis as a potential barrier to physical activity among adults with heart disease - United States, 2005 and 2007. MMWR Morb Mortal Wkly Rep. 2009;58:165–9.

38. Centers for Disease Control and Prevention (CDC). Arthritis as a potential barrier to physical activity among adults with diabetes - United States, 2005 and 2007. MMWR Morb Mortal Wkly Rep. 2008;57:486–9.

39. Hurkmans E, van der Giesen FJ, Vliet Vlieland TPM, Schoones J, Van den Ende ECHM. Dynamic exercise programs (aerobic capacity and/or muscle strength training) in patients with rheumatoid arthritis. Cochrane Database Syst Rev. 2009:CD006853. https://doi.org/10.1002/14651858.CD006853.pub2.

40. Abell J, Hootman J, Zack M, Moriarty D, Helmick C. Physical activity and health related quality of life among people with arthritis. J Epidemiol Community Health. 2005;59:380–5.

41. Sokka T, Häkkinen A, Kautiainen H, Maillefert JF, Toloza S, Mørk Hansen T, et al. Physical inactivity in patients with rheumatoid arthritis: Data from twenty-one countries in a cross-sectional, international study. Arthritis Care Res (Hoboken). 2008;59:42–50.

42. Shih M, Hootman JM, Kruger J, Helmick CG. Physical activity in men and women with arthritis: National Health Interview Survey, 2002. Am J Prev Med. 2006;30:385–93.

43. Hootman JM, Macera CA, Ham SA, Helmick CG, Sniezek JE. Physical activity levels among the general US adult population and in adults with and without arthritis. Arthritis Care Res (Hoboken). 2003;49:129–35.

44. van den Oever IAM, Heslinga M, Griep EN, Griep-Wentink HRM, Schotsman R, Cambach W, et al. Cardiovascular risk management in rheumatoid arthritis patients still suboptimal: the Implementation of Cardiovascular Risk Management in Rheumatoid Arthritis project. Rheumatology (Oxford). 2017;56:1472–8.

45. Der Ananian C, Wilcox S, Watkins K, Saunders R, Evans AE. Factors associated with exercise participation in adults with arthritis. J Aging Phys Act. 2008;16:125–43.

46. Wilcox S, Der Ananian C, Abbott J, Vrazel J, Ramsey C, Sharpe PA, et al. Perceived exercise barriers, enablers, and benefits among exercising and nonexercising adults with arthritis: Results from a qualitative study. Arthritis Care Res (Hoboken). 2006;55:616–27.

47. Baxter S, Smith C, Treharne G, Stebbings S, Hale L. What are the perceived barriers, facilitators and attitudes to exercise for women with rheumatoid arthritis? A qualitative study. Disabil Rehabil. 2016;38:773–80.

48. Khoja SS, Almeida GJ, Chester Wasko M, Terhorst L, Piva SR. Association of light-intensity physical activity with lower cardiovascular disease risk burden in rheumatoid arthritis. Arthritis Care Res (Hoboken). 2016;68:424–31.

49. Smolen JS, Breedveld FC, Burmester GR, Bykerk V, Dougados M, Emery P, et al. Treating rheumatoid arthritis to target: 2014 update of the recommendations of an international task force. Ann Rheum Dis. 2015;75:3.

50. Gossec L, Coates LC, de Wit M, Kavanaugh A, Ramiro S, Mease PJ, et al. Management of psoriatic arthritis in 2016: a comparison of EULAR and GRAPPA recommendations. Nat Rev Rheumatol. 2016;12:743–50.

20

The role of vitamin D testing and replacement in fibromyalgia

Shawn D. Ellis[1†], Sam T. Kelly[2†], Jonathan H. Shurlock[2] and Alastair L. N. Hepburn[3*]

Abstract

Background: Fibromyalgia is a debilitating condition, characterized by extensive muscular pain and fatigue. Vitamin D is essential for overall health, with ubiquitous involvement in various inflammatory and pain pathways. Little is known about its role in fibromyalgia. We performed a systematic literature review to determine if vitamin D contributes to the pathology and disability of patients with fibromyalgia, and to assess the role of vitamin D supplementation in disease management.

Methods: We searched Medline, EMBASE and the Cochrane Library for clinical studies and randomized controlled trials published in English during January 2000 to June 2017, using the terms vitamin D or hypovitaminosis D combined with fibromyalgia or FMS. References were reviewed manually and articles were only included if they were specific in their diagnosis of fibromyalgia and used appropriate control groups.

Results: Four hundred and sixty-six studies were retrieved, of which fourteen fulfilled the inclusion criteria. Six studies, of which two had the best quality evidence, found that patients with fibromyalgia have low levels of vitamin D compared to healthy controls. Conflicting results were obtained on the effect of vitamin D on pain or symptom control, with no clear consensus as to the role of supplementation in the management of fibromyalgia.

Conclusions: Our results highlight an association between vitamin D deficiency and fibromyalgia. However, its role in the pathophysiology of fibromyalgia and the clinical relevance of identifying and treating this requires further elucidation with appropriately controlled studies.

Keywords: Fibromyalgia, FMS, Vitamin D, Hypovitaminosis D, Systematic review

Background

Fibromyalgia syndrome (FMS) is a common disorder, affecting 2–3% of the population, that is characterized by chronic widespread muscular pain, generalized weakness and occasional bone pain [1]. The American College of Rheumatology (ACR) devised the 1990 criteria for FMS diagnosis based on the aforementioned symptoms being present for three months or more [1], and was updated in 2010 to include the exclusion of other disorders that might otherwise mimic FMS [2]. Interestingly, these symptoms are also found in individuals with low levels of vitamin D, particularly fatigue and widespread muscle pain and weakness [3].

Vitamin D is a pleiotropic hormone with a critical role in modulating several inflammatory and pain pathways in addition to calcium homeostasis. Observational studies suggest an association between vitamin D deficiency and chronic pain, most promisingly in fibromyalgia [4]. Indeed, it has been hypothesized that vitamin D has anti-inflammatory properties that contribute to relieving pain. In vitro studies have found that the vitamin can reduce prostaglandin E2 (PGE2) synthesis to down-regulate proinflammatory pathways [5] and its supplementation can improve musculoskeletal pain [6]. The anti-inflammatory effects of vitamin D have also been attributed to its impact on T cell differentiation and the

* Correspondence: alnhepburn@doctors.org.uk
†Shawn D. P. Ellis and Sam T. Kelly contributed equally to this work.
³Department of Rheumatology, Worthing Hospital, Worthing BN11 2DH, UK
Full list of author information is available at the end of the article

development of regulatory T cell populations that modulate pro-inflammatory Th1 and Th17 cells [7–9].

Testing for serum vitamin D levels has increased significantly in recent years [10, 11], especially in patients with musculoskeletal pain syndromes [3, 12] and those with other medically unexplained symptoms [13], presumably in the search for a potentially reversible cause. In parallel, there has been a rise in interest in this area by the pharmaceutical industry, with a corresponding increase in the number of licensed vitamin D preparations, as well as 'over the counter' supplements [14]. Taken together, these factors have significant health economic implications.

This review aims to identify and appraise the available evidence comparing vitamin D levels in FMS patients with healthy controls, and to evaluate the efficacy of supplementation in deficient FMS patients. Thus, it aims to address whether FMS patients will benefit from vitamin D deficiency testing and treatment.

Methods

This review followed the Preferred Reporting Items for Systematic Review and Meta-Analyses (PRISMA) guidelines, employing the PRISMA-TC 2015 checklist [15, 16].

Eligibility criteria

Included in the review were observational studies that prospectively compared blood serum levels of vitamin D (measured by 25(OH)D) in FMS patients with age and gender-matched healthy controls, and also randomized control trials (RCTs) that measured the correlation of vitamin D levels with changes in symptom severity in vitamin D deficient FMS patients after administration of supplementation compared with placebo. Additional inclusion criteria for these two types of studies were limited to being published in the English language, investigating human subjects of 18 years or more, diagnosis of chronic pain specific to FMS and being published between the time period of January 2000 to June 2017. Studies were excluded from the review if they had an ambiguous definition of FMS, were published before the aforementioned dates or were published in a non-English language.

Search strategy

Three independent reviewers (SE, SK and JS) performed a database search across Medline, EMBASE and the Cochrane Library, using the following terms: "vitamin D" or "hypovitaminosis D" combined with "fibromyalgia" or "FMS." Titles of retrieved studies were screened, after which abstracts and full texts of remaining studies were cross-examined according to the review inclusion criteria. A manual search of all included bibliographies was carried out to identify any omitted articles.

Quality assessment

Included studies were assessed using an adapted version of the Newcastle-Ottawa checklist [17], which is specific for the reporting of cross-sectional observational studies in order to avoid conclusions drawn from low-quality research. This comprised of three distinct areas of quality: (1) selection of the groups involved (score of: 0–4), (2) quality of the adjustment for confounding variables (score of: 0–2), and (3) ascertainment of the outcome measure of interest for the groups (score of: 0–3) thus producing a cumulative quality score for which the maximum is 9 and reflects the greatest possible methodological research quality. Similarly, RCTs were assessed against the Critical Appraisal Skills Program (CASP) which evaluates the rationale for the research, the effective randomization and blinding techniques employed, assessment of statistical techniques used, evaluation of the practical application of research population to target population who would eventually benefit from the intervention and appraisal of harms and cost-effectiveness.

Data extraction

The following information was obtained from each study: name of first author, year of publication, country in which the research was conducted, type of study design, sample size and characteristics. Outcome measures extracted included mean or median 25(OH)D or 1,25(OH)D levels, frequency of hypovitaminosis of FMS and control populations and any correlations of vitamin D levels with disease activity scores. RCTs were also searched for initial vitamin D levels, method and regimen of supplementation, post-supplementation vitamin D levels and correlation values with symptom severity measures. Information was also collected regarding the country that the research was conducted in and the gender and ethnicities of the participants.

Results

Search strategy

Four hundred and sixty-six studies were retrieved by the database and manual search, 382 of which were excluded due to title or study design. 49 duplicated articles were also removed. The full texts of the remaining 35 studies were read and their content cross-referenced with the inclusion criteria, leaving 14 relevant studies (Fig. 1). Studies were excluded for lack of control groups and non-specific diagnosis of FMS pain.

Study characteristics

Of the 14 included studies, 12 were cross-sectional [12, 18–27], comparing mean values of vitamin D in diagnosed FMS populations with healthy controls, one was a RCT [28] and one published data from both a

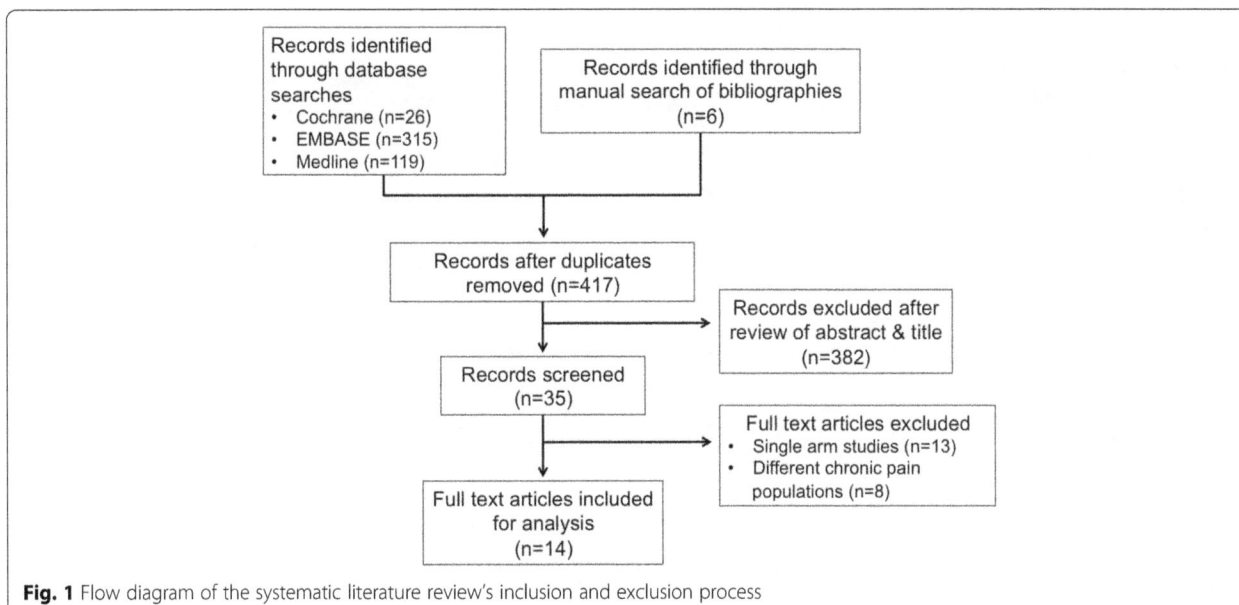

Fig. 1 Flow diagram of the systematic literature review's inclusion and exclusion process

cross-sectional study and RCT [29]. An analysis of the included studies is listed in Table 1.

The RCT was conducted as a second phase of the study that included both cross-sectional data and an RCT [28, 29]. The two aspects are discussed separately. 10 studies used the ACR 1990 diagnostic criteria to classify the FMS population [12, 18–22, 24–26, 29], while 3 studies used the 2010 criteria in conjunction with the older 1990 criteria [27, 28, 30]. One article did not specify the method of diagnosis [23]. Of the 14 studies, 13 specified the ethnic distribution of included participants, of which 5 were predominantly European populations [12, 21, 23, 24, 28], with the remainder investigating Israeli [18], Egyptian [22], Turkish [19, 25–27], Iranian [30] and Brazilian [20] populations.

Quality assessment

All thirteen included cross-sectional studies scored between 5 and 7 using the Newcastle-Ottawa score. The most frequent reasons for loss of points on the scale were an apparent lack of comparison between respondents and non-respondents, and a lack of satisfactory or justified sample size. In addition, one study did not specify the method of "ascertainment of exposure" [23], meaning the use of ACR criteria was not mentioned in its specific diagnosis of FMS. One study omitted the tender points examination from diagnosis due to a cited lack of specificity and reproducibility [29].

While the CASP checklist for RCTs is not intended to be used as a tool from which to derive a cumulative score for each study, it was observed that one RCT met 8 of the 10 [28] formative criteria, while the other met 7 [29]. Both RCTs were found to have small sample sizes, increasing the risk of an inaccurately calculated treatment effect and

misrepresentation of target population. One of the RCTs also had a 16% dropout rate [29]. The assessments were initially performed by two of the reviewers (SK and JS) and were in high concordance at 95% for cross-sectional studies and 100% for RCTs. Where there was disagreement in quality assessment, both reviewers independently re-assessed the articles until agreement was reached. A third reviewer (SE) reassessed the literature and agreed with the consensus reached by SK and JS.

Vitamin D levels in fibromyalgia patients and healthy controls

Six studies identified significantly lower vitamin D levels in FMS patients when compared with healthy controls [12, 21, 22, 24, 26, 27]. McBeth et al. investigated men, aged 40–79, in eight European cities in different countries [12]. This large cross-sectional study identified FMS patients to have significantly lower mean vitamin D levels than healthy controls (23.9 ng/ml vs. 25.6 ng/ml; $p = 0.05$) [12]. Furthermore, there were a significantly higher proportion of FMS patients who were classified as having low vitamin D levels (< 15 ng/ml) compared to healthy controls (25.5% vs. 18.6%; $p = 0.05$) [12]. Olama et al., Yildirim et al., Okyay et al. and Al-Allaf et al. also replicated this finding in their studies with smaller cohorts [22, 24, 26, 27]. Interestingly, whilst Atherton et al. also identified a positive relationship between vitamin D deficiency and FMS, they noticed the greatest contrast between FMS patients occurring with vitamin D levels < 30 ng/ml compared with patients who had vitamin D levels between 30 and 40 ng/ml; $p = 0.001$ (OR 1.57, 95% CI 1.09 to 2.26) [21].

A study by Maafi et al. in Iranian women found significantly higher vitamin D levels amongst FMS patients

Table 1 Summary of Included Studies

Author	Year	Study Design	Country	Definition of FMS	Control Characteristic	Season of Measurement	Age of Patients	Age of Controls	Sex	No. Patients	No. of Controls	Threshold of Vit D deficiency (ng/ml)	Method of Vit D measure	NC-Ottawa Scale
Al-Allaf et al.	2003	CSS	UK	ACR 1990	Age & sex matched healthy controls	No mention	42.5 ± 3.6	42.5 ± 4.3	F	40	37	8	No mention	7
Warner et al.	2008	CSS & RCT	USA	ACR 1990. Tender points exam omitted. Not age or sex matched.	Osteoarthritis affecting fewer than 3 joints.	Spring & Summer (May–Aug)	54.4 ± 11.7	66.4 ± 10.5	M + F	184	104	20	Liquid chromatography	5 N/A for RCT component
Tandeter et al.	2009	CSS	Israel	ACR 1990	Age & sex matched healthy controls	No mention	43.83 ± 7.57	40.37 ± 9.85	F	68	82	20	ELISA	6
Atherton et al.	2009	CSS	UK	ACR 1990	Participants without chronic pain in 1958 nationwide biomedical survey	Autumn–Spring (Sep–Mar)	45	45	M + F	743	5593	20	ELISA	7
Ulusoy et al.	2010	CSS	Turkey	ACR 1990	Age & sex matched healthy controls	Spring & Summer (May–June)	20–40	20–40	F	30	30	20	Liquid chromatography	7
McBeth et al.	2010	CSS	Italy, Belgium, Poland, Sweden, UK, Spain, Estonia, Hungary	ACR 1990	Individuals with no pain	No mention	40–79	40–79	M + F	263	1262	20	radioimmunoassay	7
de Rezende Pena et al.	2010	CSS	Brazil	ACR 1990	Individuals with no pain	Summer in S. hemisphere (Nov–Jan)	18–60, 44.87 ± 8.57	18–60, 32.03 ± 10.57	M + F	87	92	15	Liquid chromatography	5
Olama et al.	2013	CSS	Egypt	ACR 1990	Age & sex matched healthy controls	Spring & Summer (May–July)	32.3 ± 9.4	33.1 ± 9.7	F	50	50	20	ELISA	7
Okumus et al.	2013	CSS	Turkey	ACR1990	Mechanical low back pain; age & sex matched	Winter & Spring (Nov–Mar)	41.23 ± 4.8	39.48 ± 4.08	F	40	40	37.5	radioimmunoassay	5
Mateos et al.	2014	CSS	Spain	No mention	Age & sex matched healthy controls	Autumn & Winter (Nov–Dec)	51 ± 9.6	51.3 ± 9.9	F	205	205	8	chemiluminescence	5
Wepner et al.	2014	RCT	Austria	ACR 1990 & 2010	Individuals with FMS not receiving vit D supplement	Summer	48.37 ± 5.301	48.37 ± 5.301	M + F	15	15	32	No mention	N/A
Okyay et al.	2016	CSS	Turkey	ACR1990	Age & sex matched healthy controls	Summer	36.97 ± 8.95	35.75 ± 10.67	F	79	80	20	ELISA	7
Yildirim et al.	2016	CSS	Turkey	ACR 1990 & 2010	Age & sex matched healthy controls	No mention	49.4 ± 9.2	50.8 ± 8.8	F	99	99	20	ELISA	6
Maafi et al.	2016	CSS	Iran	ACR 1990 & 2010	Age & sex matched healthy controls	Spring–Autumn (Apr–Sep)	37.96 ± 9.8	32.63 ± 10.1	F	74	68	20	chemiluminescence	6

CSS Cross-sectional studies, RCT Randomized controlled studies, ACR American College of Rheumatology, FMS Fibromyalgia syndrome, NC Newcastle, M Male, F Female compared to healthy controls (17.2 ng/ml vs. 9.91 ng/ml; $p = 0.001$) [30]. However, the remaining cross-sectional studies found no significant difference in mean vitamin D levels between the FMS patients and healthy controls when no subgroup analysis was applied. The same studies showed no significant difference in the proportion of patients and controls that displayed vitamin D deficiency [18–20, 23, 25, 29]. Tandeter et al. found no significant difference in mean vitamin D levels between FMS patients and controls in pre-menopausal Israeli women (21.75 ng/ml vs. 19.43 ng/ml respectively), and found no significant difference in the proportion of individuals with a vitamin D deficiency between the two groups [18]. Unexpectedly, the proportion of control patients who were vitamin D deficient were found to be slightly higher at 51.2% compared to the FMS patients at 44.1% [18]. However, this was not statistically significant. No differences in vitamin D levels amongst FMS patients and healthy controls were also mirrored in another study conducted in pre-menopausal women [25], and in four other studies conducted on pre- and post-menopausal women [19, 20, 23, 29].

Interestingly, FMS patients have been found to have little seasonal variation in their vitamin D levels compared with healthy controls. A study conducted in Northern Spain by Mateos et al. found a statistically significant increase in vitamin D levels in controls compared to FMS patients after the summer months: 26.9 ng/ml and 23.3 ng/ml, ($p = 0.03$) [23]. However, there was no difference in overall vitamin D levels between FMS patients and controls throughout the year; 23.0 ng/ml vs. 24.0 ng/ml, or in PTH levels; 51.0 vs. 48.0 [23]. The lack of significant difference persisted upon subgroup analysis, finding no distinction between pre- and post-menopausal women for either measurement, although the patient-control difference did become more profound when only considering post-menopausal women ($p = 0.008$) [23].

Correlation of vitamin D with symptom scores

Unexpectedly, four studies have found an inverse correlation between pain, assessed via the visual analogue score (VAS) or tender points count (TPC), and vitamin D levels [22, 24, 26, 28]; however, the remaining studies could not identify a correlation between the two variables. Several studies have also observed further correlations between vitamin D levels and the presence of other symptoms in FMS patients. The study by Olama et al. found FMS patients with vitamin D levels ≤20 ng/ml to be more likely to have short-term memory impairment, confusion, mood disturbance, sleep disturbance, restless-leg syndrome and palpitations ($p = 0.05$) [22]. They also found inverse correlations with Beck's depression score; $r = -0.328$, $p = 0.020$, and lumbar bone

mineral density (BMD); $r = -0.052$, $p = 0.012$ [22]. Interestingly, Wepner et al. also found a significant negative correlation of vitamin D levels with the activities of daily living component of the FMS impact questionnaire (FIQ-ADL); $r = -0.344$, $p = 0.030$ [28].

Effect of vitamin D supplementation on pain scores

Warner et al. randomized 50 FMS patients with vitamin D levels between 9 and 20 ng/ml in a double-blind fashion to receive either weekly 50,000 IU vitamin D2 or placebo orally for 3 months [29]. Vitamin D levels were statistically similar at baseline for both groups ($n = 25$) and the vitamin D levels of the treatment group rose significantly higher than that of the placebo group after 3 months; 31.2 ng/ml vs 19.3 ng/ml, $p = 0.001$ [29]. This increase was not met by significant improvements in pain scores in the treated group compared to the placebo group as assessed using VAS, $p = 0.12$, or functional pain score (FPS) [29]. In fact, a significant difference in FPS after 3 months favored the placebo group, $p = 0.05$ [29].

Wepner et al. randomized 30 FMS patients with vitamin D levels < 32 ng/ml in a double-blind fashion to receive either daily 2400 IU (16,800 IU weekly) of vitamin D3 for those with vitamin D levels < 24 ng/ml, or 1200 IU (8400 weekly) for those with levels 24-32 ng/ml, or placebo in FMS patients with vitamin D levels < 32 ng/ml for 25 weeks [28]. One patient was removed from the study as they developed a mild hypercalcaemia (2.71 mmol/L) in response to supplementation. A consistent decrease in VAS score was noted for the treatment group, while remaining stable for the placebo group throughout [28]. A 2 (groups) 4 (time points) variance analysis produced a significant group effect, $p = 0.025$ [28]. No significant difference in vitamin D levels or VAS was noted 24 weeks after stopping supplementation [28]. While no time or group specific effect was noted for the short-form health survey 36 (SF-36), the physical role functioning item of this scale improved significantly from week 1 to week 25 in both supplemented groups, $p = 0.014$ [28]. No significant group-specific effects were observed in depression, anxiety, FIQ-ADL or somatization scores, although the treatment group did experience significantly better outcomes of the FIQ-ADL "morning stiffness" question than the placebo group, at week 13, $p = 0.007$ [28].

Discussion

This systematic literature review highlights evidence of vitamin D deficiency amongst certain patient populations with FMS; however, there is conflicting evidence regarding supplementation in these patients. There is also large heterogeneity in the measurement of vitamin D across the studies included in this systematic literature review. Assays used to assess 25(OH) levels, which is generally considered to be the best single marker of vitamin D status [31], included enzyme-linked immuno-sorbent assay (ELISA), radioimmunoassay, chemilumin-escent assay and liquid chromatography. This lack of standardization in the measurement of vitamin D makes it difficult to accurately interpret any relationship be-tween serum measurements and clinical deficiency. However, the Vitamin D Standardization Program (VDSP) has attempted to improve the consistency of la-boratory measurements of vitamin D and their reporting in clinical studies [32].

The highest quality available evidence indicates signifi-cantly lower vitamin D levels in FMS patients compared to healthy controls. The two largest population-based studies by McBeth et al. and Atherton et al. showed evidence of significantly lower mean vitamin D levels in FMS patients and increased odds of deficiency [12, 21], which was also found in the smaller studies by Al-Allaf et al., Olama et al., Yildirim et al. and Okyay et al. [22, 24, 26, 27]. These stud-ies confined their research to homogenous population groups. Indeed, the study by Atherton et al. represented the most robust approach in terms of exhaustively adjusting for known confounders, including BMI, social and lifestyle fac-tors, and the month of vitamin D measurement [21]. Inter-estingly, a recent meta-analysis by Hsiao et al. involving a large patient cohort of 1854 individuals with chronic pain and 7850 controls found a positive correlation between vitamin D deficiency and chronic pain (crude OR, 1.63; 95% CI, 1.20–2.23), which remained after adjusting for con-founders (pooled adjusted OR, 1.41; 95% CI, 1.00–2.00) [33]. Thus, providing strong support for a positive associ-ation between hypovitaminosis D and chronic pain condi-tions such as FMS.

Observational studies have historically implied a link be-tween hypovitaminosis D and conditions associated with chronic pain [3]. However, eight of the studies we analyzed could not draw the same conclusion [18–20, 23, 25, 28, 29], and failed to find an association between vitamin D defi-ciency and FMS. Of particular note, these studies had smaller patient and control sizes, used more heterogeneous population groups and often did not adjust for important confounders such as BMI, time spent outdoors and cloth-ing [18–20, 23, 28, 29] compared to the studies that found a positive association between lower vitamin D levels and FMS patients. Of particular note, the study by Maafi et al. found an inverse relationship between vitamin D levels in FMS patients compared to healthy controls [30]. The au-thors speculated that the study participants had easy access to over the counter vitamin D supplements and may have been self-medicating, thus confounding their findings [30].

While a higher prevalence of vitamin D deficiency in FMS patients in six cross-sectional studies has been ob-served [12, 21, 22, 24, 26, 27], these findings offer little insight into the temporal relationship between disease and deficiency. Indeed, ten of the studies we analyzed

were unable to identify a correlation between pain and vitamin D levels [12, 18–21, 23, 25, 27, 29]. Interestingly, preliminary work by Wepner et al. suggested that vita-min D supplementation reduced pain in FMS patients [28]. Warner et al. did not obtain this result or find any beneficial effects to vitamin D supplementation within a larger patient cohort [29]. This is unexpected, as vitamin D is known to modulate proinflammatory cytokine pro-duction and central pain processing, thus its deficiency has long been speculated to be involved in chronic pain conditions [34, 35]. In addition, hypovitaminosis D is as-sociated with muscle weakness and pain that improves on supplementation [36]. Both RCTs suffer from limited sample sizes in both treatment and placebo groups [28, 29], which can misrepresent a lack of treatment effect [37]. Thus, highlighting an important need for more RCTs with larger sample sizes to fully establish the role of vitamin D supplementation in treating FMS.

Another important factor to take into consideration is the seasonal and geographical impact on studies investi-gating the relationship between vitamin D and FMS. Of particular note, the RCT conducted by Warner et al. oc-curred during the summer months of the year, giving a possible explanation as to why the vitamin D levels in 50% of the placebo group were normalized at the follow up, presumably due to more exposure to sunlight [29]. Several studies have speculated that the physical and mental symptoms accompanying FMS may also dissuade patients from spending time outside in the sun, resulting in a sub-sequent reduction in their vitamin D levels [22, 30, 38]. Such a pattern has been observed in British Asian rheumatology clinic attendees within the UK [39]. Inter-estingly, the disparity observed by Olama et al. in the vita-min D levels of Egyptian women provides insight into the broad scale of deficiency among different ethnic groups. Studies suggest that ethnicities with more skin pigmenta-tion are more likely to have vitamin D deficiency [40–42]; however, the variation in vitamin D levels between pa-tients and healthy controls of darker skin tones is difficult to ascertain. This may explain the lack of associations seen in the low powered studies conducted in non-European populations [30, 41, 43].

The studies in this review have not established a clear clinical benefit to vitamin D supplementation in FMS. A recent systematic review by Gaikwad et al. also found no effect by vitamin D supplementation on chronic muscu-loskeletal pain [44]. Interestingly, the clinical trials by Wepner et al. and Warner et al. used two different forms of vitamin D supplementation (Vitamin D3 and Vitamin D2 respectively). Vitamin D3 is the naturally occurring form of vitamin D, which is also made by skin following UVB light exposure. Vitamin D2 is the derivative of vita-min D3, and commonly found in food. There is cur-rently no clear consensus regarding their efficacy in treating vitamin D deficiency; thus, further studies are needed to identify which of these is the most clinically efficacious and whether vitamin D2 or D3 should be used in future studies regarding the specific physiological benefits of vitamin D supplementation in FMS.

Conversely, as observed by Wepner et al., there is arguably a theoretical risk to supplementation with excessive vitamin D potentially increasing the risk of patient harm through the development of iatrogenic hypercalcaemia [28]. However, this risk is likely minimal. A recent large meta-analysis of vitamin D supplementation in 11,321 participants found that the incidence of adverse events were similar in both treated and placebo groups [45]. In addition, a review of vitamin D supplementation and pain management also concluded that the risks of supplementation in people with deficient levels (defined as 25-hydroxyvitamin levels < 30 nmol/L) are negligible; however, individuals with sufficient levels (25-hydroxyvitamin levels > 50 nmol/L) are unlikely to benefit from additional supplementation [4].

The variation in vitamin D dosages is a particular issue that future studies also need to address. The two RTCs in this review differed in their dosing regimens for supplementation, with Wepner et al. trialing doses of 2400 IU and 1200 IU of vitamin D daily [28] compared with Warner et al. who used 50,000 IU of vitamin D once per week in their RCT [29]. With the European Food Safety Authority suggesting that adults should not exceed 4000 IU (100 micrograms) per day [46], regimens described by Wepner et al. should be sufficient to maintain treatment effect while keeping under the toxic effects threshold of 142 ng/ml [28].

Conclusion

In summary, the evaluation of the literature suggests a positive association between the diagnoses of FMS and vitamin D deficiency. The evidence is inconsistent, owing to large heterogeneity between studies and the majority of studies possibly being too low powered to display a true effect. Furthermore, treating vitamin D deficiency in FMS has not consistently shown to be of clinical benefit, and excessive supplementation poses a theoretical risk of harm through the development of iatrogenic hypercalcemia. Nevertheless, the limited research into the effect of supplementation on symptom severity in patients with FMS reflects encouraging results that should be repeated in larger studies with a consistent treatment regimen. Future research should focus upon prospective study designs that exhaustively account for confounders, to ascertain any causative nature of vitamin D in the development of FMS. If this tenuous link is developed into a resilient association, vitamin D replenishment represents a cheap, cost-effective method of symptom improvement in patients with FMS. However, for now, the true risk versus benefit of vitamin D supplementation in FMS has not been fully ascertained and should be assessed by clinicians on an individual patient basis.

Abbreviations
ACR: American College of Rheumatology; CASP: Critical Appraisal Skills Program; FIQ-ADL: FMS impact questionnaire - Activities of daily living; FMS: Fibromyalgia syndrome; PRISMA: Preferred Reporting Items for Systematic Review and Meta-Analyses; RCT: Randomized control trial; TPC: Tender points count; VAS: Visual analogue score

Funding
No specific funding was received from any bodies in the public, commercial or not-for-profit sectors to carry out the work described in this article.

Authors' contributions
SE, SK, JS and AH were involved in the design of the study and in the analysis and discussion of the results. SE and SK wrote the manuscript. AH participated in the manuscript writing and provided final approval of the manuscript. SE, SK, JS and AH read and approved the final manuscript.

Competing interests
The authors declare that they have no competing interests.

Author details
[1]Department of Oncology, Royal Berkshire Hospital, Reading RG1 5AN, UK. [2]Department of Medicine, Royal Sussex County Hospital, Brighton BN2 5BE, UK. [3]Department of Rheumatology, Worthing Hospital, Worthing BN11 2DH, UK.

References
1. Wolfe F, Smythe HA, Yunus MB, Bennett RM, Bombardier C, Goldenberg DL, et al. The American College of Rheumatology 1990 criteria for the classification of fibromyalgia. Report of the multicenter criteria committee. Arthritis Rheum. 1990;33(2):160–72.
2. Wolfe F, Clauw DJ, Fitzcharles MA, Goldenberg DL, Katz RS, Mease P, et al. The American College of Rheumatology preliminary diagnostic criteria for fibromyalgia and measurement of symptom severity. Arthritis Care Res. 2010;62(5):600–10.
3. Plotnikoff GA, Quigley JM. Prevalence of severe hypovitaminosis D in patients with persistent, nonspecific musculoskeletal pain. Mayo Clin Proc. 2003;78(12):1463–70.
4. Helde-Frankling M, Bjorkhem-Bergman L. Vitamin D in Pain Management. Int J Mol Sci. 2017;18(10):2170–8.
5. Liu X, Nelson A, Wang X, Farid M, Gunji Y, Ikari J, et al. Vitamin D modulates prostaglandin E2 synthesis and degradation in human lung fibroblasts. Am J Respir Cell Mol Biol. 2014;50(1):40–50.
6. Gendelman O, Itzhaki D, Makarov S, Bennun M, Amital H. A randomized double-blind placebo-controlled study adding high dose vitamin D to analgesic regimens in patients with musculoskeletal pain. Lupus. 2015;24(4–5):483–9.
7. Hewison M. Vitamin D and immune function: an overview. Proc Nutr Soc. 2012;71(1):50–61.
8. Ellis SD, McGovern JL, van Maurik A, Howe D, Ehrenstein MR, Notley CA. Induced CD8 FOXP3 regulatory T cells in rheumatoid arthritis are modulated by p38 phosphorylation and monocytes expressing membrane TNF-alpha and CD86. Arthritis Rheumatol. 2014;66(10):2694–705.

9. Lu D, Lan B, Din Z, Chen H, Chen G. A vitamin D receptor agonist converts CD4+ T cells to Foxp3+ regulatory T cells in patients with ulcerative colitis. Oncotarget. 2017;8(32):53552–62.

10. Sattar N, Welsh P, Panarelli M, Forouhi NG. Increasing requests for vitamin D measurement: costly, confusing, and without credibility. Lancet. 2012; 379(9811):95–6.

11. Zhao S, Gardner K, Taylor W, Marks E, Goodson N. Vitamin D assessment in primary care: changing patterns of testing. London J Prim Care. 2015;7(2):15–22.

12. McBeth J, Pye SR, O'Neill TW, Macfarlane GJ, Tajar A, Bartfai G, et al. Musculoskeletal pain is associated with very low levels of vitamin D in men: results from the European male ageing study. Ann Rheum Dis. 2010;69(8): 1448–52.

13. Roy S, Sherman A, Monari-Sparks MJ, Schweiker O, Hunter K. Correction of low vitamin D improves fatigue: effect of correction of low vitamin D in fatigue study (EViDiF study). N Am J Med Sci. 2014;6(8):396–402.

14. Rooney MR, Harnack L, Michos ED, Ogilvie RP, Sempos CT, Lutsey PL. Trends in use of high-dose vitamin D supplements exceeding 1000 or 4000 international units daily, 1999-2014. JAMA. 2017;317(23):2448–50.

15. Moher D, Liberati A, Tetzlaff J, Altman DG, Group P. Preferred reporting items for systematic reviews and meta-analyses: the PRISMA statement. Int J Surg. 2010;8(5):336–41.

16. Moher D, Shamseer L, Clarke M, Ghersi D, Liberati A, Petticrew M, et al. Preferred reporting items for systematic review and meta-analysis protocols (PRISMA-P) 2015 statement. Syst Rev. 2015;4(1) https://doi.org/10.1186/2046-4053-4-1.

17. Stang A. Critical evaluation of the Newcastle-Ottawa scale for the assessment of the quality of nonrandomized studies in meta-analyses. Eur J Epidemiol. 2010;25(9):603–5.

18. Tandeter H, Grynbaum M, Zuili I, Shany S, Shvartzman P. Serum 25-OH vitamin D levels in patients with fibromyalgia. Isr Med Assoc J. 2009;11(6): 339–42.

19. Ulusoy H, Sarica N, Arslan S, Ozyurt H, Cetin I, Birgul Ozer E, et al. Serum vitamin D status and bone mineral density in fibromyalgia. Bratisl Lek Listy. 2010;111(11):604–9.

20. de Rezende Pena C, Grillo LP, das Chagas Medeiros MM. Evaluation of 25-hydroxyvitamin D serum levels in patients with fibromyalgia. J Clin Rheumatol. 2010;16(8):365–9.

21. Atherton K, Berry DJ, Parsons T, Macfarlane GJ, Power C, Hypponen E. Vitamin D and chronic widespread pain in a white middle-aged British population: evidence from a cross-sectional population survey. Ann Rheum Dis. 2009;68(6):817–22.

22. Olama SM, Senna MK, Elarman MM, Elhawary G. Serum vitamin D level and bone mineral density in premenopausal Egyptian women with fibromyalgia. Rheumatol Int. 2013;33(1):185–92.

23. Mateos F, Valero C, Olmos JM, Casanueva B, Castillo J, Martinez J, et al. Bone mass and vitamin D levels in women with a diagnosis of fibromyalgia. Osteoporos Int. 2014;25(2):525–33.

24. Al-Allaf AW, Mole PA, Paterson CR, Pullar T. Bone health in patients with fibromyalgia. Rheumatology. 2003;42(10):1202–6.

25. Okumus M, Koybasi M, Tuncay F, Ceceli E, Ayhan F, Yorgancioglu R, et al. Fibromyalgia syndrome: is it related to vitamin D deficiency in premenopausal female patients? Pain Manag Nurs. 2013;14(4):e156–63.

26. Okyay R, Kocyigit BF, Gursoy S. Vitamin D levels in women with fibromyalgia and relationship between pain, tender point count and disease activity. Acta Medica Mediterranea. 2016;32(1):243–7.

27. Yildirim T, Solmaz D, Akgol G, Ersoy Y. Relationship between mean platelet volume and vitamin D deficiency in fibromyalgia. Biomed Res. 2016;27(4): 1265–70.

28. Wepner F, Scheuer R, Schuetz-Wieser B, Machacek P, Pieler-Bruha E, Cross HS, et al. Effects of vitamin D on patients with fibromyalgia syndrome: a randomized placebo-controlled trial. Pain. 2014;155(2):261–8.

29. Warner AE, Arnspiger SA. Diffuse musculoskeletal pain is not associated with low vitamin D levels or improved by treatment with vitamin D. J Clin Rheumatol. 2008;14(1):12–6.

30. Maafi AA, Ghavidel-Parsa B, Haghdoost A, Aarabi Y, Hajiabbasi A, Shenavar Masooleh I, et al. Serum vitamin D status in Iranian fibromyalgia patients: according to the symptom severity and illness invalidation. Korean J Pain. 2016;29(3):172–8.

31. Holick MF. Vitamin D deficiency. N Engl J Med. 2007;357(3):266–81.

32. Durazo-Arvizu RA, Tian L, Brooks SPJ, Sarafin K, Cashman KD, Kiely M, et al. The vitamin D standardization program (VDSP) manual for retrospective laboratory standardization of serum 25-Hydroxyvitamin D data. J AOAC Int. 2017;100(5):1234–43.

33. Hsiao MY, Hung CY, Chang KV, Han DS, Wang TGI, Serum Hypovitaminosis D. Associated with chronic widespread pain including fibromyalgia? A meta-analysis of observational studies. Pain physician. 2015;18(5):E877–87.

34. von Kanel R, Muller-Hartmannsgruber V, Kokinogenis G, Egloff N. Vitamin D and central hypersensitivity in patients with chronic pain. Pain Med. 2014; 15(9):1609–18.

35. Cutolo M, Paolino S, Sulli A, Smith V, Pizzorni C, Seriolo B. Vitamin D, steroid hormones, and autoimmunity. Ann N Y Acad Sci. 2014;1317:39–46.

36. Gloth FM 3rd, Lindsay JM, Zelesnick LB, Greenough WB 3rd. Can vitamin D deficiency produce an unusual pain syndrome? Arch Intern Med. 1991; 151(8):1662–4.

37. Schulz KF, Altman DG, Moher D, Group C. CONSORT 2010 statement: updated guidelines for reporting parallel group randomised trials. BMJ. 2010;340:c332.

38. Kool MB, van Middendorp H, Boeije HR, Geenen R. Understanding the lack of understanding: invalidation from the perspective of the patient with fibromyalgia. Arthritis Rheum. 2009;61(12):1650–6.

39. Serhan E, Newton P, Ali HA, Walford S, Singh BM. Prevalence of hypovitaminosis D in indo-Asian patients attending a rheumatology clinic. Bone. 1999;25(5):609–11.

40. Looker AC, Dawson-Hughes B, Calvo MS, Gunter EW, Sahyoun NR. Serum 25-hydroxyvitamin D status of adolescents and adults in two seasonal subpopulations from NHANES III. Bone. 2002;30(5):771–7.

41. Harris SS. Vitamin D and African Americans. J Nutr. 2006;136(4):1126–9.

42. Harris SS, Dawson-Hughes B. Seasonal changes in plasma 25-hydroxyvitamin D concentrations of young American black and white women. Am J Clin Nutr. 1998;67(6):1232–6.

43. Mitchell DM, Henao MP, Finkelstein JS, Burnett-Bowie SA. Prevalence and predictors of vitamin D deficiency in healthy adults. Endoc Pract. 2012;18(6): 914–23.

44. Gaikwad M, Vanlint S, Mittinity M, Moseley GL, Stocks N. Does vitamin D supplementation alleviate chronic nonspecific musculoskeletal pain? A systematic review and meta-analysis. Clin Rheumatol. 2017;36(5):1201–8.

45. Martineau AR, Jolliffe DA, Hooper RL, Greenberg L, Aloia JF, Bergman P, et al. Vitamin D supplementation to prevent acute respiratory tract infections: systematic review and meta-analysis of individual participant data. BMJ. 2017;356:i6583.

46. EFSA Panel on Dietetic Products NaAN. Scientific opinion on the tolerable upper intake level of vitamin D. EFSA J. 2012;10(7):2813–58.

21

General practitioners' views on managing knee osteoarthritis: a thematic analysis of factors influencing clinical practice guideline implementation in primary care

Thorlene Egerton[1*] (iD), Rachel K Nelligan[1], Jenny Setchell[2], Lou Atkins[3] and Kim L Bennell[1]

Abstract

Background: Osteoarthritis (OA) is diagnosed and managed primarily by general practitioners (GPs). OA guidelines recommend using clinical criteria, without x-ray, for diagnosis, and advising strengthening exercise, aerobic activity and, if appropriate, weight loss as first-line treatments. These recommendations are often not implemented by GPs. To facilitate GP uptake of guidelines, greater understanding of GP practice behaviour is required. This qualitative study identified key factors influencing implementation of these recommendations in the primary-care setting.

Methods: Semi-structured interviews with eleven GPs were conducted, transcribed verbatim, coded by two independent researchers and analysed with an interpretive thematic approach using the COM-B model (Capability/Opportunity/Motivation-Behaviour) as a framework.

Results: Eleven themes were identified. Psychological capability themes: knowledge gaps, confidence to effectively manage OA, and skills to facilitate lifestyle change. Physical opportunity themes: system-related factors including time limitations, and patient resources. Social opportunity theme: influences from patients. Reflective motivation themes: GP's perceived role, and assumptions about people with knee OA. Automatic motivation themes: optimism, habit, and unease discussing weight. The findings demonstrated diverse and interacting influences on GPs' practice.

Conclusion: The identified themes provide insight into potential interventions to improve OA management in primary-care settings. Key suggestions include: improvements to OA clinical guidelines; targeting GP education to focus on identified knowledge gaps, confidence, and communication skills; development and implementation of new models of service delivery; and utilising positive social influences to facilitate best-practice behaviours. Complex, multimodal interventions that address multiple factors (both barriers and facilitators) are likely to be necessary.

Keywords: Knee osteoarthritis, Primary care, Clinical guidelines, General practitioner, Qualitative

Background

Osteoarthritis (OA) is a highly prevalent, disabling condition ranked the eleventh highest contributor to global disability [1, 2]. Knee OA is mostly diagnosed and managed in family practice settings [3] and principally by general practitioners (GPs, i.e. family doctors) [4]. Clinical practice guidelines (CPGs) recommend diagnosing OA using clinical criteria without imaging, and facilitating self-management through education and the provision of advice on weight management and increasing physical activity [5]. However, care inconsistent with these recommendations has been identified in several countries and health care settings [6–11]. GPs tend to over-rely on imaging for diagnosing OA [12, 13], under-emphasise exercise and weight loss options in favour of drug and surgical management [6, 9, 14], frequently refer for ineffective arthroscopic surgery [15], or refer for joint replacement

* Correspondence: thor@sutmap.com
[1]Centre for Health, Exercise and Sports Medicine, The University of Melbourne, Melbourne, Australia
Full list of author information is available at the end of the article

surgery before an adequate trial of recommended conservative treatments [10, 14].

There is a need to develop effective strategies that facilitate GPs' uptake of recommended OA management practice. Detailed behavioural analysis of the reasons behind the inadequate uptake will help inform implementation interventions [16]. There have been previous qualitative studies asking primary care practitioners about topics related to the provision of care for people with knee osteoarthritis [7, 17, 18] and osteoarthritis more generally [19–21]. Common findings include trivialising or normalising the problem, lack of knowledge/skills, and resource issues [22]. However, previous studies on the topic have not focussed in any depth on the barriers and facilitators to implementation of the priority recommendations currently identified as being the most underutilised in care globally [22]. The aim of this study was therefore to identify barriers and facilitators influencing whether GPs perform the activities of: 1) making a clinical diagnosis without imaging, 2) engaging patients in exercise and physical activity, and 3) engaging patients in weight loss. The study involved the systematic and comprehensive identification of behavioural drivers related to providing this care for people with knee osteoarthritis with the hope of uncovering new and useful additional findings. We used a novel framework to guide our classification and labelling of themes, and included a discussion of the results in the context of previous findings.

Methods

This study is part of a larger project (PARTNER) to increase delivery of recommended knee OA management within Australian primary health care. All GPs provided informed consent to be interviewed and recorded. The reporting of this study adheres to the COnsolidated criteria for REporting Qualitative studies (COREQ) 32-item checklist [23].

Design and theoretical framework

Semi-structured telephone interviews were used for data collection. An interpretive thematic analysis methodology was adopted with reference to the COM-B (Capability/Opportunity/Motivation-Behaviour) model [24] as a comprehensive framework for theme development. The COM-B model explains behaviour as resulting from interactions between physical and psychological capabilities, social and environmental opportunities, and motivators that can be either reflective (deliberate, conscious thought processes) or automatic (emotional or reactive). COM-B component definitions are provided in Table 4. The COM-B model has been used extensively in the design of behavioural interventions in a range of settings [25–27]. The COREQ-checklist was used to ensure transparent reporting of this study [23].

Participants

A purposive sample of eleven GPs ensuring a range of practice sizes, age, metropolitan/regional locations and years of practice was recruited. Initially, GPs from The Victorian Primary Care Research Network database were provided with information on study aims and invited to volunteer. Snowballing was later used to identify additional participants to approach. During recruitment, the investigators iteratively monitored participant characteristics to ensure sufficient diversity for the purposive sampling. All eligible GPs ($n = 11$) who expressed interest in volunteering were included. GPs were eligible if they were practicing in a primary care setting and saw at least one patient with knee OA per month. The sample size was determined by the concept of theoretical saturation when iterative review of the data showed sufficient repetition and depth of COM-B and inductive themes [28].

Procedure

The semi-structured interview guide, developed in collaboration with a behaviour change expert experienced in applying the COM-B model (LA) and a qualitative research expert (JS), incorporated all components of COM-B model (Table 1) and allowed further exploration of topics raised by participants.

A physiotherapist trained in qualitative interviewing (RN), conducted all interviews. Interviews were audio recorded, transcribed by an external company and checked for accuracy by RN. Field notes were taken. Digital transcripts were de-identified and stored securely. GPs were offered a $50 voucher for their participation. Interviewed GPs did not review their finalised transcripts.

Data were analysed by TE and RN and overseen by JS and LA. The systematic iterative approach used is detailed in Table 2. In summary, TE and RN both independently read all transcripts and generated codes, themes were inductively generated and revised, and these were then organised according to the COM-B model components. Data collection and analysis occurred concurrently.

Results

Table 3 outlines participant characteristics. Interviews ranged from 30 to 54 min. Analysis identified eleven themes (Table 4) from five of the six COM-B components. No themes were identified in the physical capability component.

Psychological capability

Three themes were identified within the COM-B component 'psychological capability'. These were 'knowledge

Table 1 Semi-structured interview guide

Key activity	Questions and potential probes
GP makes, communicates and documents a diagnosis of osteoarthritis clinically (without imaging)	*How do you currently arrive at a diagnosis of knee OA?* *– Are you aware that guidelines recommend making a diagnosis clinically and without imaging?* *– How do you feel about making a clinical diagnosis of knee OA (without imaging)?* *– What would you or GPs in general need to know more about in order to be comfortable with making a clinical diagnosis of knee OA?* *– What would help encourage or support GPs in making a clinical diagnosis of knee OA?* *How do you think receiving a diagnosis of knee OA impacts on patients?* *Are there any issues around patient expectations that influence how you diagnose knee OA and how you communicate the diagnosis with patients?* *Do you currently document diagnosis of "knee OA" in patients' records?*
GP provides education/advice to patients about the importance of general physical activity and regular strengthening and/or aerobic exercise during the consultation which is reinforced at later opportunities.	*What physical activity or exercise advice do you currently give to patients with knee OA?* *How confident do you feel when giving this advice?* *How important do you think it is to talk to your knee OA patients about physical activity and strengthening exercises?* *How do you think this information impacts on patients?* *Do you think GPs are familiar with the latest recommendations for physical activity in general and for exercise specifically for people with knee OA?* *Are there any additional skills or training that you would like to have regarding physical activity or exercise advice?* *Are there any other things that make it difficult for GPs to give this advice?* *Can you suggest any measures that would assist or support GPs in discussing general physical activity and targeted exercises with their knee OA patients?*
GP provides education/advice to patients either about the importance of maintaining a healthy weight or weight loss in the initial consultation which is reinforced at later opportunities (includes BMI measurement)	*What weight management advice do you currently give to patients with knee OA?* *How important do you think weight loss is for knee OA symptoms?* *How confident do you feel when giving weight loss advice?* *How do you think this information impacts on patients?* *Do you think GPs feel motivated to talk to patients about weight management / weight loss? What would increase or decrease their motivation?* *Are there any other things that make it difficult for GPs to give effective weight loss advice?* *Can you suggest any measures that would assist or support GPs in talking to patients about weight management / weight loss?* *Do you currently assess BMI with your knee OA patients?* *– How important is it that GPs assess BMI for knee OA patients?* *– What, if any, are the benefits to patients?* *– If you think GPs do not currently routinely assess BMI, what are the reasons for this? What shift of thinking is required?* *– What help or support would make it easier for GPs to assess BMI for their knee OA patients?* *– Are there any issues around patient expectation that influence whether BMI is assessed?*

Table 2 Thematic analysis stages

Stage	Description
I.	Initial familiarisation with the data – by RN and TE who listened to all audio files and read transcripts as they became available.
II.	Inductive coding of the data - RN and TE independently coded the data to identify recurrent patterns, common beliefs, barriers and enablers.
III.	Codes were discussed, and consensus reached - discussion between RN and TE, agreement reached on themes by grouping segments of code into broader categories (themes). Microsoft Excel spreadsheets used to help manage the data. In the instance of differing opinions input from JS (qualitative expert) was sought.
IV.	Themes refined and anchored to COM-B model framework – RN and TE jointly revised themes into overarching themes with codes within themes, and anchored these to the COM-B components through several iterations.
V.	Themes and codes reviewed, revised and agreed upon by all members of the research team and results summarised.

Table 3 Demographic characteristics of participating general practitioners

GP	Sex	Years in practice	Metropolitan / regional	Size of practice (number of GPs)	Approximate number of knee OA patients per month
GP1	F	32	Regional	4	6
GP2	F	26	Metropolitan	6	10–20
GP3	F	22	Metropolitan	13	2
GP4	M	44	Regional	1	40
GP5	F	5	Regional	15	20
GP6	M	31	Regional	4	6
GP7	M	30	Regional	4	4
GP8	F	26	Metropolitan	3	30
GP9	F	6	Metropolitan	24	3 to 4
GP10	F	10	Metropolitan	5	1
GP11	M	6	Metropolitan	4	3 to 10

gaps', 'confidence to effectively manage OA', and 'skills to facilitate lifestyle change'.

The first theme 'knowledge gaps' was based on GP comments relating to their knowledge about disease processes, diagnosis and best practice. In contrast to contemporary understandings [29], most GPs said they described OA to their patients as simply a problem of cartilage degeneration, joint space narrowing (on x-ray) or *"wear and tear" [GP11]* and frequently expressed beliefs that symptoms will progress, and that surgery is inevitable:

Table 4 Themes within the COM-B model

COM-B component	Theme	Code
Definition		
Psychological Capability	Knowledge gaps	Knowledge of OA disease processes and progression
Knowledge or psychological skills to engage in the necessary mental processes		Adequate knowledge about making diagnosis without imaging
		Knowledge of effective exercise and weight loss treatments
	Skills to facilitate lifestyle change	Communication skills
		Facilitation of behaviour change
	Confidence to effectively manage OA	Making the diagnosis without x-ray
		Delivering lifestyle interventions
Physical Opportunity	System-related factors	Time availability
Opportunity afforded by the environment		Access to other services for exercise and weight management advice (including cost and ease of referral)
		Clinic software
		Lifestyle treatments recommended for all chronic disease patients
	Patient resources	Ease of access
Social Opportunity	Influences from patients demands and expectations	
Opportunity afforded by interpersonal influences, social and cultural norms that impact the way we think about things		
Reflective Motivation	GP's perceived role	Paternalistic role
Reflective processes involving self-conscious intentions, beliefs regarding good and bad, self-talk		Use patient-centred approaches
	Assumptions about people with knee OA	Diagnosis of OA may foster fear avoidance behaviours
		Patient motivation to adopt lifestyle change
Automatic Motivation	Optimism	Effectiveness of non-drug conservative treatment options
Automatic processes involving emotion, desires, impulses	Habit	
	Unease discussing weight	

"They know it's permanent and...we're looking at knee replacements in the future" [GP10].

While most GPs demonstrated an understanding that x-ray findings do not typically match clinical presentation, and some were aware that imaging is not needed to reach a diagnosis of knee OA, some had a knowledge gap in this area. Some GPs reported referring for x-ray whenever knee OA is suspected, for example: *"(I) wouldn't make a diagnosis without confirmatory imaging" [GP4].* The same GP stated a belief imaging was required for diagnosis: *"Not without imaging...there can be other causes of the knee pain..." [GP4].* Despite their statements to the contrary, most of the interviewed GPs also stated a preference to use imaging to "confirm" diagnosis, and some said that imaging helps clarify disease severity.

Several comments indicated that GP knowledge of exercise and weight-loss treatments is sometimes inaccurate or inadequate. For example, in contrast to current guidelines, some GPs thought land-based exercises and joint-loading activities are detrimental, that exercise in water is the only option they can recommend, and people with knee OA considered overweight may be unable to exercise at all:

"There's a really difficult group...they can't exercise... they're so overweight...unless they're prepared to go to a pool there's often many barriers for them." [GP3].

A few GPs were dubious about the effect of exercise and weight-management advice on reducing symptoms:

"I haven't found that it [exercise] is particularly helpful. I haven't had anyone coming and raving to me saying 'Oh I felt brilliant after a swim – my knee feels amazing'. It never happens." [GP9].

The second psychological capability theme identified was 'confidence to effectively manage OA'. A few GPs demonstrated reduced *confidence* with making a diagnosis without imaging, despite having the *knowledge* that x-ray findings are not needed. For example, they said they relied on x-ray investigations for knee OA diagnosis due to low trust in their own diagnostic abilities and to *"confirm"* diagnosis: *"I have to admit that I'm not that confident" [GP9].* Reduced confidence with providing suitable exercise and weight loss advice was also demonstrated with some reporting it as their reason for referring to allied health professionals. Most recognised a need for tailored GP education to improve their confidence:

"A physio showing us a few exercises...that would be a very good thing... for us to feel a bit more confident." [GP1].

The final psychological capability theme was about having 'skills to facilitate lifestyle change'. All GPs reflected on the importance of having highly effective communication skills. For example:

"Most of a GP's life is about understanding the patient's difficulties and barriers and motivations and then acting out your advice in a way that, hopefully, helps that patient" [GP6].

The interviewed GPs acknowledged challenges of facilitating behaviour change and most felt they lacked skill in promoting readiness and motivation for these lifestyle treatments:

"The problem is how do you actually get people to do this stuff...how do you tell them what the right thing to do is?" [GP3].

Physical opportunity

Two physical opportunity themes were identified: 'system-related factors' and 'patient resources'. Regarding 'system-related factors', time pressure was discussed as a major barrier. Most GPs said they felt unable to individualise weight management and develop exercise plans within the appointment time. For example:

"The bigger issue is, I feel I don't have enough time to really give it in a way that I'm completely satisfied with" [GP5].

All interviewed GPs said that OA was often only one part of a patient's complex multi-morbidity and having time to devote to discussing OA management feels like a *"luxury" [GP3].* However, most GPs also acknowledged that lifestyle treatments benefited other chronic conditions, which they said was a facilitator to finding the time for such treatments. One GP stressed the importance of longer consultations:

"I'm a very passionate believer that long consults are of great benefit to taking a comprehensive history...and making a confident diagnosis" [GP8].

Another system-related factor identified by the interviewed GPs was limited access to other services and their associated costs. All participants expressed concerns regarding financial cost to patients when considering referral to other services:

"There may be costs for patients to engage in these programs and obviously that can be a barrier" [GP11].

Others stated barriers to utilisation of support services such as community-based rehabilitation programs included lack of availability in remote locations and long waiting lists. Most of the GPs saw government-subsidised allied health visits as a system-related facilitator to utilisation of services that support exercise and weight loss. For example:

"It's only through a chronic disease management plan that a patient can get funded allied health" [GP3].

Most participating GP's identified changes to clinical practice information technology as potential system-related facilitators, particularly to diagnosing knee OA without imaging. Suggestions offered included building specific prompts into clinic software. In contrast, one GP was sceptical about the benefit of such tools:

"The reality is those tools [checklists] exist for lots of conditions and we never use them, you know, because they're not really practical" [GP3].

'Patient resources' was the other physical opportunity theme. Having access to customisable, printable patient resources was suggested as a facilitator to GP-patient communication about both diagnosis and management options. Interestingly, one GP thought that suitable patient resources are already available (e.g. Arthritis Australia resources) commenting the issue is not a lack of resources but awareness of them:

"The resources that are already out there, are they actually being used appropriately... I'm not convinced" [GP5].

Some suggested that having patient resources embedded within current practice software or routines would increase their use by GPs.

Social opportunity

One social opportunity theme was identified: 'influences from patients demands and expectations'. Interviewed GPs expressed concern that poor patient health literacy in chronic disease management and patients' beliefs about knee OA treatment efficacy negatively influenced how exercise and weight management were discussed. Some mentioned patients often have their own ideas on management, gained from media sources, family or friends. This could understandably be problematic if they primarily involve passive treatments such as supplements and injections. Shifting patients' mind-sets to active participation in management and making lifestyle changes was reported as challenging and time consuming for GPs:

"They often come in not wanting to talk about exercise and losing weight. They want to come in and say what they've read in a recent article" [GP3].

In addition, interviewed GPs reported patient *"expectation"* [GP11] and *"pressure"* [GP6] had substantial influence on their decision to order x-ray investigations. One GP reflected:

"I do agree with the guideline...but it is hard when patients demand" [GP9].

Reflective motivation

Two themes were identified: 'GPs' perceived role' and 'assumptions about people with knee OA'. Those interviewed had varied beliefs about the GP role in OA management. Different beliefs appeared to influence the level of engagement in providing exercise and weight management advice. Some GPs demonstrated a paternalistic approach to care, seeing their role as diagnosing and giving specific treatment advice:

"I take a history...I might do further investigations. If the history and the physical examination fitted, [I] tell the patients this is what they have..." [GP3].

A few GPs said they managed OA with a patient-centred approach, discussing the benefit of working with patients to make decisions about lifestyle change:

"We certainly want to play our role and help improve [their] symptoms but [they] are actually going to be the most important person in terms of determining what happens from here" [GP5].

The second theme was 'assumptions about people with knee OA'. Interviewed GPs stated concerns with giving patients a knee OA diagnosis because they *assumed* patients would have negative connotations associated with the label:

"It's a difficult diagnosis to receive. Patients have a fear of being diagnosed. It's disappointing for them" [GP10].

One GP said a diagnosis can foster fear-avoidance behaviours, including reduced activity, as patients may believe that activity/exercise will cause further damage. Most GPs were pessimistic about their patients' abilities to make lifestyle changes to address their knee OA, assuming patients are not capable of making the required changes. One GP said firmly:

"There are a lot of patients who are lazy...won't carry out instructions and the recommendation to exercise" [GP4].

Another reflected:

"Giving people information is important but how much of it do they take on board? I guess it just varies according to the motivation of the patient" [GP3].

As a result of these assumptions, the interviewed GPs demonstrated reduced motivation to communicate the diagnosis and pursue exercise and weight-loss conversations with their knee OA patients.

Automatic motivation

Three themes were identified from the GPs' discussions: 'optimism', 'habit' and 'unease discussing weight'. GP optimism about OA management was suggested to facilitate provision of exercise and weight loss advice. A few of the GPs interviewed said they believed knee OA is a condition that can be successfully managed. They discussed the importance of conveying to patients that the diagnosis is not all negative, and try to promote management options with optimism and *"hope"* [GP3]. They argued that delivering a relatively positive prognosis to patients facilitated uptake of lifestyle changes:

"Acknowledging that it's difficult but that even in the face of difficulty there are many things that can help slow the progression" [GP3].

The influence of 'habit' was conveyed as a barrier. For example, the GPs discussed that referral for x-ray was the way things had always been done:

"It's usually a two-step process: the patient comes in and you get the history, then they come back to discuss the investigations" [GP3].

A sense of 'unease discussing weight' with patients was conveyed by all but one GP. GPs interviewed acknowledged that weight loss (when someone is overweight) is important but felt that it was a sensitive topic. Most said they were afraid of upsetting their patients and this resulted in a temptation to avoid the discussion:

"It's very demoralising for some patients. It creates an avoidance. I'm sure that's why we don't raise it with people every time" [GP3]

"I think sometimes doctors will not raise it because they don't want to annoy the patient" [GP7].

This factor is, of course, related to the knowledge gaps and confidence issues described under the psychological capability component.

Discussion

Using a theoretical model of behaviour, this study identified eleven key drivers of GP behaviour that impact implementation of recommended practice for diagnosis and non-drug, conservative management of knee OA in the Australian primary care setting.

Our findings suggest whilst GPs mostly know that knee OA can be diagnosed without imaging and that exercise and weight loss are recommended, their described behaviours in practice were often discordant with their own knowledge. We identified several barriers that lead to this discordance. Despite participating GPs describing OA diagnosis and management as straightforward, comments indicated incomplete or inaccurate *knowledge* of OA disease processes and prognosis, and low *confidence* with diagnosing knee OA without x-ray. Knowledge that goes beyond the general guideline recommendation to the what and why of exercise and weight loss interventions, and confidence in their ability to facilitate these interventions effectively, also appeared insufficient. Most, but not all, GPs were aware of their lack of knowledge and confidence. Feelings of being ill prepared to manage OA are consistent with other studies [7, 18, 22, 30, 31]. GPs in our study tended to adopt a simplistic model of OA which neglects the involvement of joint structures other than cartilage, promotes a biomedical model of the disease and its consequences, and may contribute to a fatalistic attitude among patients. Understanding knee OA as a problem of chronic pain involving broader psychosocial factors and as a condition that affects multiple joint structures [32] and therefore not requiring imaging for diagnosis [29], is likely to require a substantial shift in long-held beliefs and habits for many GPs.

GPs' reflections on conversations with their patients about OA identified a reliance on terms that normalise OA (e.g. OA is to be expected with aging), and a preference for vague, general terminology such as 'wear and tear' to communicate the diagnosis to patients. Previous research suggests a dissonance between GPs' rationale for avoiding articulating the diagnosis and how a vague diagnosis is perceived by patients. Clinicians play down an OA diagnosis in an attempt to facilitate acceptance and avoid upsetting patients [30]. However, using dismissive or reassuring terms over factual explanations and empathy can be interpreted by patients as the GP trivialising their problem [18, 30, 33] and lacking interest in their debilitating symptoms [30, 34]. GPs may therefore unintentionally be acting as a barrier to patients making beneficial lifestyle changes, communicating in a more top-down rather than collaborative way with patients about OA diagnosis and treatment options.

Time pressure was identified in our findings and has been widely cited previously as a barrier to GPs ability to implement CPG recommendations including facilitating lifestyle changes [22, 30, 31, 33–36]. The problem is exacerbated when patients with OA have multiple co-morbidities and GP consultation length averages only 14–15 min [37]. A UK study found limited time (13 min) and the presence of multiple co-morbidities (3 conditions on average) led to GPs spending minimal time on OA management and prioritising other conditions they perceived as greater threats to patient health [33]. However, OA imposes a substantial burden on individuals and impacts health-related quality of life to at least the same degree as other common chronic diseases [38, 39]. GPs placing less importance on OA management than the patients themselves may lead to under-management in primary care and patients feeling unsupported and dissatisfied [40].

While some of the barriers to evidence-based management found in this study may be specific to managing OA, many of the barriers have also been found in previous qualitative and quantitative (survey) studies on other chronic conditions including, for example, low back pain [41–43], diabetes [44, 45], chronic kidney disease [46, 47], chronic pain [48], depression [49] and obesity [50, 51]. Frequently occurring barriers include incongruency between patient wishes and guideline recommendations [41–43, 48, 49], suboptimal practitioner skills for patient education [42, 45–47, 50] – in particular, the difficulty communicating a non-biomedical explanation of a biopsychosocial problem [41, 43, 48], difficulty 'selling' lifestyle change and providing support for better self-management [42, 45–48, 50, 51], frustration with patients [45, 47, 50, 51], lack of time [41, 43, 45–49, 51], limited access to other services to help with management [41, 42, 46–49], and resistance to changing practice habits [44, 49]. Collectively, these problems may reflect the challenges in managing chronic conditions within a system designed primarily to manage acute illnesses [52, 53]. On the plus side, the commonality across many conditions, especially around lacking skills and confidence in having conversations about obesity and supporting patients to increase physical activity, means that addressing some of the barriers to optimal OA care will be transferable to improving management of many other conditions and vice versa, particularly given many patients have multi-morbidity.

Our findings identified multiple interacting barriers influence GPs' implementation of OA guideline recommendations, suggesting complex, multimodal solutions may be required. Targeted GP education and training interventions to build motivation and confidence were

potential facilitators to clinical guideline adherence identified by the GPs in ours and other studies [54, 55]. Changes to the guidelines themselves may be beneficial. Currently, OA guidelines lack specific exercise and weight management recommendations and are open to variable interpretation [56, 57] potentially resulting in GPs feeling ill equipped to deliver lifestyle interventions [22]. Further research to identify optimal exercise types and dosage, and effective weight loss interventions is required, however it is currently feasible to suggest specific exercise programs based on existing exercise science and general exercise and physical activity recommendations [58, 59], and to provide guidance on how to have effective conversations with patients to facilitate adoption of lifestyle change recommendations based on principles of patient-centred care and health behaviour change [29, 60]. Guidelines could also provide clear, plain-language statements that can be readily used by GPs during consultations to help with OA management discussions [61]. This type of communication guidance has been demonstrated to facilitate GP uptake of CPG recommendations [34]. Finally, incentivisation and/or coercion-based interventions may help address motivational barriers. This is based on the work of Michie et al. who developed the Behaviour Change Wheel [16], which is an evidence-based framework for planning behaviour change interventions [24]. The framework provides a systematic and theoretically guided method for identifying the types of interventions that could be expected to be effective. Incentivisation and coercion are behaviour change intervention 'functions' that are suggested for addressing some of the types of barriers we found among our GP sample, namely reflective and automatic motivation barriers [16]. Incentivisation has previously been used to drive GP adoption of patient-centred care; however, results have been varied [62]. Costly pay-for-performance interventions appear to influence short-term GP behaviour change, but not long-term, and do not appear to translate to improved patient outcomes [63, 64]. Coercion in this context means creating an expectation of cost. Costs could include financial loss or negative feelings about the undesired behaviour(s). Thus, examples of coercion in our context could include reducing rebates for care consistent with the undesired behaviour, providing education about the negative consequences to patients when sub-optimal care is provided, or portraying those behaviours as 'old fashioned'. Michie et al. [16] note that whether these functions are effective or not depends on the behaviour and the circumstances and should be thought of as options for consideration. Coercive interventions seem not to have been investigated as yet, and it may be that they are not perceived to be acceptable in this context. Utilising social influences via communities of practice or local opinion leaders, or diffusion of innovations aimed at shifting practice behaviours may be better options for addressing reflective and automatic motivation barriers [65].

Several strengths and limitations should be considered when interpreting the findings beyond the context of this study. The attitudes and beliefs of GPs willing to participate in research may not be representative of all GPs. Most GPs interviewed had at least 20 years experience and the views and practices may differ amongst GPs with less experience and/or those who completed training more recently. These, and other location-related contextual factors, including system-related findings pertaining specifically to the Australian healthcare system, should be considered when transferring findings to other contexts. However, it is likely that many findings will be relevant across contexts. In addition, the data represent only the version of GP's perceived reality they wanted to share with the interviewer, and interpretation is influenced by the analysis team. Thus, there may be important factors that influence GP practice behaviour not detected by the study.

Conclusion

In summary, our analysis of Australian GPs' discussion of implementing core underutilised CPG recommendations for knee OA management identified multiple influences that impact practice behaviour. Key negative influences identified were knowledge gaps, low confidence and skill deficiencies, time and other system constraints, and the GPs' perceived role, assumptions about patients and established habits. Positive influences include the benefits of healthy lifestyle changes for all patients, GP optimism and using a patient-centred approach. The complexity of these influences suggests complex, multi-model solutions may be necessary including changes to clinical guidelines, targeted education and training, the implementation of new models of service delivery and exploitation of positive social influences. Such interventions may help bridge the evidence-to-practice gap, which is almost certainly needed if the individual and societal burden of knee OA is to be reduced.

Abbreviations

COM-B: Capability/opportunity/motivation - behaviour; COREQ: Consolidated criteria for reporting qualitative studies; GP: General practitioner; OA: Osteoarthritis

Acknowledgements
The authors which to acknowledge the contribution of Marie Pirotta and Natalie Appleby who assisted with participant recruitment. We also acknowledge with gratitude the 11 general practitioners who participated in the interviews and generously provided their thoughtful and insightful comments.

Funding
This research was funded from the National Health & Medical Research Council (NHMRC) Centre of Research Excellence (CRE) in Translational Research in Musculoskeletal Pain (#1079078). KB is funded by an NHMRC Principal Research Fellowship. The NHMRC had no role in the design of the study and collection, analysis, and interpretation of data, or in writing the manuscript.

Authors' contributions
TE and KLB conceived the study. TE, RN, JS and LA designed the study and contributed to analysis and interpretation of results. RN carried out the interviews. TE and RN carried out the data coding from transcripts. KLB and RH provided content expertise to the analysis findings. All authors contributed to the writing of the manuscript and read and approved the final version.

Competing interests
The authors declare that they have no competing interests.

Author details
[1]Centre for Health, Exercise and Sports Medicine, The University of Melbourne, Melbourne, Australia. [2]School of Health and Rehabilitation Sciences, The University of Queensland, Brisbane, Australia. [3]Centre for Behaviour Change, University College London, London, UK.

References
1. Cross M, Smith E, Hoy D, Nolte S, Ackerman I, Fransen M, Bridgett L, Williams S, Guillemin F, Hill CL, et al. The global burden of hip and knee osteoarthritis: estimates from the global burden of disease 2010 study. Ann Rheum Dis. 2014;73:1323–30. https://doi.org/10.1136/annrheumdis-2013-204763.
2. Murphy LB, Sacks JJ, Brady TJ, Hootman JM, Chapman DP. Anxiety and depression among US adults with arthritis: prevalence and correlates. Arthritis Care Res. 2012;64(7):968–76. https://doi.org/10.1002/acr.21685.
3. Peat G, McArney R, Croft P. Knee pain and osteoarthritis in older adults: a review of community burden and current use of primary health care. Ann Rheum Dis. 2001;60(2):91–7.
4. Arthritis Australia: Time to move: osteoarthritis. A national strategy to reduce a costly burden. 2014.
5. Nelson AE, Allen KD, Golightly YM, Goode AP, Jordan JM. A systematic review of recommendations and guidelines for the management of osteoarthritis: the chronic osteoarthritis management initiative of the U.S. bone and joint initiative. Semin Arthritis Rheum. 2014;43:701–12. https://doi.org/10.1016/j.semarthrit.2013.11.012.
6. Basedow M, Williams H, Shanahan EM, Runciman WB, Esterman A. Australian GP management of osteoarthritis following the release of the RACGP guideline for the non-surgical management of hip and knee osteoarthritis. BMC Res Notes. 2015;8:536. https://doi.org/10.1186/s13104-015-1531-z.
7. Cottrell E, Roddy E, Foster NE. The attitudes, beliefs and behaviours of GPs regarding exercise for chronic knee pain: a systematic review. BMC Fam Pract. 2010;11:4. https://doi.org/10.1186/1471-2296-11-4.
8. Brand CA, Ackerman IN, Bohensky MA, Bennell KL. Chronic disease management: a review of current performance across quality of care domains and opportunities for improving osteoarthritis care. Rheum Dis Clin N Am. 2013;39(1):123–43. https://doi.org/10.1016/j.rdc.2012.10.005.
9. DeHaan MN, Guzman J, Bayley MT, Bell MJ. Knee osteoarthritis clinical practice guidelines - How are we doing? J Rheumatol. 2007;34(10):2099–105.
10. Porcheret M, Jordan K, Jinks C, Croft P. Primary care treatment of knee pain - a survey in older adults. Rheumatology. 2007;46(11):1694–700. https://doi.org/10.1093/rheumatology/kem232.

11. Steel N, Bachmann M, Maisey S, Shekelle P, Breeze E, Marmot M, Melzer D. Self reported receipt of care consistent with 32 quality indicators: national population survey of adults aged 50 or more in England. BMJ. 2008;337: a957. https://doi.org/10.1136/bmj.a957.

12. Glazier RH, Dalby DM, Badley EM, Hawker GA, Bell MJ, Buchbinder R, Lineker SC. Management of common musculoskeletal problems: a survey of Ontario primary care physicians. CMAJ. 1998;158(8):1037–40.

13. Brand CA, Harrison C, Tropea J, Hinman RS, Britt H, Bennell K. Management of osteoarthritis in general practice in Australia. Arthritis Care Res. 2014;66(4): 551–8. https://doi.org/10.1002/acr.22197.

14. Hunter DJ. Quality of osteoarthritis care for community-dwelling older adults. Clin Geriatr Med. 2010;26(3):401–17. https://doi.org/10.1016/j.cger. 2010.03.003.

15. Bohensky M, Barker A, Morello R, De Steiger RN, Gorelik A, Brand C. Geographical variation in incidence of knee arthroscopy for patients with osteoarthritis: a population-based analysis of Victorian hospital separations data. Intern Med J. 2014;44(6):537–45. https://doi.org/10. 1111/imj.12438.

16. Michie S, Atkins L, West R. The behaviour change wheel. A guide to designing interventions. Great Britian: Silverback Publishing; 2014.

17. Poitras S, Rossignol M, Avouac J, Avouac B, Cedraschi C, Nordin M, Rousseaux C, Rozenberg S, Savarieau B, Thoumie P, et al. Management recommendations for knee osteoarthritis: how usable are they? Joint Bone Spine. 2010;77(5):458–65. https://doi.org/10.1016/j.jbspin.2010.08.001.

18. Alami S, Boutron I, Desjeux D, Hirschhorn M, Meric G, Rannou F, Poiraudeau S. Patients' and practitioners' views of knee osteoarthritis and its management: a qualitative interview study. PLoS One. 2011;6(5):e19634. https://doi.org/10.1371/journal.pone.0019634.

19. Mann C, Gooberman-Hill R. Health care provision for osteoarthritis: concordance between what patients would like and what health professionals think they should have. Arthritis Care Res. 2011;63(7):963–72. https://doi.org/10.1002/acr.20459.

20. Rosemann T, Wensing M, Joest K, Backenstrass M, Mahler C, Szecsenyi J. Problems and needs for improving primary care of osteoarthritis patients: the views of patients, general practitioners and practice nurses. BMC Musculoskelet Disord. 2006;7:48. https://doi.org/10.1186/1471-2474-7-48.

21. Barozzi N, Tett SE. Perceived barriers to paracetamol (acetaminophen) prescribing, especially following rofecoxib withdrawal from the market. Clin Rheumatol. 2009;28(5):509–19. https://doi.org/10.1007/s10067-008-1077-8.

22. Egerton T, Diamond LE, Buchbinder R, Bennell KL, Slade SC. A systematic review and evidence synthesis of qualitative studies to identify primary care clinicians' barriers and enablers to the management of osteoarthritis. Osteoarthr Cartil. 2016. https://doi.org/10.1016/j.joca.2016.12.002.

23. Tong A, Sainsbury P, Craig J. Consolidated criteria for reporting qualitative research (COREQ): a 32-item checklist for interviews and focus groups. Int J Qual Health Care. 2007;19(6):349–57. https://doi.org/10.1093/ intqhc/mzm042.

24. Michie S, van Stralen MM, West R. The behaviour change wheel: a new method for characterising and designing behaviour change interventions. Implement Sci. 2011;6:42. https://doi.org/10.1186/1748-5908-6-42.

25. McSharry J, Murphy PJ, Byrne M. Implementing international sexual counselling guidelines in hospital cardiac rehabilitation: development of the CHARMS intervention using the behaviour change wheel. Implement Sci. 2016;11(1):134. https://doi.org/10.1186/s13012-016-0493-4.

26. Barker F, de Lusignan S, Cooke D. Improving collaborative behaviour planning in adult auditory rehabilitation: development of the I-PLAN intervention using the behaviour change wheel. Ann Behav Med. 2016. https://doi.org/10.1007/s12160-016-9843-3.

27. Fulton EA, Brown KE, Kwah KL, Wild S. StopApp: using the behaviour change wheel to develop an app to increase uptake and attendance at NHS stop smoking services. Healthcare (Basel). 2016;4(2). https://doi.org/10. 3390/healthcare4020031.

28. Gibbs L, Kealy M, Willis K, Green J, Welch N, Daly J. What have sampling and data collection got to do with good qualitative research? Aust N Z J Public Health. 2007;31(6):540–4. https://doi.org/10.1111/j.1753-6405.2007.00140.x.

29. National Clinical Guideline Centre. Osteoarthritis. Care and management in adults. Clinical guideline CG177. Methods, evidence and recommendations. London: National Institute for health and care excellence; 2014.

30. Paskins Z, Sanders T, Hassell AB. Comparison of patient experiences of the osteoarthritis consultation with GP attitudes and beliefs to OA: a narrative review. BMC Fam Pract. 2014;15:46. https://doi.org/10.1186/1471-2296-15-46.

31. Ashman F, Sturgiss E, Haesler E. Exploring self-efficacy in Australian general practitioners managing patient obesity: a qualitative survey study. Int J Family Med. 2016;2016:8212837. https://doi.org/10.1155/2016/8212837.

32. Neogi T. The epidemiology and impact of pain in osteoarthritis. Osteoarthr Cartil. 2013;21(9):1145–53. https://doi.org/10.1016/j.joca.2013.03.018.

33. Paskins Z, Sanders T, Croft PR, Hassell AB. The identity crisis of osteoarthritis in general practice: a qualitative study using video-stimulated recall. Ann Fam Med. 2015;13(6):537–44. https://doi.org/10.1370/afm.1866.

34. Baumann M, Euller-Ziegler L, Guillemin F. Evaluation of the expectations osteoarthritis patients have concerning healthcare, and their implications for practitioners. Clin Exp Rheumatol. 2007;25(3):404–9.

35. Cuperus N, Smink AJ, Bierma-Zeinstra SM, Dekker J, Schers HJ, de Boer F, van den Ende CH, Vliet Vlieland TP. Patient reported barriers and facilitators to using a self-management booklet for hip and knee osteoarthritis in primary care: results of a qualitative interview study. BMC Fam Pract. 2013; 14:181. https://doi.org/10.1186/1471-2296-14-181.

36. Lau R, Stevenson F, Ong BN, Dziedzic K, Treweek S, Eldridge S, Everitt H, Kennedy A, Qureshi N, Rogers A, et al. Achieving change in primary care - causes of the evidence to practice gap: systematic review of reviews. Implement Sci. 2016;11:40. https://doi.org/10.1186/s13012-016-0396-4.

37. Britt H, Miller G. BEACH program update. Aust Fam Physician. 2015; 44(6):411–4.

38. Parker L, Moran GM, Roberts LM, Calvert M, McCahon D. The burden of common chronic disease on health-related quality of life in an elderly community-dwelling population in the UK. Fam Pract. 2014;31(5):557–63. https://doi.org/10.1093/fampra/cmu035.

39. Hunter DJ, Schofield D, Callander E. The individual and socioeconomic impact of osteoarthritis. Nat Rev Rheumatol. 2014;10(7):437–41. https://doi. org/10.1038/nrrheum.2014.44.

40. Arthritis Australia: The ignored majority. The voice of arthritis. A national survey to discover the impact of arthritis on Australians. 2011.

41. Bishop FL, Dima AL, Ngui J, Little P, Moss-Morris R, Foster NE, Lewith GT. "Lovely pie in the sky plans": A Qualitative Study of Clinicians' Perspectives on Guidelines for Managing Low Back Pain in Primary Care in England. Spine (Phila Pa 1976). 2015;40(23):1842–50. https://doi.org/ 10.1097/BRS.0000000000001215.

42. Chenot JF, Scherer M, Becker A, Donner-Banzhoff N, Baum E, Leonhardt C, Keller S, Pfingsten M, Hildebrandt J, Basler HD, et al. Acceptance and perceived barriers of implementing a guideline for managing low back in general practice. Implement Sci. 2008;3:7. https://doi.org/10.1186/1748-5908-3-7.

43. Slade SC, Kent P, Patel S, Bucknall T, Buchbinder R. Barriers to primary care clinician adherence to clinical guidelines for the management of low back pain: a systematic review and metasynthesis of qualitative studies. Clin J Pain. 2016;32(9):800–16. https://doi.org/10.1097/AJP.0000000000000324.

44. Havele SA, Pfoh ER, Yan C, Misra-Hebert AD, Le P, Rothberg MB. Physicians' views of self-monitoring of blood glucose in patients with type 2 diabetes not on insulin. Ann Fam Med. 2018;16(4):349–52. https://doi. org/10.1370/afm.2244.

45. Rushforth B, McCrorie C, Glidewell L, Midgley E, Foy R. Barriers to effective management of type 2 diabetes in primary care: qualitative systematic review. Br J Gen Pract. 2016;66(643):e114–27. https://doi. org/10.3399/bjgp16X683509.

46. van Dipten C, van Berkel S, de Grauw WJC, Scherpbier-de Haan ND, Brongers B, van Spaendonck K, Wetzels JFM, Assendelft WJJ, Dees MK. General practitioners' perspectives on management of early-stage chronic kidney disease: a focus group study. BMC Fam Pract. 2018;19(1):81. https:// doi.org/10.1186/s12875-018-0736-3.

47. Vest BM, York TR, Sand J, Fox CH, Kahn LS. Chronic kidney disease guideline implementation in primary care: a qualitative report from the TRANSLATE CKD study. J Am Board Fam Med. 2015;28(5):624–31. https://doi.org/10. 3122/jabfm.2015.05.150070.

48. Becker WC, Dorflinger L, Edmond SN, Islam L, Heapy AA, Fraenkel L. Barriers and facilitators to use of non-pharmacological treatments in chronic pain. BMC Fam Pract. 2017;18(1):41. https://doi.org/10.1186/s12875-017-0608-2.

49. Aakhus E, Oxman AD, Flottorp SA. Determinants of adherence to recommendations for depressed elderly patients in primary care: a multi-methods study. Scand J Prim Health Care. 2014;32(4):170–9. https://doi.org/ 10.3109/02813432.2014.984961.

50. Henderson E. Obesity in primary care: a qualitative synthesis of patient and practitioner perspectives on roles and responsibilities. Br J Gen Pract. 2015; 65(633):e240–7. https://doi.org/10.3399/bjgp15X684397.

51. Hiddink GJ, Hautvast JG, van Woerkum CM, Fieren CJ, Van 't Hof MA. Nutrition guidance by primary-care physicians: perceived barriers and low involvement. Eur J Clin Nutr. 1995;49(11):842–51.

52. Wagner EH. Managed care and chronic illness: health services research needs. Health Serv Res. 1997;32(5):702–14.

53. Rothman AA, Wagner EH. Chronic illness management: what is the role of primary care? Ann Intern Med. 2003;138(3):256–61.

54. Tzortziou Brown V, Underwood M, Mohamed N, Westwood O, Morrissey D. Professional interventions for general practitioners on the management of musculoskeletal conditions. Cochrane Database Syst Rev. 2016;5:Cd007495. https://doi.org/10.1002/14651858.CD007495.pub2.

55. Mostofian F, Ruban C, Simunovic N, Bhandari M. Changing physician behavior: what works? Am J Manag Care. 2015;21(1):75–84.

56. Codish S, Shiffman RN. A model of ambiguity and vagueness in clinical practice guideline recommendations. American Medical Informatics Association. AMIA Annu Symp Proc. 2005;2005:146.

57. Gupta S, Rai N, Bhattacharrya O, Cheng AY, Connelly KA, Boulet LP, Kaplan A, Brouwers MC, Kastner M. Optimizing the language and format of guidelines to improve guideline uptake. CMAJ. 2016;188(14):E362–e368. https://doi.org/10.1503/cmaj.151102.

58. American College of Sports Medicine, Chodzko-Zajko WJ, Proctor DN, Fiatarone Singh MA, Minson CT, Nigg CR, Salem GJ, Skinner JS. American College of Sports Medicine position stand. Exercise and physical activity for older adults. Med Sci Sports Exerc. 2009;41(7):1510–30. https://doi.org/10.1249/MSS.0b013e3181a0c95c.

59. American Geriatrics Society Panel on Exercise and Osteoarthritis. Exercise prescription for older adults with osteoarthritis pain: consensus practice recommendations. J Am Geriatr Soc. 2001;49:808–23.

60. Dwamena F, Holmes-Rovner M, Gaulden CM, Jorgenson S, Sadigh G, Sikorskii A, Lewin S, Smith RC, Coffey J, Olomu A. Interventions for providers to promote a patient-centred approach in clinical consultations. Cochrane Database Syst Rev. 2012;12:CD003267. https://doi.org/10.1002/14651858.CD003267.pub2.

61. Mickan S, Burls A, Glasziou P. Patterns of 'leakage' in the utilisation of clinical guidelines: a systematic review. Postgrad Med J. 2011;87(1032):670–9. https://doi.org/10.1136/pgmj.2010.116012.

62. Scott A, Sivey P, Ait Ouakrim D, Willenberg L, Naccarella L, Furler J, Young D. The effect of financial incentives on the quality of health care provided by primary care physicians. Cochrane Database Syst Rev. 2011;9:CD008451. https://doi.org/10.1002/14651858.CD008451.pub2.

63. Flodgren G, Eccles MP, Shepperd S, Scott A, Parmelli E, Beyer FR. An overview of reviews evaluating the effectiveness of financial incentives in changing healthcare professional behaviours and patient outcomes. Cochrane Database Syst Rev. 2011;7:Cd009255. https://doi.org/10.1002/14651858.cd009255.

64. Chauhan BF, Jeyaraman M, Mann AS, Lys J, Skidmore B, Sibley KM, Abou-Setta A, Zarychanksi R. Behavior change interventions and policies influencing primary healthcare professionals' practic - an overview of reviews. Implement Sci. 2017;12(1):3. https://doi.org/10.1186/s13012-016-0538-8.

65. Grol R, Grimshaw J. From best evidence to best practice: effective implementation of change in patients' care. Lancet. 2003;362(9391):1225–30. https://doi.org/10.1016/S0140-6736(03)14546-1.

22

Identifying the unmet information and support needs of women with autoimmune rheumatic diseases during pregnancy planning, pregnancy and early parenting

Rhiannon Phillips[1]*[iD], Bethan Pell[2], Aimee Grant[2], Daniel Bowen[1], Julia Sanders[3], Ann Taylor[4], Adrian Edwards[1], Ernest Choy[5] and Denitza Williams[1]

Abstract

Background: Autoimmune rheumatic diseases (ARDs) such as inflammatory arthritis and Lupus, and many of the treatments for these diseases, can have a detrimental impact on fertility and pregnancy outcomes. Disease activity and organ damage as a result of ARDs can affect maternal and foetal outcomes. The safety and acceptability of hormonal contraceptives can also be affected. The objective of this study was to identify the information and support needs of women with ARDs during pregnancy planning, pregnancy and early parenting.

Methods: This mixed methods study included a cross-sectional online survey and qualitative narrative interviews. The survey was completed by 128 women, aged 18–49 in the United Kingdom with an ARD who were thinking of getting pregnant in the next five years, who were pregnant, or had young children (< 5 years old). The survey assessed quality-of-life and information needs (Arthritis Impact Measurement Scale Short Form and Educational Needs Assessment Tool), support received, what women found challenging, what was helpful, and support women would have liked. From the survey participants, a maximum variation sample of 22 women were purposively recruited for qualitative interviews. Interviews used a person-centered participatory approach facilitated by visual methods, which enabled participants to reflect on their experiences. Interviews were also carried out with seven health professionals purposively sampled from primary care, secondary care, maternity, and health visiting services.

Results: Survey findings indicated an unmet need for information in this population (ENAT total mean 104.85, SD 30.18). Women at the pre-conception stage reported higher needs for information on pregnancy planning, fertility, giving birth, and breastfeeding, whereas those who had children already expressed a higher need for information on pain and mobility. The need for high quality information, and more holistic, multi-disciplinary, collaborative, and integrated care consistently emerged as themes in the survey open text responses and interviews with women and health professionals.

Conclusions: There is an urgent need to develop and evaluate interventions to better inform, support and empower women of reproductive age who have ARDs as they navigate the complex challenges that they face during pregnancy planning, pregnancy and early parenting.

Keywords: Autoimmune rheumatic disease, Pregnancy, Family planning, Parenting, Infant feeding, Information, Support, Timeline, Qualitative, Visual methods

* Correspondence: PhillipsR19@cardiff.ac.uk
[1]Division of Population Medicine, School of Medicine, Cardiff University, Cardiff, UK
Full list of author information is available at the end of the article

Background

When Autoimmune Rheumatic Diseases (ARDs) affect women of reproductive age, this raises a range of issues around family planning, pregnancy, and early parenting [1, 2]. Both ARDs and their treatments can cause problems with fertility, complications during pregnancy, and impact on contraceptive choices [1, 3]. Many women with ARDs will have positive pregnancy and parenting outcomes but there are risks involved [4, 5]. Women with ARDs who are of childbearing age face complex choices about starting (or enlarging) a family now or sometime in the future [6], but they struggle to get enough information and support [2].

Nearly half of pregnancies in Britain are not planned [7]. Choices of contraception can be complicated for women with ARDs, for example the combined progesterone and oestrogen oral contraceptive pill is not recommended for women with more severe forms of Lupus, particularly when they have renal involvement or test positive for antiphospholipid antibodies [3]. Nonetheless, the vast majority of women with rheumatic diseases have viable contraceptive options, including barrier methods, intra-uterine devices and progesterone-only medication [8]. In a survey completed by 212 women of reproductive age who had Systemic Lupus Erythematous in the United States, 97 (46%) women were at risk of unplanned pregnancy (unprotected sex or unreliable method of contraception) in the past three months. A survey in Switzerland ($n = 170$ women) found that around a third of women with inflammatory arthritis who are taking medication that is contraindicated in pregnancy, such as methotrexate and leflunomide, use ineffective or no contraception [9].

In an Australian mixed methods study ($n = 27$), women with Rheumatoid Arthritis (RA) reported that they struggled to find enough information about family planning, pregnancy and early parenting [2]. The study indicated that there was a high demand for more information on the safety of medications during pregnancy and breastfeeding in particular [2]. While Rheumatologists were the primary source for information, women also placed a high value on patient-facing arthritis organisations and on learning from the personal experiences of other women [2]. A systematic review [10] of interventions to improve knowledge and self-management skills around contraception, pregnancy and breastfeeding in women with RA identified only one well designed evaluation of education or self-management focused on pregnancy [11]. In that study, a decision aid for women with Rheumatoid Arthritis to support their decision making about starting (or enlarging) a family improved knowledge about RA and pregnancy and decisional conflict [11]. A further eight studies that were identified in the review of general Rheumatoid Arthritis self-management interventions included a minor component on family planning [10]. Three

of these contained information about methotrexate use in pregnancy and/or breastfeeding [12–14], one included a warning about lack of evidence with regard to the safety of biological therapy use during pregnancy [15], three provided advice on relationship, family, and/or sexual issues [16–18], and one involved a discussion about contraception and fertility [19]. Only four of these studies included an outcome measure relevant to family planning or pregnancy [12–14, 19].

More integrated care and better information and counselling around pregnancy and early parenting for women with ARD and other chronic diseases have been recommended [2, 10, 20–23]. However, there is little high quality evidence on how to meet the educational, self-management or broader non-pharmacological health and social care needs of women with ARDs in this context [10]. The objectives of this study were to establish what the unmet information and support needs of women in the UK who have ARDs are during pregnancy planning, pregnancy and early parenting, and to identify opportunities to better meet these needs.

Method

Design

We used a mixed methods design, which incorporated a cross-sectional online survey and qualitative interviews with women with ARDs and health professionals. To enable comparisons between this UK study and a previous Australian study [2], we used similar sampling methods and inclusion criteria, and included a modified version of the Educational Needs Assessment Tool [24, 25] to assess information needs.

Online cross-sectional survey

Participants and recruitment

The survey was made available using the Bristol Online Surveys system. The patient survey was advertised through the study website, social media (Twitter & Facebook), via UK arthritis patient organisations (Lupus UK, Arthritis Care, Vasculitis UK), peer-support groups (Facebook groups for people trying to conceive/pregnancy in Lupus and vasculitis), and online networks for parents (Netmums and Mumsnet). We also used Facebook and Twitter advertising systems to promote the study. To facilitate recruitment, we offered the following incentives: a donation of 50p for each questionnaire completed to UK arthritis charities, and an option to enter a prize draw to win a £100 in gift vouchers.

Inclusion criteria

Women aged 18–49 years, who have an ARD (i.e. inflammatory arthritis or auto-immune connective tissue disease for which people would normally be under the care of a rheumatologist), and were: planning to become pregnant in the next 5 years; and/or currently pregnant;

and/or had been pregnant within the last 5 years; and/or had a child (or children) under 5 years of age.

Exclusion criteria

Disease not classified as an ARD (e.g. joint hypermobility, fibromyalgia).

Measures

Information needs A modified version of the Educational Needs Assessment Tool (ENAT) [24, 25] was used, which is a validated measure with 39 items to assess educational needs in seven domains; pain management, movement, feelings, the arthritis process, treatment from health care professionals, self-management and support from others. An international study [24] demonstrated that the ENAT is a valid tool for identification of information needs relating to rheumatic diseases, with high internal consistency. The items are scored on a five point Likert scale, providing total score ranging from 0 (lowest educational need) to 156 (highest educational need) [24]. While uploading the modified ENAT for use in the current study to the online survey software, one response category ('fairly important') was omitted, and consequently items were scored on a four-point scale: 1-not at all important, 2-a little important, 3-very important, 4-extremely important. To retain as much comparability as possible with previous studies, the individual item scores were transformed from a four point (1–4) to a five point (0–4) scale prior to calculation of the total score, so that its overall range would correspond with the original ENAT (0–156). The subscale total scores were Rasch transformed to provide interval rather than ordinal level data [25].

Additional items were included in the information needs section of the survey, using the four-point Likert scales to assess information needs in relation to: sex and relationships, contraception, preparation for pregnancy, how to increase chances of getting pregnant naturally, fertility treatments, options for giving birth, managing pain during childbirth, and breastfeeding. These items were developed by the research team based on the educational needs identified through previous studies [2, 10, 11], and guided by two Patient and Public Involvement representatives (both women with young children who had ARDs) who highlighted which issues were most important to them from a patient perspective. The patient representatives also requested items be included on the use of transcutaneous electrical nerve stimulation (TENS) as this may be useful for pain management, and how they could get access to their test results, which could prove difficult between appointments. The additional items from the family planning, pregnancy, and early parenting were scored separately from the original

ENAT items and were not included in the total ENAT score.

Disease-related quality of life This was assessed using the Arthritis Impact Measurement Scale Version 2 Short Form (AIMS2-SF) [26]. The AIMS2-SF is a validated 26-item measure with five factors; physical symptoms, mobility, role (work), social interaction, and affect. The AIMS2-SF has similar psychometric properties to the AIMS2, good test-retest reproducibility and sensitivity to change. Items are scored on a 5-point Likert scale from 0 to 4, and in each component scores are normalised so that they range from 0 (perfect health to 10 (worst possible health) [26]. Thus, higher scores indicate a greater impact of arthritis on each of these domains.

Lived experience and expressed support needs Using open-response items, participants were asked what they found: i) most challenging; ii) most helpful; and; iii) what support they would have wanted while planning a family, being pregnant, or having young children. Participants were asked whether they were currently having, had previously had, or wanted the following types of support: access to a health professional to act as their main point of contact and care coordinator; physiotherapy; opportunity to talk to other people with similar experiences and to get advice (i.e. peer-support); talking therapies (e.g. counselling, Cognitive Behavioural Therapy); alternative and complementary therapies (e.g. acupuncture, aromatherapy, herbal remedies). These items were developed by the research team based on sources of information and support for women with long-term illnesses while they are building a family that were identified in the literature [2, 4, 10, 21]. The items were reviewed by two patient representatives to assess relevance, clarity and acceptability of the questions.

Clinical and demographic information The survey included questions on type of ARD (drop down list); years since onset of ARD; current medication (drop down list); co-morbidities (open text), and; family situation (currently pregnant, planning to try to get pregnant within the next 5 years, and/or had a pregnancy in the last 5 years, had children already, and if so, how many and what their ages are). Demographic data were collected on date of birth, highest educational qualification, geographical location (postcode), marital status, ethnicity, and current employment status.

Survey data analysis

Analysis of the quantitative data was carried out using SPSS v23. Analysis was primarily descriptive, providing an overview of the information and support needs. To identify differences in information needs (ENAT) and quality of life (AIMS2-SF) of women by family status (had or did not have children) and disease group, independent t-tests were carried out, and 95% confidence intervals were calculated. Between-group differences in support received/desired, which were binary categorical variables, were calculated using Chi-square tests. To ensure that there were sufficient numbers for analysis, and due to the differences between rheumatic diseases in disease processes and pregnancy outcomes [1, 4, 5], diseases were broadly categorised as: inflammatory arthritis (rheumatoid arthritis, psoriatic arthritis, ankylosing spondylitis, idiopathic juvenile arthritis, and non-specific inflammatory arthritis), connective tissue diseases (Systemic Lupus Erythematous, systemic sclerosis, and non-specific autoimmune connective tissue disease), and vasculitis. The Holm-Bonferroni correction for multiple comparisons can be used on both parametric and non-parametric tests [27]. The Holm-Bonferroni correction included both the t-tests and Chi-square tests as these tests were conducted on the same data set. Using this method, alpha was set at 0.005. Open text data from the survey were coded thematically using an inductive approach to identify frequent, dominant, and significant themes that emerged from the data [28].

Qualitative interviews

We adopted a person-centered ethos. As women were being asked about emotional and complex issues in this study, a flexible narrative approach was used to encourage them to talk about their 'lived experiences' in their own words, focusing on things that were important to them, rather than being guided by a researcher-generated topics [29]. A timeline-assisted method was used, where participants were asked to create a visual representation of their histories before the interview [30]. Women were sent a 'What to expect' sheet was posted to participants along with stationary items, which provided guidance on some of the topics that were of interest to the research team (see Additional file 1). The timelines were used as an elicitation tool in interviews to provide cues and prompt discussion [30]. A topic guide was not used by the researchers during the interviews as the objective of the interviews was to learn about the lived experiences of women, rather than to determine the frequency of predetermined events [31]. The use of participatory approaches such as this in qualitative research can empower participants by allowing them to navigate the conversation, increase their level of comfort in discussing sensitive topics, provide positive moments and opportunities for closure, and can thereby improve the quality of data collected [30, 32].

Participants

Women who had expressed interest in being contacted for an interview through the survey were purposively sampled based on their family situation. The aim was to achieve a broadly equal representation of women who were: (i) thinking about getting pregnant; (ii) currently pregnant, or; (iii) had young children, so that the views of women who were at different stages of starting a family could be captured. Women were contacted through e-mail or telephone, based on the contact details provided in the survey. Women who expressed interest in being interviewed were sent a study information pack containing participant information sheet, consent form and stamped return envelope.

Healthcare professionals were identified through professional networks (e.g. Welsh Arthritis Research Network) and were purposively sampled for key professional groups who were involved in the care of women with ARDs in primary care (GPs), secondary care (Rheumatologists, Nephrologists, and Nurse Specialists), and maternity and children's services (Midwives and Health Visitors – i.e. National Health Service nurses who provide advice and assistance to parents with young children). Healthcare professionals who expressed an interest in participating were e-mailed a participant information sheet and consent form.

Interview procedure

Interviews were conducted face-to-face at women's homes, at Cardiff University, or by telephone. For pragmatic reasons, babies and young children were present during some interviews with women, but no other adults were present. Before the interviews, women were sent a resource pack, which included various items of stationary, an exemplar blank timeline template, and some examples of the themes that we were interested in covering during the interview. This encouraged participants to reflect on their experiences and to guide the discussion during the interview. The timelines provided a visual tool to enable women to map out their journey towards starting a family, noting key events and their physical and emotional responses to these. Women who had prepared timelines could use these as prompts for topics they wanted to discuss during the interviews. Women had the flexibility to use a timeline template provided by the research team, generate their own, or tell their story in their own way if they preferred.

Interviews with healthcare professionals were guided by an interview schedule (Additional file 2), which focused on the health professional's role, challenges in providing care for women with ARDs who are starting a family, and how care could be improved. Visual timelines were drafted by the researcher at the end of the interview to map out what health professionals had talked about in terms of how healthcare services were provided along women's journeys through pre-conception, pregnancy and early parenting, and to identify at which points extra support might be needed. The timelines were sent to the healthcare professional after the interview for participant validation, to ensure that they captured the conversation accurately, and healthcare professionals were encouraged to amend the timelines if needed.

Interviews were carried out by Denitza Williams PhD (DW) and Bethan Pell BSc (BP). DW was a post-doctoral researcher and BP a research assistant at the time the interviews were carried out, and both researchers are female. Both researchers had previous experience of carrying out qualitative interviews, and were provided with additional training and supervision in study specific procedures by the lead author (Rhiannon Phillips, PhD) and qualitative lead for this project (Aimee Grant, PhD). The interviewers had no relationship with the participants prior to the interviews and had no prior knowledge of their goals or characteristics, other than the participant information pack provided as described above. Where participants asked the interviewers about their background during interviews, the interviewers explained that they were researchers that were not from a medical background, nor were they experts in rheumatic diseases, but rather that they were interested in hearing about women's experiences to inform further research on better meeting their information and support needs. Interviews were audio-recorded and interviewers made field notes as soon as possible after interviews. The interviewers requested a copy of the completed versions of the timelines to provide context during the analysis, although this was voluntary. Transcripts were not returned to participants for comment and participants did not comment on the findings. Health professionals were given an opportunity to review and comment on the timelines produced by the researcher to summarise their discussions. No repeat interviews were carried out.

Qualitative analysis

All interviews were audio-recorded and transcribed verbatim. The data were analysed thematically using a hybrid approach of inductive and deductive analysis, based primarily on social phenomenology [33]. The analysis focused primarily on the data-driven process of understanding how people make sense of and interpret the phenomena of their everyday world [33]. The deductive component of the analysis was far less pronounced in this study, seeking only to identify themes relating to information and healthcare needs of this and similar populations that had been highlighted in previous research [1, 2, 21]. NVivo V10 was used to facilitate analysis. DW carried out the data coding. Our protocol did not include dual coding of the data. Instead we used regular qualitative research team meetings to discuss data production, the development of the coding framework and data analysis, with each member of the qualitative research group (DW, BP, RP, AG) adding their own unique

perspective to the analysis through these meetings. This approach has been identified as appropriate in qualitative research [34]. We were guided by the concept of 'information power' [35] rather than 'saturation'; the research team judged the sample to provide a sufficient depth and range of knowledge to meet the study objectives.

Results
Survey findings

The online survey was completed by 131 women. Two of these had diagnoses that were not classified as ARDs and one did not provide information on her diagnosis, so 128 responses were included in analysis. Demographic and clinical characteristics of participants are shown in Table 1. There were no statistically significant differences between women who had children already and those who did not for any of the AIMS2-SF disease related quality of life domains. Women with inflammatory arthritis reported a greater impact of their disease on their physical mobility than those with connective tissue disease (mean difference 0.89, 95%CI 0.23 to 1.56, $p = 0.009$) or vasculitis (mean difference 1.23, 95%CI 0.36 to 2.09, $p = 0.006$), but no other differences were found between disease groups for disease related quality of life.

Descriptive statistics for information and support needs are shown in Table 2 for all participants, and for those who already have children compared with those do not have children. Women who had children already had higher information needs in the ENAT movement domain than those who did not have children. Information needs relating to the reproductive health items were higher across the board for women who had not yet had children compared with those who had children, with the exception of the sex and relationships item. No statistically significant differences were found in information and support needs by disease group (inflammatory arthritis, connective tissue diseases, or vasculitis).

Qualitative findings

Of the 128 survey participants, 118 (92.2%) provided a response to one or more of the open-text questions. Twenty-two out of 88 women approached (25%) took part in interviews. Six women were interviewed face-to-face and 16 were interviewed by telephone. Interview duration ranged from 20 to 85 min, with a mean duration of 48 min for telephone interviews and 64 min for face-to-face interviews. A higher proportion of interview participants had a university degree (72.7% vs. 55.5%) and were in employment (either full or part time) (86.4% vs. 69.5%) than those who were not interviewed. Women who took part in an interview also had a lower AIMS-2 impact of arthritis on physical functioning score than those who did not (95% CI 0.37, 1.95, $p < 0.005$). Three of

Table 1 Clinical and demographic characteristics of survey and interview participants

Variable	Category	Survey (*n* = 128) Number (%)	Patient interviews (*n* = 22) Number (%)
Primary diagnosis	Systemic Lupus Erythematosus	42 (32.8)	7 (13.6)
	Rheumatoid Arthritis	23 (18)	3 (31.8)
	Vasculitis	23 (18)	6 (27.3)
	Non-specific inflammatory arthritis/connective tissue disease	18 (14.1)	4 (18.2)
	Idiopathic Juvenile Arthritis	9 (7)	1 (4.5)
	Psoriatic Arthritis	7 (5.5)	1 (4.5)
	Other ARD	6 (4.7)	0 (0)
Duration of illness	Up to 1 year	6 (4.7)	2 (9.1)
	1 to 5 years	41 (32)	6 (27.3)
	More than 5 years	79 (61.7)	14 (63.6)
	Missing data	*2 (1.6)*	*0 (0)*
Family situation: (number and % responding 'yes')	Have children already	71 (55.5)	13 (59.1)
	Thinking about getting pregnant in the next five years	77 (60.2)	7 (31.8)
	Currently trying to get pregnant	9 (7)	2 (9.1)
	Currently pregnant	8 (6.3)	2 (9.1)
	Have been pregnant in the last 5 years	63 (49.2)	11 (50)
Education	Have a university degree	71 (55.5)	16 (72.7)
Employment status	Full time paid work	51 (39.8)	8 (36.4)
	Part time paid work	38 (29.7)	11 (50)
	Unemployed & seeking work	4 (3.1)	0 (0)
	Not employed & currently not seeking work	25 (19.5)	2 (9.1)
	In full or part time education	6 (4.7)	1 (4.5)
	Rather not say	4 (3.1)	0 (0)
Relationships	Married, civil partnership, or living together	107 (83.6)	18 (81.8)
	Other	21 (16.4)	4 (12.2)
	Missing data	*2 (1.6)*	*1 (4.5)*
Ethnic group	British, English, Welsh, Scottish, or Irish	114 (89)	19 (86.4)
	Other: non-European	12 (9.4)	2 (9.1)
	Other: European	2 (1.6)	0 (0)
	Missing data	*1 (0.8)*	*1 (4.5)*
		Mean (SD)	Mean (SD)
Age	Range: 21 to 48 years	32.75 (6.1)	33.86 (5.3)
Disease-related Quality of Life (AIMS2-SF normalised scores)	Physical	3.52 (1.8)	2.56 (1.38)
	Symptoms	5.41 (3.22)	4.24 (3.51)
	Affect	4.57 (2.4)	4.12 (2.42)
	Social	5.74 (1.76)	6.02(1.64)
	Role	7.79 (3.0)	7.29 (2.80)

the women interviewed produced visual timelines, while 12 had prepared notes, prompts, diagrams, or brought along medical records to use in the discussion. Seven healthcare professionals of 25 (28%) invited to interview were recruited. These were two midwives, one health visitor, two consultant rheumatologists, one general practitioner, and one nephrologist. Only one of the health professionals suggested minor changes to the timeline visual produced following their interview to accurately reflect their views.

Table 2 Information and support reported in the online survey ($n = 128$)

Variable		All ($n = 128$)	Women who have children ($n = 71$)	Women who don't have children yet ($n = 57$)	Between group comparisons for women who already have vs. don't have children		
Information needs		Mean (SD)	Mean (SD)	Mean (SD)	Mean difference	95% CI	P value
ENAT (Rasch-transformed scores)	Pain	15.4 (4.94)	16.3 (4.84)	14.2 (4.84)	2.13	(0.42 to 3.84)	0.015
	Movement	13.7 (4.47)	14.6 (4.30)	12.4 (4.40)	2.23	(0.69 to 3.77)	0.005
	Feelings	10.8 (4.44)	11.1 (4.51)	10.5 (4.38)	0.63	(−0.95 to 2.02)	0.431
	Arthritis	20.1 (6.49)	20.3 (6.36)	19.8 (6.48)	0.50	(−1.77 to 2.76)	0.666
	Treatments	18.2 (8.36)	19.1 (8.15)	17.1 (8.56)	2.02	(−0.94 to 4.97)	0.180
	Self-help	16.3 (6.05)	16.3 (6.05)	16.3 (6.11)	−0.05	(−2.20 to 2.10)	0.963
	Support	10.6 (3.41)	10.7 (3.34)	10.4 (3.52)	0.33	(−0.88 to 1.54)	0.587
	Total	104.9 (30.18)	108.2 (29.20)	100.6 (31.14)	7.51	(−3.12 to 18.15)	0.164
Reproductive health information needs (single items, range 0–4)	Sex and relationships	1.8 (1.44)	1.5 (1.33)	2.2 (1.52)	−0.67	(−1.17 to −0.16)	0.01
	Contraception	1.7 (1.66)	1.3 (1.56)	2.2 (1.66)	−0.93	(−1.50 to −0.35)	0.002
	Preparing for pregnancy	2.2 (1.76)	1.3 (1.65)	3.4 (1.02)	−2.12	(−2.62 to −1.63)	< 0.001
	Increasing chances of pregnancy naturally	2.1 (1.74)	1.2 (1.60)	3.4 (1.02)	−2.06	(−-2.56 to −1.55)	< 0.001
	Fertility treatments	1.6 (1.71)	0.8 (1.35)	2.7 (1.53)	−1.90	(−2.40 to −1.39)	< 0.001
	Options for giving birth	2.1 (1.81)	1.2 (1.68)	3.2 (1.38)	−1.89	(−2.44 to −1.34)	< 0.001
	Managing pain during childbirth	2.0 (1.79)	1.2 (1.65)	3.0 (1.43)	−1.79	(−2.34 to −1.24)	< 0.001
	Breastfeeding	1.9 (1.75)	1.3 (1.73)	2.6 (1.51)	−1.26	(−1.84 to −0.68)	< 0.001
Support needs		Yes: n (%)	Yes: n (%)	Yes: n (%)	Chi square		P value
Previously had/ currently having	Care planning	73 (57.0%)	45 (63.4%)	28 (49.1%)	2.62		0.111
	Care co-ordination	62 (48.4%)	33 (46.5%)	29 (50.9%)	0.245		0.722
	Peer-support	41 (32%)	19 (26.8%)	22 (38.6%)	2.034		0.184
	Physiotherapy	65 (50.8%)	39 (54.9%)	26 (40.0%)	1.098		0.374
	Talking therapies	41 (32%)	25 (35.2%)	16 (28.1%)	0.741		0.448
	Alternative/ complementary therapies	30 (23.4%)	18 (25.4%)	12 (21.1%)	0.326		0.676
	Practical help with daily activities	24 (18.8%)	19 (26.8%)	5 (8.8%)	6.716		0.012
Would like this if available	Care planning	59 (46.1%)	30 (42.3%)	29 (49.2%)	0.946		0.375
	Care co-ordination	67 (52.3%)	40 (56.3%)	27 (47.4%)	1.020		0.374
	Peer-support	80 (62.5%)	48 (67.6%)	32 (56.1%)	1.773		0.202
	Physiotherapy	53 (41.4%)	31 (43.7%)	22 (38.6%)	0.334		0.592
	Talking therapies	67 (52.3%)	37 (52.1%)	30 (52.6%)	0.003		1.000
	Alternative/ complementary therapies	72 (56.3%)	41 (57.7%)	31 (54.4%)	0.145		0.723
	Practical help with daily activities	66 (51.6%)	39 (54.9%)	27 (47.4%)	0.724		0.477

Thematic analysis of the three sources of qualitative data – the open-text survey items, interviews with women, and interviews with health professionals - revealed three overarching main themes: information needs, multi-disciplinary management, and accessing support. The three main themes and 14 sub-themes that emerged for the three sources of data are summarised in Table 3, and are discussed below.

Information needs

Women reported a range of information needs, which corresponded to five sub-themes: timing of information and planning; disease activity and safe disease management, miscarriage, birth choices, and infant feeding. Both the survey and interview data indicated that women wanted timely, high quality and accessible information about these issues. The safety of medications during pregnancy and breastfeeding were often discussed by women:

> *But nobody's told me what the side effects of steroids are during pregnancy, they just say it's kind of the safest option really and that they'll judge it when they get to it depending on how bad I am. So I'm walking into the unknown, I have no idea.*

(P13, Rheumatoid Arthritis, no children)

> *The thing that I struggled with is that nobody knows, or seems to know how rheumatology and breastfeeding works and I wanted to take the medication if possible.*

(P6, psoriatic arthritis, one child)

Where pregnancy was not an option, women expressed a desire for information about alternatives such as adoption. Health professionals also recognised that there is an unmet need for high quality, timely, written information for women and that pregnancy needs to be planned carefully.

Multi-disciplinary management

The importance of multi-disciplinary care was a prominent theme in the interviews with women and health professionals. Two sub-themes were identified within this theme: unmet need for multi-disciplinary care, and the value of multi-disciplinary care. Women's experiences varied widely, but most felt that there was a lack of well co-ordinated multidisciplinary management between different secondary care departments, as well as primary care, and this could undermine women's trust.

> *I've always been the go between, the departments don't really talk to each other and I've many a time been in a position when I, I've said to either my GP or my consultant you've lied to us because you're both telling me different things.*

(P13, Rheumatoid Arthritis, no children)

All clinicians felt that multidisciplinary management during pregnancy planning, pregnancy, and early parenting was optimal for achieving the best outcomes for women and their children. While secondary care physicians generally reported that women with ARDs who are planning a family or pregnant are already managed through multidisciplinary teams, it was also acknowledged that not all regions within the UK have a multidisciplinary set-up. For example, rheumatology centres in England were thought to be generally better funded and were encouraged to become centres of excellence, whilst in other regions of the UK (Wales, Scotland and Northern Ireland) this was not necessarily the case.

Accessing support

Women and health professionals recognised that women needed to access a range of services and support, and seven sub-themes emerged during analysis: regional differences, pre-conception counseling, care planning, social and practical support, peer-support, tailoring existing services for women with ARDs, psychological support, and support with functional symptoms. Regional variation in the availability of services, including multi-disciplinary teams, pre-conception counseling, social care, and psychological support were identified through the survey and interviews with women and health professionals, indicating that there was considerable variability in the services available to women. Travelling in order to receive specialist care was also challenging for women, as was attending frequent appointments when they were also caring for young children. Care planning, social and practical support, and psychological support were recognised by women and health professionals as important aspects of care, but were not always available to women. Women also talked about the importance of peer-support, in particular the ability to learn from the experience of others with a similar disease. However, the health professionals did not discuss peer-support.

While women acknowledged that they had a range of unmet information needs, pre-conception counseling as a service was not discussed in either the survey or interviews. Rather, they accessed what they viewed as being minimal pre-conception advice during their secondary care appointments. Health professionals felt that as well as the provision of good quality written information, women would need face-to-face discussions with health professionals because of the complexity of the disease and associated medications, and felt that pre-conception counselling would be needed. There was a discrepancy between different health professionals' views of which service should offer pre-conception counseling. Midwives felt that it should be conducted by GPs and/or sexual health clinics, whilst GPs and secondary health

Table 3 Summary of key themes from survey open text questions, interviews with women with ARDs, and interviews with health professionals

Main themes	Sub-themes	Exemplary quotes	Survey responses (n = 118)	Interviews with women (n = 22)	Interviews with health professionals (n = 7)
Information needs	Timing of information & planning	"It has to be planned because at the moment I can't just have a child you know, and that doesn't help because like most people's family they aren't planned you know, because I need to find someone who is willing for that as well" (P2, vasculitis, no children)	Timescales involved with planning a pregnancy were challenging for women: i.e. changing medication a long time in advance of trying to conceive, needing to wait until condition is stable enough to conceive. Risk of unplanned pregnancies & what to do if this happens was a concern. The importance of receiving a timely diagnosis was highlighted.	Women wanted timely, high quality and accessible information. Women recognised that starting a family is a complex process requiring planning. They felt that information about planning a family should be presented and discussed from the point of diagnosis. Some women expressed a need for information about the alternatives to pregnancy, e.g. adoption.	There is an unmet need for quality, timely, written information for women. Pregnancy needs to be planned carefully.
	Disease activity & safe disease management	"I've got my own kind've own concerns about you know being at a point where I'm well enough to become pregnant, being well during the pregnancy, can I stay well enough for 9 months that I don't need extra medication that would impact on the pregnancy?" (P10, vasculitis, no children)	Women wanted high quality condition specific evidence and advice on pregnancy with ARDs, including information on: the impact of reducing or changing medication while staring a family on disease activity; flare-ups, whether their condition was hereditary, and; what the implications of changes in serum antibody activity were for conception and pregnancy outcomes.	Several women had concerns about unpredictability of ARD following medication change and keeping 'well' long enough to conceive. The safety of medications during pregnancy and breastfeeding were often discussed by women, as they felt they had insufficient information about this.	Secondary care physicians felt that women need to be in good physical state with well-managed ARD when trying to conceive.
	Miscarriage	"You never prepare yourself for having a miscarriage, but we were working on the basis that if I had a successful pregnancy it's a bonus because the odds were against us as the doctors had said" (P16, non-specific inflammatory arthritis, two children)	Several women expressed concerns about risks, lack of support following miscarriage, not knowing the cause of miscarriages (i.e. ARD related or other factors).	Women talked about concerns about miscarriage risk, the emotional impact of miscarriage, and not knowing the cause of miscarriage.	Secondary care physicians identified that there is a risk of miscarriage associated with some medicines used to manage ARDs, and that women are likely to need more information and support with this.
	Birth choices	"I feel like I have less options" (P5, Systemic Lupus Erythematous, no children)	Challenges women faced included coping with premature births, and lack of involvement in decisions about method of delivery.	Women often experienced a lack of information, and expressed a need for collaborative conversations when discussing options for birth.	Need for collaborative conversations during discussions about birth options was highlighted by secondary care physicians and midwives.
	Infant feeding	"By about 4 weeks my mum was saying please stop breastfeeding and she'd been very pro-breastfeeding, but she could obviously see I was struggling (with mobility and pain), but I marched on and then at 6 weeks I dropped the child" (P9, non-specific inflammatory arthritis, two children)	Lack of information & evidence about efficacy and safety of medication to manage disease and pain during breastfeeding was identified as a challenge by several women.	Desire to breastfeed baby whilst also being able to manage ARD symptoms, such as impact of disease flare and pain, was often challenging for women. Women felt that there was a need for more awareness about the impact of chronic conditions on breastfeeding amongst midwives/health visitors.	Midwives identified a need to utilise midwifery expertise in supporting breastfeeding through advice on infant feeding as well as positions for holding the baby.

Table 3 Summary of key themes from survey open text questions, interviews with women with ARDs, and interviews with health professionals (Continued)

Main themes	Sub-themes	Exemplary quotes	Survey responses (n = 118)	Interviews with women (n = 22)	Interviews with health professionals (n = 7)
Multi-disciplinary management	Unmet need	"This time around I think I didn't get monitored closely enough during the pregnancy really. I think it must be resources and there's never any communication between rheumatology and the obstetricians" (P6, psoriatic arthritis, one child)	Despite requiring input from a range of health and social care services, examples of formal multi-disciplinary team input were rare. Poor communication was important to women, who reported receiving inconsistent advice, not being listened to, and not being believed as challenges. Some women were discouraged from getting pregnant due to their disease.	Several women felt that there was a lack of multidisciplinary management that included secondary and primary care services. Women felt that their clinicians often focused on the management of their disease, and that they did not view them holistically.	Secondary care physicians reported that women who are planning a family were already managed through multi-disciplinary teams, but acknowledged that this might not be available to women ion all areas of the UK
	Value of multi-disciplinary care	"And so it's actually getting everybody that might need to be involved to see it in a more holistic way." (HP1, health visitor)	Women valued care from a range of services in addition to rheumatology, including primary care physicians, obstetrics, counselling, physiotherapy, occupational therapy, and midwifery and health visiting services.	Women who received care from a multidisciplinary team with an open line of communication, usually those receiving their treatment at national centres of excellence, found the approach helpful. Women recognised the value of a multi-disciplinary approach, especially input from midwives and health visitors from the early stages of pregnancy onwards.	High level of consensus that multidisciplinary care is needed.
Accessing support	Regional differences	"So a lot of the things that are available are area specific and not needs specific you know so your need might meet the threshold but be outside of the area" (HP1, health visitor) m	Travel to specialist services, and ability to access to fertility services were challenging in some areas.	Women acknowledged that there was considerable variation between regions in the availability of services, including social care and psychological support. Some women reported that travel to secondary care/specialist services can be difficult.	Health professionals recognised that pre-conception counseling was not always available due to regional variation. It was also acknowledged that not all regions within the UK have a multidisciplinary set-up.
	Pre-conception counselling	"There are other areas of where it (pre-conception counselling) is much less developed and those sort of services tend not to be available and the general NHS approach to these patients is much more chaotic and it's very much up to the patients to try to find out, you know, the advice" (HP5, secondary care physician)	Though women talked about the need for more information and emotional support, pre-conception counseling services were not specifically discussed.	Pre-conception advice occurred during secondary care appointments, but provision of advice was minimal for most women.	Pre-conception counselling is fundamental in supporting women with ARDs, but is not universally available. There was variance between health professionals in perceptions of who is responsible for pre-conception counselling (primary or secondary care).
	Care planning	"If I had an appointment made when I was pregnant so we could've planned those early weeks and planned a best case scenario and a worst case	Concerns about the potential of disease activity flare during pregnancy/post-partum and the management options. Frequency of appointments	Some women had experienced a lack of rapid access/care planning for post-partum flare ups, but several women reported a lack of care planning. Continuity of care was felt to be particularly important during	Health professionals felt there was a need for multidisciplinary care planning, including incorporating occupational therapists.

Table 3 Summary of key themes from survey open text questions, interviews with women with ARDs, and interviews with health professionals (*Continued*)

Main themes	Sub-themes	Exemplary quotes	Survey responses (n = 118)	Interviews with women (n = 22)	Interviews with health professionals (n = 7)
		scenario (...) maybe it would've been nicer to have had a more realistic approach to what I could achieve (P9, non-specific inflammatory arthritis, two children)	and lack of co-ordination of care were challenging for women.	pregnancy and planning for birth. Women reported that they often had to explain their 'story' in relation to their ARD and pregnancy due to a lack of continuity of care.	
	Social & practical support	*The health visitor got in touch with a local council with a (...) families team and I quickly got assigned a social worker (...) she used to take children (...) to school, she'd bring them in the afternoon and she would give them to the parents in the evening* (P14, Systemic Lupus Erythematous, three children)	Social care, support from partners and family, and help with childcare were viewed as being helpful. These were areas where women felt that support needed to be improved, along with more support from employers, financial support, and greater understanding and awareness from social welfare agencies. Accessing healthcare could be challenging when caring for young children.	Social and familial support vital for practical/physical demands of parenting was a prominent theme. Views of partners were important to women in making decisions about building a family.	The provision and availability of social support was discussed by some health professionals. It was felt some social support might be available to help with practical aspects of parenting, such as getting children to school or providing care whilst the mother is attending hospital appointments or during hospital admission.
	Peer-support	*What you really want is somebody else who's been through that to say this is how they found it* (P10, vasculitis, no children) (P	Peer-support and learning from the experiences of others were valued by women. Greater availability of peer-support was identified as an area for improvement.	Women often reflected on the availability of online peer-support due to the lack of disease specific groups available. Women wanted to hear about the experiences of other women with ARDs.	Not discussed.
	Tailoring existing healthcare services for women with ARDs	*I mean we need more education, I'm thinking about health visitors but we need more education I think about attachment because it's really key in these things and understanding how if you have, whatever it is really, if something hijacks your care-giving experience as an adult, how that affects the sort of longer term outcomes for the child and the relationship.* (HP1, health visitor)	Women felt existing services should be improved by: providing more involvement in decisions about their health and building a family; provision of consistent and proactive care, and; specialist midwife/specialist nurse involvement during pregnancy. Good communication, clear advice, being open to questions, compassion, kindness, understanding, encouragement, and honesty from health professionals were viewed as being important aspects of care.	Availability and suitability of mother and baby groups as a traditional form of support was frequently discussed. Women reported that they would attempt to engage in mother and baby groups, but would often struggle to fully participate due to their limited mobility. Some women felt there was a need for specialised mother and baby groups. Some women's experiences with occupational therapy services were that they did not take into account their role as a mother who needs to look after a child.	During pregnancy, health visitors and midwives felt that clinician training in the management of chronic conditions and their potential impact on the family unit was needed to help facilitate a multidisciplinary approach.
	Psychological support	*I was again feeling totally useless because I should have been able to drive him (son), I should've been able to just get dressed, get him in the car and to the hospital	More emotional support and counseling was viewed as a way of improving care. Uncertainty about the impact of disease on pregnancy (and	Women expressed a need for more psychological support. For many women, their ARD led to them feeling restrained by their physical symptoms, and they felt that	Health professionals felt that it was important to consider the psychological support needs of women. They felt that support for anxiety and depression was needed due to the specific challenges

Table 3 Summary of key themes from survey open text questions, interviews with women with ARDs, and interviews with health professionals (*Continued*)

Main themes	Sub-themes	Exemplary quotes	Survey responses (n = 118)	Interviews with women (n = 22)	Interviews with health professionals (n = 7)
		...and I could not put one foot in front of the other, I was so tired" (P14, Systemic Lupus Erythematous, three children)	vice versa) and ability to cope with demands of parenting resulted in fear and anxiety. The impact on women's identity was often discussed, with women wanting to be a 'normal' parent and to be seen as a whole person not a disease. Having realistic parenting ideals was perceived to be helpful. Positive aspects of parenting included motivation and sense of purpose.	they were unable to do some of the things that 'normal' mothers do.	associated with planning a pregnancy, changing medication, managing a pregnancy and coping with a young child whilst also dealing with ARD symptoms.
	Support with functional symptoms	*"(Daughter) was christened in October 2015 and I couldn't even hold her, I could not stand up and hold her so when she got christened, I couldn't even hold my daughter at the font"* (P4, non-specific inflammatory arthritis, one child)	Women expressed concerns about whether they would be 'well enough' to cope with caring for young children due to fatigue, exhaustion, lack of sleep, pain and mobility.	Several women found that fatigue, pain, and mobility presented challenges when it came to caring for young children.	Health professionals acknowledged a need for the provision of social and psychological support to help women cope with these symptoms.

professionals felt that it should occur in secondary care. In particular, secondary care physicians felt that specialist nurses were best placed to offer pre-conception counselling.

I think, you know doctors are fine at giving the sort of sciencey side but I think patients are much more likely to open up to specialist nurses (...) Nurses have more time, it's easier to write that into their job description than it is to write it into doctor's job description.

(HP5, secondary care physician)

The need to tailor existing services to meet the specific needs of women with ARDs emerged as a theme. For example, women reported that they would attempt to engage in mother and baby groups, such as baby massage, but would often struggle to fully participate due to their limited mobility.

Because of course it was a baby massage course the baby's on the floor. If I was on the floor I couldn't get up so the first couple of weeks I went I was sat on a chair leaning over but then I just it started to make my back ache and everything else.

(P4, non-specific inflammatory arthritis, one child)

Women reflected on the difficulties they experienced, and highlighted the need for a modified group suitable for women with limited mobility.

So maybe, maybe there's a way of setting up an arthritic mother's group, or something like that.

(P9, non-specific inflammatory arthritis, two children)

Health professionals also felt that it was important to consider the specific support needs of women with ARDs.

I'm just thinking about the, there's very specific anxiety and concerns that come for these women in the context of their parenting role having a chronic sort of autoimmune disorder.

(HP1, Health visitor)

The need for greater awareness and education for a broader range of health professionals who would be in contact with women during pregnancy and early parenting, such as midwives and health visitors, was recognised by women and health professionals.

Recommendations for improving care from women with ARDs and health professionals

A number of recommendations were made by women and health professionals during the interviews for the improvement of care and support of women during pre-conception, pregnancy and early parenting. These focused on the need for clear and timely information about medication, clear and collaborative communication between clinicians and patients, multidisciplinary management, and increased practical as well as emotional support. Table 4 outlines the general recommendations made by both women and health professionals.

Discussion

The findings of our survey and qualitative research indicated that women with ARDs in the UK have a wide range of unmet information and support needs in relation to pregnancy planning, pregnancy, and early parenting. While some had experienced comprehensive multi-disciplinary care that met their expressed needs, others struggled to get any information or support at all with navigating the complex challenges that they faced during this important time in their lives. Health professionals echoed the views of women in many ways, and they felt that pre-conception counseling and a multi-disciplinary approach to care could be particularly useful.

Information needs

Our findings, in line with those of Ackerman et al. [2], indicated that with women with ARDs report a broad range of unmet information needs when they are building a family. A modified version of the ENAT was used in the current study. Therefore, caution should be taken in directly contrasting scores for this measure with other studies. Nonetheless, the total ENAT scores in the current study and Ackerman et al.'s [2] study with women with Rheumatoid Arthritis in Australia indicated that the overall need for information in this population is high; the total mean ENAT score was 104.9 (SD 30.18) in the current study, and 97.2 (SD 30.8) in the Ackerman et al. [2] study, with the total ENAT score having a range from range 0 (lowest need) to 156 (highest need). In the current study, the greatest expressed need for information related to information about disease processes and treatments from health professionals. Women also expressed a need for specific information in relation to family planning, conception, pregnancy, and breastfeeding. The information needs of women in our study were similar overall across the different types of rheumatic disease and family status. However, we identified statistically significant differences in the information needs of women who already had children compared with those who did not, with the former requiring more information about managing the physical limitations of their

Table 4 Recommendations from women with ARDs and health professionals for improving of care and support during pre-conception, pregnancy and early parenting

Recommendations	Women (survey and interview)	Health Professionals
Information and communication	Clear information on medication use during pregnancy planning, pregnancy and breastfeeding Patient-centered approach. More empowerment and involvement in decisions about medication	High quality written information: pre-conception, pregnancy, post-partum and pre-conception counselling The need for a patient-centered approach (shared decision-making) in consultations
Multi-disciplinary management	Multi-disciplinary, proactive and better coordinated care (mainly rheumatology, obstetrics, fertility and mental health services)	More training for health professionals such as health visitors, occupational therapists, and midwives about chronic conditions and their impact
Support	Tailoring of professionally led mother and baby groups to ensure they are suitable for women with a chronic condition which affects mobility Peer-support & information on the experiences of others in a similar situation. More practical support, such as agencies that can provide childcare and home help	Psychological support provided more widely Provision of social care support

disease, and the latter expressing a greater need for information to prepare them for conception, pregnancy, childbirth, and breastfeeding.

Our qualitative findings from the open text sections of the survey and the interviews with women also indicated that women struggled to get the information and support that they needed. Information about their disease, and specifically how it was likely to affect them (and their children) during pregnancy and early parenting was a prominent theme. Women expressed a need for more information about the safety of using medication during breastfeeding, and expressed concerns about how their disease would impact on their role as a parent. From women's reports, it seems that they were often falling into the gaps in terms of receiving the right information and support with family planning, pregnancy and early parenting. These issues were seen as being peripheral in secondary care where disease management was the main priority, but neither were women's needs being met elsewhere via services that women without ARDs would typically access.

Support needs

The AIMS2-SF scores indicated that ARDs had a wide reaching impact on quality of life for women in all the disease groups. In line with this, women reported valuing a range of healthcare, social care, and community based support for managing their disease, physical and emotional symptoms, and practical aspects of daily living. AIMS2-SF scores were broadly similar to those reported for Rheumatoid Arthritis patients in a trial of needs-based patient education [36]. However, in our study women reported a particularly high impact of their disease on work (role domain mean 7.79, SD 3.0). Functional disability and fatigue have previously been identified as having an impact on the parenting roles of women with Systemic Lupus Erythematous [37]. Women with Rheumatoid Arthritis also report that pain and fatigue impacts on their parenting roles [38]. The dual pressure of work and household/family demands can be challenging for younger women with Rheumatoid Arthritis, but employment has important health, social, and emotional benefits that should not be overlooked [39, 40]. Women with inflammatory arthritis reported a higher impact of their disease on their physical mobility than the other disease groups, which would be consistent with the pain, impaired joint mobility, and decreased aerobic fitness that is characteristic of inflammatory arthritis [41]. Nonetheless, our qualitative data indicated that physical functioning was challenging across disease groups, particularly while caring for young children, and information and support needs reported via the survey were similar for those with inflammatory arthritis, connective tissue diseases (including Systemic Lupus Erythematous), and vasculitis.

Women reported that access to health and social care support (both specialist and community-based) during early parenting was variable and fragmented, with some having difficulty even getting their basic medical needs attended to, while others felt they received excellent multi-disciplinary care.

Healthcare professionals' views

The interviews with health professionals in our study highlighted the need for a more coordinated and proactive approach to providing women with the information that they need. Physicians felt family planning should be dealt with in a secondary care setting in this context due to the complexity of these diseases, with specialist nurses being well placed to have these discussions. Midwives and health visitors thought that primary care and family planning clinics were well placed to support women with their family planning decisions. In an Australian Delphi study with rheumatologists, obstetricians and obstetric medicine physicians, and pharmacists, guiding principles for clinical practice were that information delivery needed to be: coordinated; delivered in an appropriate mode and format, at the right time, and tailored to the individual patient; based on best available evidence; delivered by the right health professionals at the right time, and; a non-judgmental approach is required for infant feeding [42].

Implications for clinicians and policy makers

A more coordinated, holistic, and equitable approach is required to ensure that information and support needs of women with ARDs are met during a time in their lives when they are likely to encounter numerous challenges and complex choices. Tailored support is required by women with ARDs at various stages during pregnancy planning, pregnancy and early parenthood, and these issues should be revisited regularly as women's circumstances change. More holistic and coordinated care could improve health and quality of life outcomes for women with ARDs and their offspring. The roles of different members of multi-disciplinary teams in supporting women of reproductive age with ARDs need to be considered [42, 43].

High quality, consistent and timely information resources need to be made available on the wide range of issues that affects this population. Clinicians' interpersonal and communication skills are important, as well as fostering a culture of openness and involvement of patients in decisions. A need for pre-conception counseling for women with long-term limiting illnesses has previously been identified [21]. Having children is a highly emotive issue and it has been suggested that women with ARDs should consult with a clinical psychologist when they are preparing for pregnancy [44]. Women in this study reported struggling with miscarriage in particular, and for many their partner's role in caring for them and their children was vitally important. Clinical psychology, counselling and family therapy services could provide support women and their families with these issues.

Community based support, including peer-support, practical help with caring for young children, raising general awareness, support with infant feeding, and social care also need to be considered to meet the complex needs of this group. Previous studies of the perceived impact of ARDs on parenting roles, including in Lupus [37], Rheumatoid Arthritis [38] and systemic sclerosis [45], have indicated that pain, fatigue and problems with mobility can have a significant impact on the daily tasks associated with parenting, such as picking up and carrying children, or getting up and down from the floor. These challenges were discussed by several mothers that we interviewed, and they highlighted the importance of community based services, such as Occupational Therapy assessments, social care services, domestic help, and support with childcare. However, mothers reported that these services were often orientated towards the mother's needs as a disabled person, but did not take into account her role as a mother and the tools and adaptations that might benefit her in caring for her child. The potential to tailor these services so that they take into account the needs of pregnant women and families with young children should be investigated.

The themes identified in this study in terms of unmet information and support needs are similar to those reported in studies carried out in Australia [2, 42] and the United States of America (USA) [37, 38, 45, 46]. However, there are differences between Australia, the USA, and the UK in the organisation and structure of healthcare systems [47]. Our study also highlighted considerable variability in the organisation and availability of healthcare services in different regions within the UK. Consequently, needs and support mechanisms are likely to vary nationally and internationally, and this needs to be taken into account in designing interventions to better meet the information and support needs of this population.

Strengths and weaknesses of the study

Using a mixed-methods approach enabled analysis of data from different sources (survey, interviews with women, and interviews with health professionals), and from people with a wide range of experiences, to identify a range of gaps in meeting the information and care needs of women with ARDs. The survey was cross-sectional, so the association between reported information and support needs and outcomes could not be assessed. The survey used a combination of validated measures and additional items relating to specific reproductive health information needs

and sources of support were included that were developed by the research team in conjunction with patient representatives to highlight areas for further research; as such, the latter were not validated measures. The modified ENAT scores provide valuable information on the unmet needs of patients in this study, but due to differences in the rating scales used, comparison with the original ENAT [24] scores reported in other studies should be treated with caution. Survey participants were self-selecting, and it was not possible to calculate response rate using the online recruitment method. Therefore, we do not know to what extent these findings will generalise beyond the study population.

Our in-depth person-centered qualitative research allowed us to understand more about women's information needs, why and how they were or weren't met, and how information and support needs could be better met from the perspectives of women with a range of ARDs and health professionals from a variety of disciplines and settings. However, women who took part in interviews were more highly educated, more likely to be employed, and had lower AIMS2 scores than the overall survey participants, which was indicative of a sampling bias that should be taken into consideration when generalising from the findings. We interviewed health professionals from primary, secondary, and maternity health care services, but we were unable to engage with some important professional groups within the confines of the time and resources available for this study, including rheumatology nurses and obstetricians. The primary reason given by health professionals for non-participation in interviews was lack of time due to other demands.

Conclusions

There is an urgent need to develop and evaluate interventions for women of reproductive age who have ARDs that will improve the quality of information, promote more collaborative decision making with regard to motherhood and healthcare choices, and re-design health and social care services to provide more accessible, timely, integrated, and holistic care.

Acknowledgements
The authors wish to thank all of the women and health professionals that took part in this research. We would like to thank our patient involvement representatives for their support in inspiring, designing and guiding this work.

Funding
This study was supported by a Wellcome Trust Institutional Strategic Support Fund grant. The lead author's fellowship at PRIME Centre Wales, Cardiff University, is funded by Health and Care Research Wales. Neither the Wellcome Trust nor Health and Care Research Wales had any role in the design of the study, collection, analysis, and interpretation of data, or in preparation of this manuscript.

Authors' contributions

RP conceived the project conducted statistical analysis and drafted and revised the manuscript, and is guarantor for this manuscript. AG led on designing the qualitative interviews, and DW & BP collected and analysed the qualitative data. DB led on survey data collection. Co-authors provided specific expertise in qualitative methods (AG, BP, DW), development and implementation of the social media communication strategies (DB), primary care (AE), rheumatology (EC), midwifery (JS), pain management and medical education (AT), and psychology (RP, DW) during study design and interpretation of findings. All authors have commented on previous drafts of the manuscript, and have approved the final version.

Authors' information

The lead author (RP) is a Health Psychologist and health services researcher with a long-standing interest in musculoskeletal complaints and in maternal and child health. RP worked with a multi-disciplinary team of co-authors, with expertise in Rheumatology (EC), General Practice (AE), pain management (AT), psychology (DW), midwifery (JS), social media communication (DB), qualitative research (AG, BP, RP, DW).

Competing interests

The authors declare that they have no competing interests.

Author details

[1]Division of Population Medicine, School of Medicine, Cardiff University, Cardiff, UK. [2]Centre for Trials Research, Cardiff University, Cardiff, UK. [3]School of Healthcare Sciences, Cardiff University, Cardiff, UK. [4]Centre for Medical Education, Cardiff University, Cardiff, UK. [5]Division of Infection and Immunity, School of Medicine, Cardiff University, Cardiff, UK.

References

1. Ostensen M, Andreoli L, Brucato A, Cetin I, Chambers C, Clowse MEB, Costedoat-Chalumeau N, Cutolo M, Dolhain R, Fenstad MH, et al. State of the art: reproduction and pregnancy in rheumatic diseases. Autoimmun Rev. 2015;14(5):376–86.
2. Ackerman IN, Jordan JE, Van Doornum S, Ricardo M, Briggs AM. Understanding the information needs of women with rheumatoid arthritis concerning pregnancy, post-natal care and early parenting: a mixed-methods study. BMC Musculoskelet Disord. 2015;16:194.
3. Julkunen HA. Oral contraceptives in systemic lupus erythematosus: side-effects and influence on the activity of SLE. Scand J Rheumatol. 1991; 20(6):427–33.
4. Ostensen M, Brucato A, Carp H, Chambers C, Dolhain RJEM, Doria A, Foerger F, Gordon C, Hahn S, Khamashta M, et al. Pregnancy and reproduction in autoimmune rheumatic diseases. Rheumatology. 2011; 50(4):657–64.
5. Ostensen M, Cetin I. Autoimmune connective tissue diseases. Best Practice & Research Clinical Obstetrics & Gynaecology. 2015;29(5):658–70.
6. Prunty MC, Sharpe L, Butow P, Fulcher G. The motherhood choice: a decision aid for women with multiple sclerosis. Patient Educ Couns. 2008; 71(1):108–15.
7. Wellings K, Jones KG, Mercer CH, Tanton C, Clifton S, Datta J, Copas AJ, Erens B, Gibson LJ, Macdowall W, et al. The prevalence of unplanned pregnancy and associated factors in Britain: findings from the third National Survey of Sexual attitudes and lifestyles (Natsal-3). Lancet. 2013; 382(9907):1807–16.
8. Clowse MEB. Managing contraception and pregnancy in the rheumatologic diseases. Best Practice & Research in Clinical Rheumatology. 2010;24(3):373–85.
9. Ostensen M, von Esebeck M, Villiger PM. Therapy with immunosuppressive drugs and biological agents and use of contraception in patients with rheumatic disease. J Rheumatol. 2007;34(6):1266–9.
10. Ackerman IN, Ngian G-S, Van Doornum S, Briggs AM. A systematic review of interventions to improve knowledge and self-management skills concerning contraception, pregnancy and breastfeeding in people with rheumatoid arthritis. Clin Rheumatol. 2016;35(1):33–41.
11. Meade T, Dowswell E, Manolios N, Sharpe L. The motherhood choices decision aid for women with rheumatoid arthritis increases knowledge and reduces decisional conflict: a randomized controlled trial. BMC Musculoskelet Disord. 2015;16:260.
12. Ciciriello S, Buchbinder R, Osborne RH, Wicks IP. Improving treatment with methotrexate in rheumatoid arthritis-development of a multimedia patient education program and the MiRAK, a new instrument to evaluate methotrexate-related knowledge. Semin Arthritis Rheum. 2014;43(4):437–46.
13. Li LC, Adam PM, Backman CL, Lineker S, Jones CA, Lacaille D, Townsend AF, Yacyshyn E, Yousefi C, Tugwell P, et al. Proof-of-concept study of a web-based methotrexate decision aid for patients with rheumatoid arthritis. Arthritis Care & Research. 2014;66(10):1472–81.
14. Mohammad A, Kilcoyne A, Bond U, Regan M, Phelan M. Methotrexate information booklet study 2008. Clin Exp Rheumatol. 2009;27(4):649–50.
15. Fraenkel L, Peters E, Charpentier P, Olsen B, Errante L, Schoen RT, Reyna V. Decision tool to improve the quality of care in rheumatoid arthritis. Arthritis Care & Research. 2012;64(7):977–85.
16. Ellard D, Barlow J, Paskins Z, Stapley J, Wild A, Rowe I. Piloting education days for patients with early rheumatoid arthritis and their partners: a multidisciplinary approach. Musculoskeletal Care. 2009;7(1):17–30.
17. Hammond A, Bryan J, Hardy A. Effects of a modular behavioural arthritis education programme: a pragmatic parallel-group randomized controlled trial. Rheumatology. 2008;47(11):1712–8.
18. Hammond A, Young A, Kidao R. A randomised controlled trial of occupational therapy for people with early rheumatoid arthritis. Ann Rheum Dis. 2004;63(1):23–30.
19. Homer D, Nightingale P, Jobanputra P. Providing patients with information about disease-modifying anti-rheumatic drugs: individually or in groups? A pilot randomized controlled trial comparing adherence and satisfaction. Musculoskeletal Care. 2009;7(2):78–92.
20. Doria A, Bajocchi G, Tonon M, Salvarani C. Pre-pregnancy counselling of patients with vasculitis. Rheumatology. 2008;47:13–5.
21. Steel A, Lucke J, Adams J. The prevalence and nature of the use of preconception services by women with chronic health conditions: an integrative review. BMC Womens Health. 2015;15:14.
22. Ngian G-S, Briggs A, Ackerman I, Van Doornum S. Safety of anti-rheumatic drugs for rheumatoid arthritis in pregnancy and lactation. International journal of Rheumatic Diseases, Online First. 2016;19:834–843.
23. Ostensen M. Connective tissue diseases: contraception counseling in SLE - an often forgotten duty? Nat Rev Rheumatol. 2011;7(6):315–6.
24. Ndosi M, Bremander A, Hamnes B, Horton M, Kukkurainen ML, Machado P, Marques A, Meesters J, Stamm TA, Tennant A, et al. Validation of the educational needs assessment tool as a generic instrument for rheumatic diseases in seven European countries. Ann Rheum Dis. 2014;73(12):2122–9.
25. Ndosi M, Tennant A, Bergsten U, Kukkurainen ML, Machado P, de la Torre-Aboki J, Vlieland T, Zangi HA, Hill J. Cross-cultural validation of the educational needs assessment tool in RA in 7 European countries. BMC Musculoskelet Disord. 2011;12:110.
26. Guillemin F, Coste J, Pouchot J, Ghezail M, Bregeon C, Sany J. The AIMS2-SF: a short form of the arthritis impact measurement scales 2. French quality of life in rheumatology group. Arthritis Rheum. 1997;40(7):1267–74.
27. Holm S. A simple sequential rejective multiple test procedure. Scand J Stat. 1979;6(2):65–70.
28. Thomas D. A general inductive approach for analyzing qualitative evaluation data. Am J Eval. 2006;27(2):237–46.
29. Gabb J, Fink J. Telling moments and everyday experience: multiple methods research on couple relationships and personal lives. Sociology. 2015;49(5):970–87.
30. Goldenberg T, Finneran C, Andes KL, Stephenson R. Using participant-empowered visual relationship timelines in a qualitative study of sexual behaviour. Global Public Health. 2016;11(5–6):699–718.
31. Snow D, Anderson L, FLofland J, Lofland L. Analyzing social settings: a guide to qualitative observation and analysis, Fourth Edition edn. Belmont: Wandsworth publishing; 2005.
32. Kolar K, Ahmad F, Chan L, Erickson PG. Timeline mapping in qualitative interviews: a study of resilience with marginalized groups. Int J Qual Methods. 2015;14(3):13–32.
33. Fereday J, Muir-Cochrane E. Demonstrating rigor using thematic analysis: a hybrid approach of inductive and deductive coding and theme development. Int J Qual Methods. 2006;5(1):80–92.
34. Barbour RS. Checklists for improving rigour in qualitative research: a case of the tail wagging the dog? BMJ. 2001;322(7294):1115–7.
35. Malterud K, Siersma VD, Guassora AD. Sample size in qualitative interview studies:guided by information power. Qual Health Res. 2016;26(13):1753–60.
36. Ndosi M, Johnson D, Young T, Hardware B, Hill J, Hale C, Maxwell J, Roussou E, Adebajo A. Effects of needs-based patient education on self-efficacy and

health outcomes in people with rheumatoid arthritis: a multicentre, single blind, randomised controlled trial. Ann Rheum Dis. 2016;75(6):1126–32.

37. Poole JL, Rymek-Gmytrasiewicz M, Mendelson C, Sanders M, Skipper B. Parenting: the forgotten role of women living with systemic lupus erythematosus. Clin Rheumatol. 2012;31(6):995–1000.

38. Katz PP, Pasch LA, Wong B. Development of an instrument to measure disability in parenting activity among women with rheumatoid arthritis. Arthritis Rheum. 2003;48(4):935–43.

39. Phillips C, Main C, Buck R, Aylward M, Wynne-Jones G, Farr A. Prioritising pain in policy making: the need for a whole systems perspective. Health Policy. 2008;88(2–3):166–75.

40. Harrison MJ. Young women with chronic disease: a female perspective on the impact and management of rheumatoid arthritis. Arthritis Care & Research. 2003;49(6):846–52.

41. Piva SR, Almeida GJM, Wasko MCM. Association of Physical Function and Physical Activity in women with rheumatoid arthritis. Arthritis care & research. 2010;62(8):1144–51.

42. Briggs AM, Jordan JE, Ackerman IN, Van Doornum S. Establishing cross-discipline consensus on contraception, pregnancy and breast feeding-related educational messages and clinical practices to support women with rheumatoid arthritis: an Australian Delphi study. BMJ Open. 2016;6(9): e012139.

43. Soh MC, Nelson-Piercy C. High-risk pregnancy and the rheumatologist. Rheumatology. 2015;54(4):572–87.

44. Kosowicz M, Ostanek L, Majdan M, Olesinska M, Teliga-Czajkowska J, Wiland P. Selected principles of proper education of women with rheumatic diseases in respect of pregnancy planning. Reumatologia (Warsaw). 2014;52(1):49–56.

45. Poole JL, Willer K, Mendelson C, Sanders M, Skipper B. Perceived parenting ability and systemic sclerosis. Musculoskeletal Care. 2011;9(1):32–40.

46. Katz PP. Childbearing decisions and family size among women with rheumatoid arthritis. Arthritis & Rheumatism-Arthritis Care & Research. 2006; 55(2):217–23.

47. Policies EOoHSa. Health Systems in Transition summary. Copenhagen: Australia: World Health Organisation (Europe); 2006.

Permissions

All chapters in this book were first published in RHEUMATOLOGY, by BioMed Central; hereby published with permission under the Creative Commons Attribution License or equivalent. Every chapter published in this book has been scrutinized by our experts. Their significance has been extensively debated. The topics covered herein carry significant findings which will fuel the growth of the discipline. They may even be implemented as practical applications or may be referred to as a beginning point for another development.

The contributors of this book come from diverse backgrounds, making this book a truly international effort. This book will bring forth new frontiers with its revolutionizing research information and detailed analysis of the nascent developments around the world.

We would like to thank all the contributing authors for lending their expertise to make the book truly unique. They have played a crucial role in the development of this book. Without their invaluable contributions this book wouldn't have been possible. They have made vital efforts to compile up to date information on the varied aspects of this subject to make this book a valuable addition to the collection of many professionals and students.

This book was conceptualized with the vision of imparting up-to-date information and advanced data in this field. To ensure the same, a matchless editorial board was set up. Every individual on the board went through rigorous rounds of assessment to prove their worth. After which they invested a large part of their time researching and compiling the most relevant data for our readers.

The editorial board has been involved in producing this book since its inception. They have spent rigorous hours researching and exploring the diverse topics which have resulted in the successful publishing of this book. They have passed on their knowledge of decades through this book. To expedite this challenging task, the publisher supported the team at every step. A small team of assistant editors was also appointed to further simplify the editing procedure and attain best results for the readers.

Apart from the editorial board, the designing team has also invested a significant amount of their time in understanding the subject and creating the most relevant covers. They scrutinized every image to scout for the most suitable representation of the subject and create an appropriate cover for the book.

The publishing team has been an ardent support to the editorial, designing and production team. Their endless efforts to recruit the best for this project, has resulted in the accomplishment of this book. They are a veteran in the field of academics and their pool of knowledge is as vast as their experience in printing. Their expertise and guidance has proved useful at every step. Their uncompromising quality standards have made this book an exceptional effort. Their encouragement from time to time has been an inspiration for everyone.

The publisher and the editorial board hope that this book will prove to be a valuable piece of knowledge for researchers, students, practitioners and scholars across the globe.

Contributors

A. Machin and C. D. Mallen
Research Institute for Primary Care and Health Sciences, Primary Care Sciences, Keele University, Newcastle-under-Lyme, Staffordshire, UK

I. C. Scott and S. L. Hider
Research Institute for Primary Care and Health Sciences, Primary Care Sciences, Keele University, Newcastle-under-Lyme, Staffordshire, UK
Department of Rheumatology, Haywood Hospital, High Lane, Burslem, Staffordshire, UK

Tore Saxne, Pierre Geborek and Meliha C. Kapetanovic
Department of Clinical Sciences Lund, Section of Rheumatology, Lund University, Skåne University Hospital, SE-221 85 Lund, Sweden.

Per Nived
Department of Infectious Diseases, Central Hospital Kristianstad, J A Hedlunds väg 5, SE-291 85 Kristianstad, Sweden

Thomas Mandl
Department of Clinical Sciences Malmö, Section of Rheumatology, Lund University, Skåne University Hospital, Malmö, Sweden

Lillemor Skattum
Department of Laboratory Medicine, Section of Microbiology, Immunology and Glycobiology, Lund University, Lund, Sweden
Clinical Immunology and Transfusion Medicine, Lund, Region Skåne, Sweden

Susan M. Goodman and Anne R. Bass
Department of Medicine, Weill Cornell Medical School, Division of Rheumatology Hospital for Special Surgery, 535 E 70th St, New York City, NY 10021, USA

Aprajita Jagpal
Division of Clinical Immunology and Rheumatology, University of Alabama at Birmingham, 836 Faculty Office Tower, 510 20th Street South, Birmingham, AL 35294, USA

Iris Navarro-Millán
Joan and Sanford I Weill Medical College of Cornell University, Division of General Internal Medicine, 525 East 68th Street, F-2019, PO Box #331, New York, NY 10065, USA
Division of Rheumatology, Hospital for Special Surgery, New York, NY, USA

Daniel F. McWilliams and Nalinie Joharatnam
Arthritis Research UK Pain Centre, NIHR Nottingham Biomedical Research Centre and Division of Rheumatology Orthopaedics and Dermatology, University of Nottingham Clinical Sciences Building, City Hospital,Nottingham NG5 1PB, UK

David A. Walsh
Arthritis Research UK Pain Centre, NIHR Nottingham Biomedical Research Centre and Division of Rheumatology Orthopaedics and Dermatology, University of Nottingham Clinical Sciences Building, City Hospital,Nottingham NG5 1PB, UK
Department of Rheumatology, Sherwood Forest Hospitals NHS Foundation Trust, Sutton-in-Ashfield, UK

Patrick D. W. Kiely
Department of Rheumatology, St Georges Healthcare NHS Trust, London, UK

Adam Young
University of West Hertfordshire, Watford, UK

Deborah Wilson
Department of Rheumatology, Sherwood Forest Hospitals NHS Foundation Trust, Sutton-in-Ashfield, UK

Rosarin Sruamsiri
Health Economics, Janssen Pharmaceutical KK, 5-2, Nishi-kanda 3-chome Chiyoda-ku, Tokyo 101-0065, Japan
Center of Pharmaceutical Outcomes Research, Naresuan University, Phitsanulok, Thailand

Jörg Mahlich
Health Economics, Janssen Pharmaceutical KK, 5-2, Nishi-kanda 3-chome Chiyoda-ku, Tokyo 101-0065, Japan
Düsseldorf Institute for Competition Economics (DICE), University of Düsseldorf, Düsseldorf, Germany

Yuko Kaneko
Division of Rheumatology, Department of Internal Medicine, Keio University School of Medicine, Tokyo, Japan

Kristen E. Castro, Kaitlyn D. Corey, Diana L. Raymond, Michael R. Jiroutek and Melissa A. Holland
Campbell University College of Pharmacy and Health Sciences, 180 Main Street PO Box 1090, Buies Creek, NC 27506, USA

Adel M. Al-Awadhi
Department of Medicine, Faculty of Medicine, Kuwait University, Jabriya, Kuwait
Rheumatic Disease Unit, Al-Amiri Hospital, Dasman, Kuwait

Mohammad Z. Haider, Jalaja Sukumaran and Sowmya Balakrishnan
Department of Pediatrics, Faculty of Medicine, Kuwait University, P. O. Box 24923, 13110 Safat, Kuwait

Annemarie Schorpion and Robin Neubauer
Hospital of the University of Pennsylvania, Philadelphia, USA

Chris T. Derk
Hospital of the University of Pennsylvania, Philadelphia, USA
Division of Rheumatology, University of Pennsylvania, 5th Floor White Building, 3400 Spruce Street, Philadelphia, PA 19107, USA

Max Shenin
Thomas Jefferson University Hospital, Philadelphia, USA

Vibeke Strand
Stanford University, Palo Alto, CA, USA

M. Elaine Husni
Cleveland Clinic, Cleveland, OH, USA

Keith A. Betts
Analysis Group Inc., 333 South Hope Street, 27th Floor, Los Angeles, CA 90071, USA

Yan Song and Jing Zhao
Analysis Group Inc., Boston, MA, USA

Rakesh Singh, Jenny Griffith, Marci Beppu and Arijit Ganguli
AbbVie Inc., Mettawa, IL, USA

Mark E. Roberts
Greater Manchester Neuroscience Centre, Salford Royal NHS Foundation Trust, Manchester Academic Health Science Centre, Stott Lane, Salford, UK

James B. Lilleker
Greater Manchester Neuroscience Centre, Salford Royal NHS Foundation Trust, Manchester Academic Health Science Centre, Stott Lane, Salford, UK
NIHR Manchester Biomedical Research Centre, Central Manchester University Hospitals NHS Foundation Trust, The University of Manchester, Manchester, UK

Hector Chinoy
NIHR Manchester Biomedical Research Centre, Central Manchester University Hospitals NHS Foundation Trust, The University of Manchester, Manchester, UK
Rheumatology Department, Salford Royal NHS Foundation Trust,Manchester Academic Health Science Centre, Stott Lane, Salford, UK

Patrick Gordon
King's College Hospital NHS Foundation Trust, London, UK

Janine A. Lamb
Centre for Integrated Genomic Medical Research, School of Health Sciences, Faculty of Biology Medicine and Health, The University of Manchester, Manchester, UK

Robert G. Cooper
Centre for Integrated Genomic Medical Research, School of Health Sciences, Faculty of Biology Medicine and Health, The University of Manchester, Manchester, UK
MRC-ARUK Institute for Ageing and Chronic Disease, University of Liverpool, Liverpool, UK

Heidi Lempp
Academic Rheumatology, Faculty of Life Sciences and Medicine, King's College London, London, UK

Paula Jordan
Myositis UK, Southampton, UK

Ben Darlow, Melanie Brown and Eileen McKinlay
Department of Primary Health Care and General Practice, University of Otago - Wellington, Wellington, New Zealand

Bronwyn Thompson
Department Orthopaedic Surgery and Musculoskeletal Medicine, University of Otago - Christchurch, Christchurch, New Zealand

Ben Hudson
Department of General Practice, University of Otago - Christchurch, Christchurch, New Zealand

Rebecca Grainger
Department of Medicine, University of Otago - Wellington, Wellington, New Zealand

J. Haxby Abbott
Department of Surgical Sciences, University of Otago, Dunedin, New Zealand

Julia Held, Birgit Mosheimer-Feistritzer and Johann Gruber
Department of Internal Medicine II, Infectious Diseases, Immunology,Rheumatology, Pneumology, Medical University of Innsbruck, Anichstr. 35,A-6020 Innsbruck, Austria

Günter Weiss
Department of Internal Medicine II, Infectious Diseases, Immunology,Rheumatology, Pneumology, Medical University of Innsbruck, Anichstr. 35,A-6020 Innsbruck, Austria
Christian Doppler Laboratory for Iron Metabolism and Anemia Research, Innsbruck, Austria

Erich Mur
Department for Physical Medicine and Rehabilitation, University of Innsbruck, Innsbruck, Austria

Matthew J. Koster and Kenneth J. Warrington
Division of Rheumatology, Mayo Clinic College of Medicine and Science, 200 1st St SW, Rochester, MN 55905, USA

Elisabeth Mogard and Elisabet Lindqvist
Department of Clinical Sciences Lund, Rheumatology, Lund University, Skane University Hospital, Lund, Sweden

Ann Bremander
Department of Clinical Sciences Lund, Rheumatology, Lund University, Faculty of Medicine, Lund, Sweden
School of Business, Engineering and Science, Rydberg Laboratory for Applied Science, Halmstad University, Halmstad, Sweden

Spenshult Research and Development Center, Halmstad, Sweden

Stefan Bergman
Department of Clinical Sciences Lund, Rheumatology, Lund University, Faculty of Medicine, Lund, Sweden
Spenshult Research and Development Center, Halmstad, Sweden
Primary Health Care Unit, Department of Public Health and Community Medicine, Institute of Medicine, Sahlgrenska Academy, University of Gothenburg, Gothenburg, Sweden

William Masson, Sara Muller, Rebecca Whittle, James Prior, Toby Helliwell and Christian Mallen
Arthritis Research UK Primary Care Centre, Primary Care Sciences, Keele University, Keele, Staffordshire ST5 5BG, UK

Samantha L. Hider
Arthritis Research UK Primary Care Centre, Primary Care Sciences, Keele University, Keele, Staffordshire ST5 5BG, UK
Rheumatology Department, Haywood Rheumatology Centre, Staffordshire ST6 7AG, UK

Seoyoung C. Kim and Daniel H. Solomon
Division of Pharmacoepidemiology and Pharmacoeconomics, Department of Medicine, Brigham and Women's Hospital, Harvard Medical School, 1620 Tremont St, Suite 3030, Boston, MA 02120, USA
Division of Rheumatology,Immunology, and Allergy, Department of Medicine, Brigham and Women's Hospital, Harvard Medical School, Boston, MA, USA

Kathleen Vanni, Penny Wang, Alyssa Wohlfahrt, Zhi Yu, Fengxin Lu and Anarosa Campos
Division of Rheumatology, Immunology, and Allergy, Department of Medicine, Brigham and Women's Hospital, Harvard Medical School, Boston, MA, USA

Courtney F. Bibbo
Division of NuclearMedicine, Department of Radiology, Brigham and Women's Hospital, Harvard Medical School, Boston, MA, USA

Marcelo F. Di Carli
Division of NuclearMedicine, Department of Radiology, Brigham and Women's Hospital, Harvard Medical School, Boston, MA, USA
Division of Cardiovascular Medicine,Department of Medicine, Brigham and Women's Hospital, Harvard Medical School, Boston, MA, USA

Rajesh K. Garg
Division of Endocrinology, Diabetes and Hypertension,Department of Medicine, Brigham and Women's Hospital, Harvard Medical School, Boston, MA, USA

Stacy Smith
Department of Radiology, Brigham and Women's Hospital, Harvard Medical School, Boston, MA, USA

Gwenda Simons and Marie Falahee
Institute for Inflammation and Aging, Rheumatology Research Group,College of Medical and Dental Sciences, University of Birmingham,Birmingham B15 2TT, UK

Rebecca J Stack
Institute for Inflammation and Aging, Rheumatology Research Group,College of Medical and Dental Sciences, University of Birmingham,Birmingham B15 2TT, UK
Department of Psychology, Nottingham Trent University, 50 Shakespeare St, Nottingham NG1 4FQ, UK

Christopher D Buckley and Karim Raza
Institute for Inflammation and Aging, Rheumatology Research Group,College of Medical and Dental Sciences, University of Birmingham,Birmingham B15 2TT, UK

Department of Rheumatology, Sandwell and West Birmingham Hospitals NHS Trust, Birmingham, UK
Arthritis Research UK Rheumatoid Arthritis Pathogenesis Centre of Excellence, MRC Arthritis Research UK Centre for Musculoskeletal Ageing Research and NIHR Biomedical Research Centre, College of Medical and Dental Sciences, University of Birmingham, Birmingham, UK

Michaela Stoffer-Marx
Section for Outcomes Research, Center for Medical Statistics, Informatics, and Intelligent Systems, Medical University of Vienna, Spitalgasse 23, BT88/E 031090 Vienna, Austria
University of Applied Sciences FH Campus Wien, Vienna 1100, Austria

Erika Mosor and Tanja Stamm
Section for Outcomes Research, Center for Medical Statistics, Informatics, and Intelligent Systems, Medical University of Vienna, Spitalgasse 23, BT88/E 031090 Vienna, Austria
Division of Rheumatology, Department of Internal Medicine III, Medical University of Vienna, Vienna, Austria

Kanta Kumar
The Institute of Clinical Sciences, College of Medical and Dental Sciences, University of Birmingham, Birmingham B15 2TT, UK
Faculty of Biology,Medicine and Health, School of Health Sciences, University of Manchester, Manchester M13 9PL, UK

Mats Hansson
Centre for Research Ethics and Bioethics, Uppsala University, Box 564, SE-751 22 Uppsala, Sweden

Premarani Sinnathurai and Lyn March
Institute of Bone and Joint Research, Kolling Institute, Northern Sydney Local Health District, Sydney, NSW, Australia

Department of Rheumatology,Royal North Shore Hospital, Reserve Road, St Leonards, NSW 2065, Australia
Sydney Medical School, University of Sydney, Sydney, NSW, Australia

Alexandra Capon
Department of Rheumatology,Royal North Shore Hospital, Reserve Road, St Leonards, NSW 2065, Australia

Lyndall Henderson
Sydney Medical School, University of Sydney, Sydney, NSW, Australia

Rachelle Buchbinder
Monash Department of Clinical Epidemiology, Cabrini Institute, Malvern, VIC, Australia
Department of Epidemiology and Preventive Medicine, School of Public Health and Preventive Medicine, Monash University, Clayton, VIC, Australia

Vibhasha Chand
Centre of Cardiovascular Research and Education in Therapeutics, School of Public Health and Preventive Medicine, Monash University, Clayton, VIC, Australia

Marissa Lassere
School of Public Health and Community Medicine, University of New South Wales, Sydney, NSW, Australia
Department of Rheumatology, St George Hospital, Kogarah, NSW, Australia

Shawn D. Ellis
Department of Oncology, Royal Berkshire Hospital, Reading RG1 5AN, UK

Sam T. Kelly and Jonathan H. Shurlock
Department of Medicine, Royal Sussex County Hospital, Brighton BN2 5BE, UK

Alastair L. N. Hepburn
Department of Rheumatology, Worthing Hospital, Worthing BN11 2DH,UK

Thorlene Egerton, Rachel K Nelligan and Kim L Bennell
Centre for Health, Exercise and Sports Medicine, The University of Melbourne, Melbourne, Australia

Jenny Setchell
School of Health and Rehabilitation Sciences, The University of Queensland, Brisbane, Australia

Lou Atkins
Centre for Behaviour Change, University College London, London, UK

Rhiannon Phillips, Daniel Bowen, Adrian Edwards and Denitza Williams
Division of Population Medicine, School of Medicine, Cardiff University, Cardiff, UK

Bethan Pell and Aimee Grant
Centre for Trials Research, Cardiff University, Cardiff, UK

Julia Sanders
School of Healthcare Sciences, Cardiff University, Cardiff, UK

Ann Taylor
Centre for Medical Education, Cardiff University, Cardiff, UK

Ernest Choy
Division of Infection and Immunity, School of Medicine, Cardiff University, Cardiff, UK

Index

www.ingramcontent.com/pod-product-compliance
Lightning Source LLC
Chambersburg PA
CBHW080644200326
41458CB00013B/4730